=2-50

7-1-23

AGE LATER

AGE LATER

How to look seven years younger

in just seven weeks.

Marc A. Ronert, M.D., Ph.D.

Ronert Health, LLC

FIRST EDITION

Dr. Marc A. Ronert with Janna Ronert

Photos and illustrations by shutterstock.com and istock.com

Cover and portrait photography by Gary James

ISBN 978-1-7326762-0-6

Published by Ronert Health, LLC Publishing   Palm Beach and Berlin

www.agelaterbook.com
For more information, news and frequent updates, please visit agelaterbook.com.

www.hushandhush.com

www.imageskincare.com

Ronert Health, LLC can bring authors to your live event. For more information, or to book an event, contact Ronert Health at admin@ronerthealth.com.

To my wife, Janna, who supports me in anything I do,

my parents, without them nothing would be possible,

the best kids in the world, Zurich and Milana

who teach me more than anybody can imagine

and finally COCO for inner peace.

CONTENTS

Chapter 4

Chapter 5

Chapter 6

Chapter 7

Chapter 8

Chapter 9

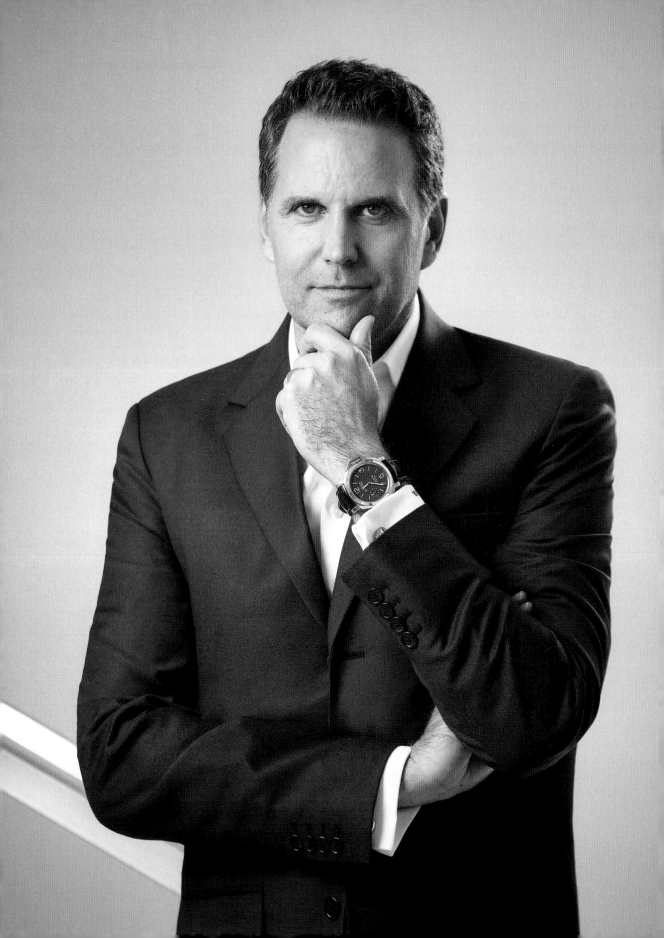

PREFACE

As far back as I can remember, I always wanted to become a physician.

Apart from a grandmother from Russia who died before I was born, my family had no real connection to the health-care industry. Yet, early on, I had this intrinsic fascination with how the body functions, how all the cells in our body communicate with one another, and why animals and people get sick. The question never occurred to me what I wanted to be when I grew up.

The answer was always there.

After finishing high school in Germany, and after a short year in the United States as an exchange student, I started medical school in Dusseldorf, Germany. I had a passion for anatomy and physiology (the normal functions of living organisms), but I quickly learned something about myself. It was tough for me, emotionally, to deal with very sick or chronically ill patients and often not see improvement in the treatment they received. Shortly after finishing medical school I received my Ph.D.

When I came in contact with the field of plastic surgery, it was like a light bulb went on. The direction I wanted to pursue became crystal clear. The idea of helping people achieve or regain a normalized appearance after tumors, genetic defects or burns—sometimes through simple and short procedures—excited me like nothing else in my life.

I was fortunate enough to have a great mentor, the former president of the German Association of Plastic Surgeons, Professor R.R. Olbrisch, who taught me everything that I know about plastic surgery—and who offered me a full residency program at his university-affiliated clinic.

We covered the spectrum of major plastic surgery: reconstruction of the face and body after traumas, tumors, burns, genetic deformities, breast reconstruction after cancer and radiation. We also learned about aesthetic plastic surgery: liposuction, facelifts, eyelid surgery and tummy tucks. It was an amazing experience.

As young physicians in the clinic, my colleagues and I had tremendous responsibility to care for thousands of patients a year. When we worked in the clinic for long hours, weekends and holidays, I never considered it work. It became my life—my mission—to help people in need, to restore their self-confidence after an accident, to normalize their appearance after a debilitating cancer removal, to help alleviate pain and restriction in mobility after a burn contracture.

In 2004, during an International Society of Aesthetic Plastic Surgery Conference in Houston, Texas, a turn of events occurred. It was August, and Professor Olbrisch and I were traveling from Germany to present a novel research project that we were spearheading at our clinic.

Back then, we implanted small little tissue expanders into the skin of patients, and these tissue expanders would absorb body fluids, swell and create new skin at that area. We then would utilize the newly formed skin to recreate breasts after breast amputations, or for defect coverage after tumor excisions.

Little did I know that my future wife, Janna, would be attending the same conference. She was in Houston to show off a newly created line of skin-care products, which she called Image International. Our stories differ on how we met for the first time, but along with showing me her newly created products, she also ended up showing Houston to a German guy who had never been to Texas. We quickly developed a deep connection that exists to this day.

After I returned to Germany, we stayed in contact. It was my good fortune that Janna later decided to spend a good year with me in Germany while I was finishing my residency program.

After that, I would fly to Houston to see her while she was busy building her business. We discovered that our mutual attraction didn't just exist on an emotional level. We had similar ideas and the same ambitious plans about business and aging later.

At any given moment we would brainstorm about how we could expand the Image name—and create something together that could potentially change the world. Since, back then, I was the only "International" at Image International, we renamed the company Image Skincare, and I started to become more involved in the business.

The first thing we did was to get European approval, translate the product descriptions into German, and sell Image Skincare products at our clinic (as well as distribute them throughout Germany). We created new products and product lines, and substantiated our claims about their clinical effectiveness through clinical studies.

In a few short years, we developed an internationally recognized brand that is now one of the leading and most innovative professional skin-care companies in the world, one that focuses on how to help our clients and patients to *Age Later*.

Many of the concepts we developed through our skin-care line can be found in this book. Many of the aging processes that happen within our skin also affect other cells in our body.

Part of the reward of being a board-certified plastic surgeon, a profession that I've been fortunate enough to practice now for the better part of two decades, involves addressing issues over which my patients have no control.

Since earning my Ph.D. in 2001 and launching my career in Germany (before later moving to South Florida), I've been able to use my skills to correct aesthetic concerns caused by injuries or that people have had since birth. Such cases often involve reconstructing skin and tissue; depending on the severity of the condition, this can require multiple procedures.

In recent years, however, I've been thinking more and more about issues where, I'm convinced, every person's own actions can make a difference—issues where they do have control.

Many of my clients seek surgical remedies for aesthetic concerns that have nothing to do with physical injuries or conditions present since birth. Instead, they're concerns related to the passage of time. On the one hand, we all know aging is an inevitable part of life—and that there is no magical fountain of youth.

But why, then, do some people do it so much more gracefully than others?

This is the question that began my quest to better understand the process of aging. I wanted to learn how skin, muscles and other tissues change over time. Why people who are young in years appear much older. And why people who've already lived rich lives still maintain a youthful appearance.

Naturally, there is a genetic component to aging. Your inner biological clock ticks on, no matter what you do. This is largely determined by the biological coding in your DNA. Your cells cannot replicate forever, and eventually cell damage leads to apoptosis, or cell death. Your DNA also determines your susceptibility to certain illnesses, and those illnesses can further accelerate cell aging.

Skin always is a great indicator of age. Your skin is a mirror that reveals the state of health of your entire body. The same genetic mechanisms, and the same exposures to an aggressive environment, drive the deterioration of cells inside and on the surface of the body. Healthy skin reflects a healthy body. And a healthy body has healthy skin.

That said, as I researched the various causes of tissue degeneration, I became more aware that there is much we can do to slow down the aging process—and that aging, to a large extent, is something that human beings do to ourselves. We can accelerate or curtail the aging process depending on the choices we make and how we live our lives.

Visible signs of aging are caused by years of damage to our body and skin cells simply by living in the world. But so many other factors play into aging.

Our food consumption and nutrition choices can create and sustain healthy cells or accelerate their deterioration. Lack of exercise can create significant health issues, while adequate exercise of the right type makes us healthier and extends our lives. Neglecting our skin and exposing it to sun damage can cause it to age; worse still, unhealthy skin becomes a weaker barrier against disease, toxins and allergens. If your skin is sick, you're going to get sick. Psychological stresses can impact the brain and nervous system, and there are positive actions we can all take to reduce stress and acquire a calmer mental condition.

These topics form the pillars of this book: food, exercise, skin care and inner peace.

I started my career with a focus on skin care and appearance, and I quickly learned that true skin health cannot be achieved with great skin care alone. Each one of these dimensions is important if you want to have attractive, youthful and healthy skin.

 I wrote this book to share those insights with readers—and to help anyone who wants to look and feel younger achieve that goal. As you improve skin health and appearance, as you find an inner calm and get yourself into the best physical and mental shape possible, your overall health and energy levels will receive a boost as well.

You will *Age Later*, by staying younger, longer.

Chapter 1

GROWING OLDER, STAYING YOUNGER

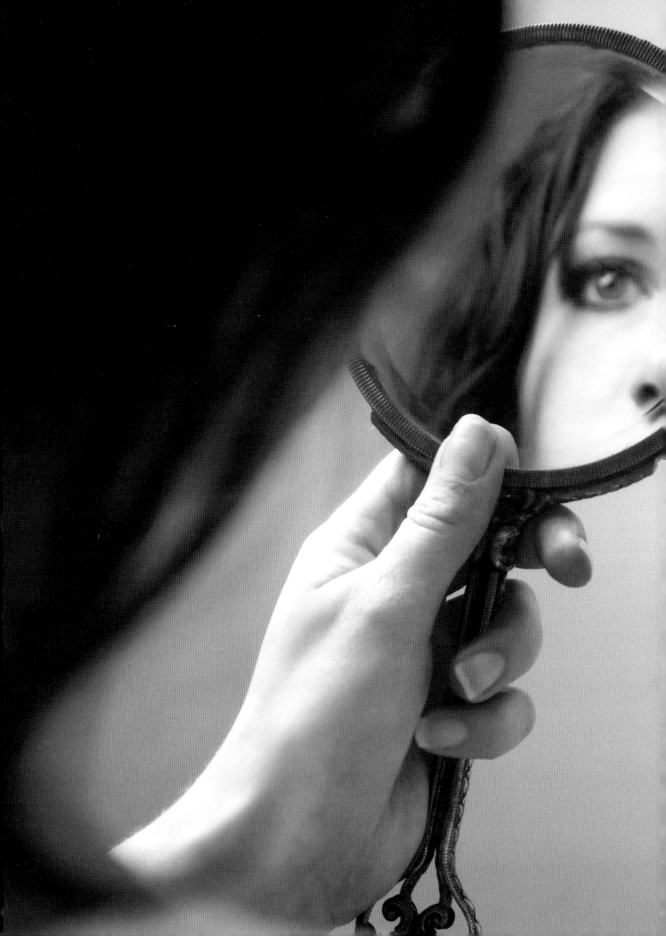

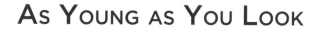

AS YOUNG AS YOU LOOK

Despite all the advances of modern science, and our ability to understand how the human body works, too many people today feel that they're aging too fast.

What's happening?

It doesn't help that we're both beneficiaries and victims of the modern world. When the hard-wiring inside our bodies starts to misfire, modern medical technology often can fix it, or at least make it more bearable. At the same time, modern life offers all kinds of roadblocks that prevent us from truly nurturing our bodies and minds. Our working lives are hectic and stressful. We struggle to turn off our laptops and put down our cellphones. We're consistently tempted by food and drink that undermines our nutritional needs. And we barely have time to decompress, let alone follow a dedicated daily exercise routine.

But as many people have discovered, it doesn't need to be like this. You can take more control of these aspects of your life—and countless others—if you make the necessary commitment. The healthy living choices described in this book encourage you to do just that. I also will provide you with medical insights into the inner workings of the human body, knowledge that will help you take better care of your physical and mental health.

Age Later helps you understand the human aging process; it explains the importance of informed food choices and healthier ways of eating. You will learn how to take care of your skin, that critically important physical boundary between you and the environment you live in. You will learn the importance of exercise—activity both for your body and for your mind. All of this will enable you to take effective action to improve your health, which will make you look and feel younger.

Everyone counts the years at the same rate, according to the calendar. But there is no reason for that calendar to place limits on your health, capabilities and energy. There are many things we can do to delay or eliminate some of the biological problems of growing older—and this book will help you do just that.

Age Later will enable you to improve the quality of your life no matter how old you are (or how old you feel), but the sooner you start, the better. Ideally, everyone should be introduced to a healthy and sustainable lifestyle when they are children. Good habits formed in childhood are likely to be long-lasting and effective. It's better to avoid damage than to have to fix it.

Still, even if you haven't taken the best care of yourself so far in life, it's not too late to chart a new course. You can start at any age and obtain some benefits. You can add years to your life. And those years can be useful, productive and pleasurable.

It's been my experience that getting started is the biggest hurdle for the kind of life changes that *Age Later* proposes. But trust me: When you begin to experience the benefits of looking better, feeling stronger, being more active and thinking with greater clarity, then these healthy living choices will no longer feel like hard work.

They'll feel like a blessing.

This book can help you plan and implement these life changes, so it's primarily about the actions you need to take. Some of you will want to know more than just what to do—you'll also want to know why and what evidence supports these recommendations. Although this book is not intended to be a textbook, I will provide you with information about the important and interesting scientific research that makes it possible for everyone (including me) to do far more than just prolong your life span.

Looking younger is great, and living longer is wonderful too, as long as you're healthy enough to enjoy your extended life. But don't forget about the real payoff: The guidelines that lead to looking younger and living longer also should lead to a more productive and fulfilling life.

What is "Growing Old"?

Why do humans age? Aging is not just the result of the passage of time. It's the result of what happens to our bodies during that passage of time.

Our skin and body tissues are constantly fighting a battle against the assaults of the environment in which we live. We benefit from sunlight, but direct sun also damages our skin. Our skin and body cells must cope with wind, snow, heat, cold, rain, drought, radiation, toxins and chemicals. Bacteria and viruses, fungi and toxins are all around us, and many of these microorganisms damage our cells. Sometimes that damage can be permanent. This is nothing new: bugs, toxins and radiation[1] have been around longer than human beings. Mostly, we have learned to fend off these attacks. But humans still wear out.

We have to eat food to fuel our activities and build our bodies. In the developed world we generally overeat, and some of that food harms our bodies. We evolved over a long period, possibly 200,000 years, to thrive on a wide range of complex plants, plus many different kinds of animal meat.

Today, we consume a record amount of meat. According to the U.S. Department of Agriculture, the average American consumer was on track to devour 222.2 pounds of red meat and poultry in 2018, more than any recorded year in history. Conversely, people are not eating enough vegetables; this has happened mostly in the last couple of hundred years. In addition, many modern foods do us more harm than good, and that too contributes to the aging process inside our bodies.

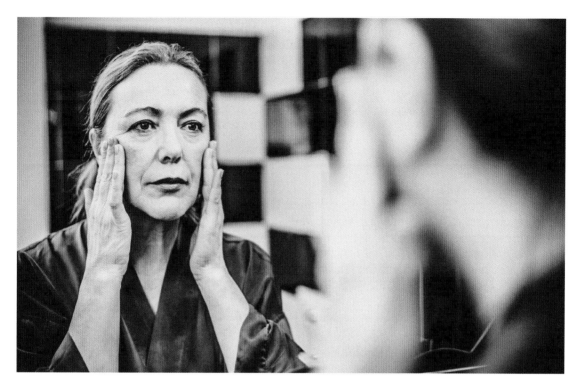

Humans are by nature active mammals, yet modern humans, with some exceptions, move their bodies and limbs far less than they should. That means that as the years go on, our muscles and skeletons deteriorate: If we don't use it, we lose it. Lack of exercise is a huge contributor to unnecessary early aging. In the U.S., 70 percent of the adult population is now overweight or obese. [2] That's a staggering number that has wide and profound consequences for the health and youthfulness of this generation.

As a result of the accumulation of damage from the environment, poor nutrition and lack of exercise, our cells degrade over time, and our bodies wilt.

We tend to describe this wearing out process as "growing old." The longer we live, the more we expect to decay. Historically, it seemed that this was simply inevitable. But now we have unlocked many of the secrets of the aging process and discovered that there are several ways in which we can help our skin and body maintain much of the vigor and healthiness of youth. Although we may not uncover the secret of eternal life any time soon, it might be closer than you think.

Over the years, different theories have been put forward to explain aging. Those theories focus on different body processes and conditions, including inflammation, cell deterioration, DNA mutations, glycation, telomere shortening, oxidation and more. It is now becoming clear that no single theory adequately explains everything to do with aging: It's complicated. Yet, despite differences in scientific detail, these multiple theories all point to similar conclusions concerning the good habits that will maintain health and prolong life. My recommendations will enable you to tackle aging on multiple fronts, and not with faddish methods and potions. *Age Later* offers proven habits—good habits—that will soon come to feel natural and normal.

COUNTING YEARS IS NOT HELPFUL

It's not easy to consider aging without counting years. Our established practice is to measure the age of people by the calendar. How many years, months, days, hours, minutes and seconds have they been alive on this planet? But this is chronological age, which is just a number. What we should focus on instead is biological age. This is our age as measured by health, appearance and physical capabilities.

Look around. We've all come across a 50-year-old person who looks 70. On the other hand, we've all met 55-year-olds who look and act like they're only 40. They're not only attractive, but they're also alert and active. What makes it possible for people to look so much younger than their chronological years? Why do others age much faster?

The choices we make over the years correlate with outcomes in our lives. Only a fraction of how we look, how we feel and how we age has to do with our genetic makeup; it's much more about the lifestyle choices we make.

If you're unhealthy and overweight, your biological age will be older than your chronological age. On the other hand, if you're mentally and physically fit, your biological age may be years younger than your chronological age. People who invest in a healthy lifestyle—and all that implies—delay getting older. That's what the *Age Later* program is all about.

People who are younger than their year count really do possess skin and body tissues that are similar to people who are younger, chronologically. This is true for their muscles, and it's even true at the cellular level within the body. Some people think this is mostly about having "good genes," but that's not the case. People who are biologically younger than their chronological age achieve this result mainly by making deliberate choices—healthy choices—about their lifestyle.

Age Later will explain how to maintain a higher level of youthful healthiness than any previous generation of humans could hope to experience. Being healthy means more than just avoiding disease; it also means having organs that function and tissues that respond like those of a young person. Maintaining that kind of youthful health involves understanding and combatting the natural processes that cause aging. This book will redirect your focus. It's not about counting years and taking short cuts. It's about understanding how your body works, eliminating destructive patterns, establishing new routines and building a healthy, happy and harmonious lifestyle—one smart and informed decision at a time.

GROWING OLD IS NOT FATAL

Did you know that in the United States it's not possible to die of old age? At least, not in an official capacity. Old age is not regarded as a fatal disease that can be written on a death certificate.

People who are "old" generally die of one or more of the following conditions: heart disease, cancer, respiratory disease, stroke, diabetes, dementia (including Alzheimer's); that is, if they don't die in an accident, or by murder or suicide.

Nevertheless, the process of "growing older" is a real thing. There are changes to the body—internal and external—that reflect the wear and tear on it, even though those changes are not usually the cause of death. What typically happens is that the cellular and structural changes caused by the aging process tend to gradually make us more vulnerable to the sort of illnesses that eventually lead to death. Lack of mental and physical resilience also can make us more vulnerable to accidents.

Growing old is in itself not fatal, but the diseases often associated with the aging process are. In order to live a longer and healthier life, we need to delay the aging process—and also to build up resistance to diseases. The good news is that both of these amount to the same thing. The healthy eating habits and other good routines needed to prolong the life of your body and skin tissues are mostly the same habits that will protect you against life-terminating diseases.

Depending on when you start taking your health and lifestyle choices more seriously, it's possible, in my opinion, to add 10, 20, even 30 years to your life.

In medieval England, life expectancy at birth was no more than 30 years on average.[3] By 1900, things had improved. Average life expectancy in the U.S. was around 47 years at the beginning of the 20th century.[4] Living to the ripe age of 47 may not sound like much by today's standards, but it represented a more than 50-percent improvement over the previous 700 years. By 2015, life expectancy at birth had soared to an average of 77 years; that's more than a 60-percent improvement over a period of some 100 years. That's serious progress. (Unfortunately, in 2016 and 2017, life expectancy dropped in consecutive years, with previous improvements in nutrition and exercise leveling off, and the opioid epidemic cutting a significant number of lives short.)

Our DNA doesn't evolve very quickly. The DNA in our bodies today is not much different from the DNA of our ancestors from a thousand years ago. So, this massive increase in life expectancy has little to do with pre-determined genetic factors—and almost everything to do with the way we lead our lives. Humans have made improvements in personal hygiene, public sanitation, food quality, illness prevention, childbirth practices, surgical procedures, and effective treatments for many ailments that were once regarded as certain death sentences. The reason many of us today can expect to live until we're 70 or older is because of these dramatic and comparatively recent advancements in our everyday life, not because our genetic makeup has improved by leaps and bounds.

That process of change continues, and we can now predict a further extension of life expectancy—but only for those who pay attention and make the kinds of choices that we now understand can lead to a longer, healthier existence. Unfortunately, the population as a whole doesn't always see the bigger picture, especially when it's being bombarded by messages that promote unhealthy foods and unwise lifestyle choices.

Is Aging An Illness?

Most of us don't really think of "growing old" as an illness. Nor should we. Growing old doesn't mean that we automatically will become sick or ravaged by disease. We tend to view aging merely as a manifestation of the natural course of events. That said, there are parallels to draw when it comes to aging and illness. In both, there may be intrinsic and extrinsic factors at play. Genes can influence the aging process, just as they can influence susceptibility (or resistance) to certain illnesses. External agents—the environment, the quality of the foods we eat, microscopic organisms around and inside us—can accelerate the aging process, just as they can cause illness. The impact of aging, just like the impact of illnesses, in some ways impairs the performance of our bodies. Unhealthy people and old people alike are never quite operating at their peak.

Above all, aging is related to actual changes happening to our bodies: our cells, organs and chemical balances.

We expect, in this day and age, that medicine can prevent or cure almost any illness, or at least reduce the associated pain and distress. If it can't be addressed now, we trust that it may be curable in the future as scientific advances create options for treatments. We should think of aging in a similar way—as something, given the resources at our disposal, that we should be able to curb. Over the last few decades we have successfully built an understanding of the many interacting processes involved in aging. More importantly, we're developing additional ways of intervening in the aging process.

I am confident that we can delay aging in predictable ways by encouraging a regimen of behavior and nutrition based on sound evidence. Just as we learn how to prevent specific illnesses, we can learn how to prevent the aging process. In some ways it amounts to the same thing.

Some experts will go further and suggest that it will be possible to extend life beyond normal spans, using all that we know today plus some new therapies that are within our grasp. Many plants and animals live much longer than humans, and we are gaining an understanding of how those organisms maintain cellular integrity over such long periods. Perhaps we can use some of that knowledge to further extend our lives.

Unquestionably, we can do a lot to live longer. We don't need to accept that advancing years inevitably lead to diminishing health, performance and mental acuity. Being old in years, while remaining young in health and appearance, could (and should) become the norm for us all.

Seed and Soil

More than 120 years ago, toward the end of the 19th century, a doctor named Stephen Paget popularized the expression "seed and soil" as a simple way of describing the relationship between the human body and disease. His specific area of study was cancer and how it spreads throughout the body.[5]

He reasoned, based on autopsies of many patients who died of the disease, that the chance of a cancer spreading from its original location to other parts of the body is only partly based on the aggressiveness of the cancer—and that it's more about the receptiveness of the host tissue itself.

Paget talked about "seed and soil" as a useful metaphor to explain this effect. Every farmer, gardener and window-box owner knows that the success of a crop depends on the caliber of seeds—as well as the quality of the soil in which those seeds are planted. Not all plants thrive in the same type of soil, so seeds from the same plant that land in different soils produce dramatically different results.

When a cancer appears somewhere in the body, there is a chance that it will migrate to some other organ. (We call this migration process metastasis.) Paget showed that certain body organs are more susceptible than others to metastasis, and that cancer does not move steadily through the body cell by cell, which was the accepted wisdom at the time. Instead, cancers spread rapidly in some people, more slowly in others. Over the 100-plus years since Paget wrote his famous paper, many research projects have established the soundness of the idea[6], and no research has led to results that undermine it.

We now know that one of the ways cancers spread to other organs is by shedding cells into the bloodstream and lymphatic system in vast numbers, which allows them to reach every part of the body. Most of these cancerous cells will be destroyed by the body defenses (if those defenses are working well), and only a few of the cancerous cells land in fertile soil, in an organ that is predisposed and welcoming to cancers.[7] A better understanding of this mechanism led to an avalanche of research on predisposition, to identify what makes our tissues "predisposed." Why do some people provide a welcoming environment for illness, when others are not so vulnerable?

We know now that certain genetic characteristics can, in different ways, predispose our bodies to certain ailments, but non-genetic factors can similarly create a predisposition and also affect the incidence of cancer. We now understand that the risk of cancer is increased for people who smoke, drink excessive amounts of alcohol, are overweight, are routinely exposed to certain chemicals, or are exposed to excessive sunlight and radiation. Cancer is linked to chronic inflammation and a suppressed immune system.

So, it is clear that the condition of your body (the "soil" in Paget's metaphor) is highly relevant to cancer. For cancer, an unhealthy body provides optimal growing conditions. The same principle applies to cardiovascular disease, to diabetes and to some neurological conditions. To resist illness, you must improve your body's internal environment and defenses so that it can fight off those illnesses from the moment they try to take root.

Modern life tends to push people toward unhealthy food, lack of exercise, exposure to environmental hazards, and high levels of stress and anxiety. You can clear all of those hurdles. All it takes is knowledge, awareness and a desire to design a lifestyle that meets your goals of looking younger and aging later.

How We Make Progress

The history of medicine, as it pertains to the human species, is primarily a story of trial and error, mixed with some rituals, guesswork and superstition. Medical intervention once was considered useless or even damaging. Think about it. We're only a handful of generations removed from the prevailing belief that people weren't meant to live long lives. Gradually, we moved beyond guesswork to adopt methods that involved careful observation, analysis and deduction. Physicians, scientists and researchers began to understand the underlying mechanisms of disease and contagion. We learned about bacteria and viruses and their life cycles, and how they interacted with our bodies. Our growing knowledge enabled us to develop new medical treatments and techniques—and to make improvements in nutrition, personal hygiene and public health measures. Over time, a combination of effective treatments and preventive measures significantly increased the average human life expectancy.

Today, we know so much about how to prevent illness and how to slow the aging process that when someone becomes seriously ill, or "old" too early, it often means they haven't paid attention to what we already know about good nutrition, exercise and self-care. We are still adding to that foundation of knowledge.

There are some diseases, of course, that we can't completely fix. Once the damage is done, the body stays damaged. But prevention is better than cure, as your grandmother always told you. Consequently, *Age Later* is more about maintaining and improving health and youthfulness, and less about curing ailments.

Does This Really Work?

Some people reading this book will be skeptical, convinced that we don't know enough about the aging process. They'll point out that humans find ways every day of polluting the world in which we live, which makes it even harder to avoid the cell damage that leads to aging. Environmental hazards from human-generated chemicals, constantly evolving pathogens, fast food, and high-stress situations—it's not easy to avoid the numerous factors that can accelerate aging. While civilization has blessed us with countless benefits, it's also brought about challenges that our forefathers never could have imagined. I also accept that we don't yet have all the answers when it comes to the causes of aging and illness.

But there's a flip side to that skepticism—and it's bright and brimming with potential. We know much more than we did just a few years ago, and every year brings new insights.

Today, we have access to well-researched evidence on how to delay aging and look younger, but it's tough for people to sort out the facts when the online and media outlets offer so much health and wellness "advice," much of it conflicting. Some advice is based on authentic research, but much of it is assertion based on nothing more than guesswork. In this book, every recommendation is based on valid research—some recent, some long-standing—with no wild conjectures or proposals based on hunches.

We already have reached the point where we can, with confidence, suggest ways of changing life habits to increase the chances of looking younger, feeling younger, extending life and embracing it. In the not-too-distant future, it's likely that current lines of scientific research will deliver results that will help us fine-tune lifestyle choices based on each individual's unique physical characteristics and genetic dispositions.

In the meantime, there's more than enough fact-based information in *Age Later* to change lives right now—even though it stands to reason that the program may not work exactly the same way for every person.

Everyone can, however, benefit from making the healthy living choices suggested in this book—no matter their age, ethnicity, skin color or cultural background.

Some of you already may be following a lifestyle similar to the one I describe. For you, the road to living younger longer will be easier—although I hope you'll be motivated to do even more to boost your health (and to help others do the same). On the other hand, if, having read the book, you feel that this program is going to be tough work, then you probably are one of the people who will benefit most.

While biologically we are all very much alike, we are still different. We have different genes, our body chemistry is not all the same, and our social contexts vary widely. Some people will have strong support from others, some will not. Some people form habits more quickly than others and will find it easier to adhere to the program. Some people will struggle to remain diligent about the changes to their lifestyle; staying power always is an important factor in achieving a successful outcome.

People sometimes don't realize that aging is interfering with their well-being until someone else points it out. Because of that, people unknowingly live sub-optimal lives for years, accumulating damage to their body tissues and feeling older than they need to feel. No matter how old you are (or feel), you can undo some of the harm that has accumulated and slow the aging process over the years to come.

Those of you still young enough to feel somewhat invincible should remember that aging begins from the moment you're born and continues for the rest of your life. It's easier to learn new habits early in your journey; every year you delay will make future reversal more difficult.

There is only one way to find out how well it will turn out for you: Follow the program—and see for yourself if you don't notice a difference in only seven weeks.

THE CHRISTMAS TREE OF HEALTHY LIVING CHOICES

The life expectancy in the USA is an average of 78.7 years, 1.5 years lower than the Organization for Economic Development (OECD) estimates. Shocking is the fact that the life expectancy in the USA is going down due to decline of emotional wellbeing and increase in addiction. There is a 137% increase in opioid related deaths between 200 and 2014 in the USA. For the second year in the row in 2016 and 2017, life expectancy is dropping in the US, while in many countries the life expectancy continues to increase for decades of years. Japan leads the world ranking with 83.7 year, while even though much better than the USA, Germany lags behind many other European Countries with 80.6 years, with most common deaths due to cardiovascular disease and cancer. The EU commission calculated that 28% of the burden of disease in Germany in 2015 could be attributed to behavioral risk factors, like diet, smoking, alcohol and low physical activity.

In my own calculation and assumption, based on research and hard scientific evidence, I am calculating that depending on your own healthy living choices you make, your individual life expectancy can fluctuate in a range of 30 years. Think about this twice: Depending on your own, deliberate choices your make for yourself, regardless of genetics, environment and other outside factors that you cannot control, you can decide for yourself to live 30 years longer! And the end result of how long you will live depend on decisions you make every single day. Each healthy or unhealthy living choice will either move you a tap to the left, or a tap to the right of your own life line. I illustrated the correlation of your choices you make every day in the following "Christmas Tree of Living Choices":

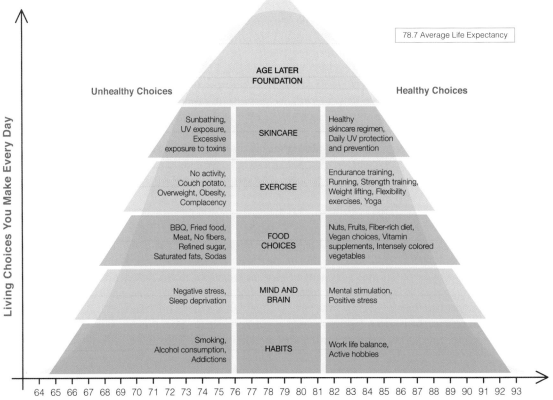

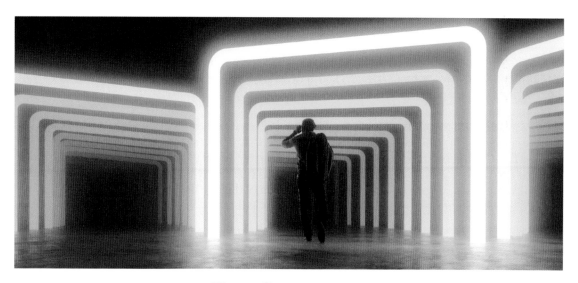

THE CHALLENGE

In this book, I challenge you to build a set of healthy habits, creating a day-to-day routine that will enhance your well-being, and make you look and feel more youthful. This requires commitment. And patience. And trust in the process. Changing bad habits into good habits—when it comes to eating, exercise, skin care and peace of mind—isn't an overnight process.

But I encourage you to give *Age Later* a try—even if it seems daunting at first. Stick with the program for at least seven weeks, and you'll stand a great chance of retaining your healthy habits as part of a new—and permanent—lifestyle.

Throughout the book, I'll encourage you to start taking the initiative. Many people don't get serious about becoming healthy until a doctor expresses concern. By that time, the challenges are even greater. No one should wait. Be proactive and start now.

Of course, you should consult your medical advisors if you have concerns, but don't wait for them to tell you to make life changes. Talk about this with your friends, but don't allow pressure from others to slow you down. Tell your family what you're doing, but make it clear that their job is to support you, unequivocally. Take matters into your own hands. Do it for yourself, for those you love and for those who love you.

Today, we can seriously challenge aging, thanks to our continuously improving understanding of how the human body works and how aging takes place inside it. That understanding can help us make informed decisions about our health, our diet, our fitness and even our mindset.

Looking and feeling seven years younger within seven weeks is just the start. By adopting the practices outlined in *Age Later* into your daily routine, until it becomes second nature, you'll begin to view life, and all of its possibilities, like you never have before.

Chapter 2

HEALTH, AGING
AND THE HUMAN BODY

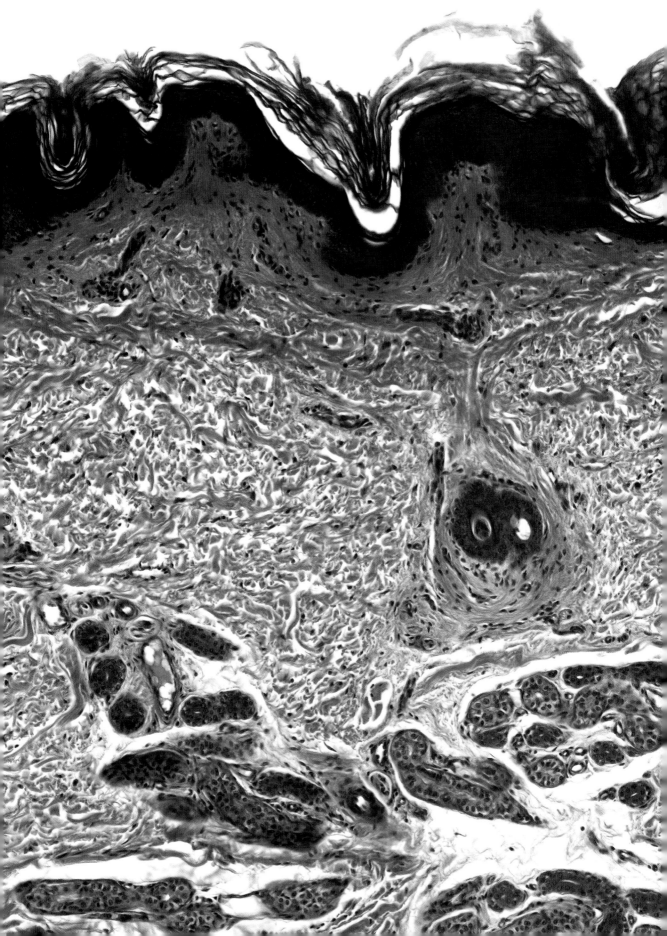

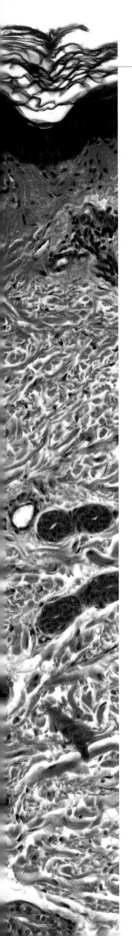

HEALTH, AGING AND THE HUMAN BODY

Aging can be linked to microscopic parts of our bodies that wear out or become damaged. If we want to slow down the aging process, it helps to understand what some of those body parts are, how genetics and the environment can cause deterioration, and how the process of deterioration takes place at the cellular level.

For those of you already having a panicked flashback to that high school biology class, don't worry. There won't be a quiz at the end of this chapter. In fact, if you want to fast-forward through this section, and perhaps revisit it later, it's fine.

That said, the healthy living choices recommended in *Age Later* have everything to do with what's going on deep inside your body. A little knowledge about your cellular self will go a long way toward connecting the dots between day-to-day decisions and staying younger longer.

CELLS: THE BUILDING BLOCKS OF LIFE

THE MIRACLE OF CELLS

Every human life starts with a cell, the smallest unit of organization in all living things. Some organisms, like bacteria, consist of one single cell. Humans are multicellular life forms: millions of cells joined together to make a complex living entity. Cells form the structure of your body and also carry out specific tasks. Every part of your body, including your brain and skin, contains its own set of specially adapted cells.

As you no doubt recall from your sex education classes, a woman contributes a special cell during conception, a human egg that contains a copy of her chromosomes; a man, meanwhile, contributes a sperm that contains a copy of his chromosomes. The merging of the female egg and the male sperm during fertilization results in a fertilized egg (or zygote) that contains a full set of DNA (deoxyribonucleic acid) from both parents. The fertilized egg undergoes a process (meiosis) during which the strands of DNA from the man and woman are rearranged and recombined to produce a new set of chromosomes with genetic information from each parent.[8] In the human embryo, all cells descend from that initial clump of cells formed during the merging of the female egg and the male sperm. The embryonic cells multiply by division (mitosis): Each cell, when it is ready, divides into two cells, and so on.

Each new cell contains its own copy of a unique personal genome that defines in great detail the genetic inheritance of this new human. Cell division continues after birth, into adulthood, until we die.

Cells are made of proteins, with each cell containing thousands or millions of protein molecules. There are several varieties of proteins, each made of different combinations of amino acids. Throughout our lives, the DNA in our cells informs the way that proteins are put together from amino acids and how cells are assembled from proteins.

Your nervous system features cells adapted for use as neurons. There are different kinds of neurons used for sensing, communication and controlling muscles. The cells in your nervous system link everything together, allowing humans to operate as well-integrated mega-organisms instead of a sack of proteins.

Skin cells are another special type of cell. They form the fabric of the different layers of skin that encase human bodies. They also carry out vital functions involving skin health, damage repair and resistance against harmful organisms.

There are at least a hundred different types of cells in the human body. All told (excluding red blood cells[9]), an adult human contains at least eight trillion individual cells.[10]

And, yet, cells are the ultimate team players. One individual cell seems rather insignificant, but together they work seamlessly to form a functioning human being. In a healthy body, they protect themselves when under attack, they replicate for growth—and they even die when that's the right thing to do for the team.

As a team, cells cooperate to build all the organs of the body: organs that process and digest food, circulate blood, distribute oxygen, manage waste—and much more.

What's Inside the Cell?

Structural cells of the human body each contain a nucleus. Inside each nucleus are 23 pairs of chromosomes, which in turn host our genes, the molecular units of heredity that allow us to pass along characteristics from parents to children. Think about that for a second: There's a copy of your own personal set of chromosomes inside every one of the human body's eight trillion cells. The 23 pairs of chromosomes contain all of your personal genetic information, coded in long stranded molecules of your DNA.

That personal DNA code records our genetic inheritance,[11] defining a multitude of personal characteristics, from the color of our eyes to our likelihood of succumbing to a neurodegenerative disease as we grow older.

Under the microscope,[12] a string of DNA looks something like a ladder that's been twisted into a spiral, often described as a double helix.

The two sides are made of a sugar-based substance, and the millions of rungs of ladder are made from combinations of just four chemicals.[13] Each rung consists of a pair of those chemicals, called a nucleotide pair or a base pair.[14] The sequences of these chemical pairs form various patterns, and some of those patterns are called genes. There are around three billion of these base pairs forming around 20,000 genes, so there's room for variety. A string of DNA may contain the coded information for one gene or for several genes.[15] Those sequences of chemicals define your genetic inheritance.

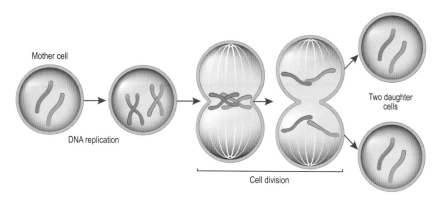

Mother cell

DNA replication

Cell division

Two daughter cells

The Importance of Mitochondria

Inside each cell there are essential components called mitochondria that are responsible for maintaining proper functioning of every cell in your body. Mitochondria are specialized subunits (organelles) located in the region around the nucleus. This region (called the cytoplasm) consists of a glob of a jelly substance (cytosol) in which thousands of mitochondria and other kinds of organelles exist.

Mitochondria perform a range of tasks for the cell, responding to chemically coded messages from inside and outside the cell. They convert varieties of food and oxygen into a standard type of fuel (adenosine triphosphate, ATP[16]), which is used by the cell to perform its many functions, including building proteins. In some types of cells, mitochondria also make cholesterol and blood components. Mitochondria play a role in "retiring" cells when they have served their purpose or when the cell is damaged. The process of regulated cell death, or apoptosis, is fundamental to building and maintaining a healthy body. Apoptosis disposes of cells that are too old or damaged, thus preventing defects from spreading throughout the body. Typically, mitochondria do that quietly and efficiently.

Mitochondria lead busy and complex lives. It's almost as if they are independent creatures working selflessly to keep our cells healthy and active. They even have their own DNA (mitochondrial DNA or mtDNA), which is quite different from the DNA in our chromosomes; it's even shaped differently (circular, with no free ends, instead of in long strands). Every mitochondrion in every cell has its own exact copy of your mtDNA.

Mitochondrial DNA contains the genetic instructions to control all the production and management processes carried out by the mitochondria. The mtDNA genetic code specifies everything to do with building proteins, cholesterol and blood components, not to mention making life-or-death decisions about each and every cell.

Your mtDNA contains all that information in just 37 genes, not a large number compared to the estimated 20,000 genes contained in your chromosomal DNA. There's another major difference. Your chromosomal DNA comes from each parent: 23 chromosomes, totaling around 10,000 genes from each. In contrast, your mitochondrial DNA comes entirely from your mother. And your mother received her mtDNA from her mother, all the way back through the generations.

In performing such a wide range of essential functions for our cells, mtDNA creates waste products[17] along the way. If waste products accumulate they can damage mitochondrial DNA leading to neurological problems and accelerated aging.

The health of these trillions of tiny organelles inside our cells is tightly linked to the health of our entire body. We still have much to learn about the intrinsic and extrinsic factors that affect mitochondrial health, but it's becoming clear that healthy living choices play a vital role. Avoiding refined sugar,[18] maintaining a balanced and nutritious diet, and exercising all play a part.

How We Grow and Develop

Cell fission continues as a baby grows into an adult. Cells continue to replicate by splitting when they reach a certain size or condition. Even as adults, we need to add to the number of cells in our body so we can grow and so we can replace damaged cells. The replication process never ends during our lifetimes. It's estimated that an adult creates more than 20 million new cells each day.

The splitting process, mitosis, is not as simple as it sounds. Before division can start, the valuable DNA must be replicated: The DNA of each chromosome is divided down the middle, the basis for a creation of two identical copies. That requires some internal construction work and consumption of energy. Then, during fission, one copy of the DNA goes to each of the two new cells. Also, all the other cell material must be divided between the two new cells and used to reconstruct all the cell components.

At the end of mitosis, we end up with two cells to replace the one original cell. The two together contain all the material from the original cell, so the new cells (daughter cells) each start off about half the size of the old cell (mother cell). Most importantly, each daughter cell has a complete copy of the DNA, so each contains an instruction set for doing its job in the body— and, at some future point, the ability to split once again into two new daughter cells.

Our Friendly Microbes

Bacteria and yeasts (and other tiny creatures called archaea) densely populate our entire planet. They also densely populate human beings—to an extent that may surprise you. Different types are on our skin and in our digestive systems and other organs. The number of bacteria in a 155-pound human being is somewhere around 40 trillion. Compare that to the estimated number of cells of all types in the human body, which is roughly 30 trillion.[19]

Microbes have been with us for millions of years.[20] New babies inherit a starter pack at birth, some of which have been passed down for many generations. These long-inherited families of microbes are part of what makes us human beings.

Healthy infants, children and adults have acquired microbe populations that are friendly to human existence. These bacteria populations play essential roles in digesting food to extract or create nutrients,[21] converting food to energy, protecting us against diseases, and repairing external and internal damage. Our bodies could not function without these microbes.

We're also exposed to different microbes through our interactions with food, the environment and our contact with other people. Unlike with genes, our mix of microbes can change from time to time. In fact, you can change the mix in your body and on your skin within days just by altering what you eat. Antibiotics and other drugs, meanwhile, can shift the balance internally by killing or weakening friendly microbes along with unfriendly bugs. As a result, the differences in microbe populations from person to person can be dramatic—both in overall number and types.

People long have noted that there were connections between certain microbe populations and human health, but studying these connections has not been easy.

Fortunately, scientists now know much more about the microbes on our skin and through-out our bodies thanks to a powerful new tool: the Human Microbiome Project.[22] One of the early findings of this research was a confirmation that human health and longevity is linked not only to our genes and the environment but also to the health and capabilities of those trillions of microbes. Some microbes are more beneficial than others, and some populations are damaging to health. A healthy, friendly microbial population tends to fight off unfriendly microbes, or at least keep their populations at levels low enough to prevent significant damage. But if too many dangerous microbes reside in or on your body, they can make you ill.

Microbes have short lives (hours or days), so the colony renews itself rapidly using the food we share with them. This means we must constantly provide our digestive system with foods that nurture our internal microbiome. We need to encourage the beneficial bacteria and dis-courage the bad flora.

This is where the brain comes into play. Your brain and your stomach communicate in so-phisticated ways.[23] There are neural cells in your digestive system that are in constant conversa-tion with neural cells in your brain. There are about as many neurons managing your digestive system as there are in the brain of a small dog. In the same way that dogs can be trained, so can your stomach-brain connection—if you persist gently but firmly.

The chemicals that our gut microbes produce can use this communications channel to trigger signals to the brain. These signals can influence our mental processes. Thus, what we eat and drink can affect our mood and behavior. Conversely, our changing moods can give us indigestion, create an urge to eat or suppress our appetite. When you suddenly feel like eating something unhealthy, is it your brain sending you this message, or some not-so-friendly sug-ar-loving internal bacteria?

Microbes have their own genes—and their environment is us, their human hosts. The vigor, healthiness and variety of these microbes can affect our well-being and longevity.

THE INS AND OUTS OF AGING

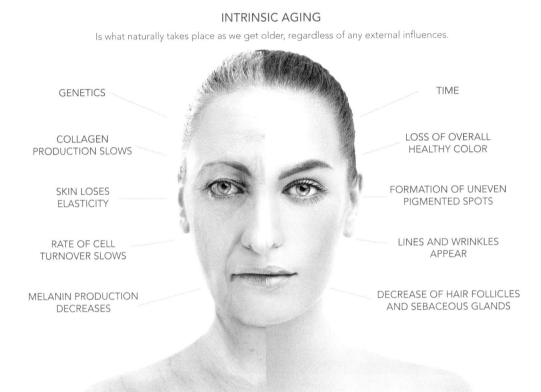

INTRINSIC AGING

Is what naturally takes place as we get older, regardless of any external influences.

GENETICS

COLLAGEN PRODUCTION SLOWS

SKIN LOSES ELASTICITY

RATE OF CELL TURNOVER SLOWS

MELANIN PRODUCTION DECREASES

TIME

LOSS OF OVERALL HEALTHY COLOR

FORMATION OF UNEVEN PIGMENTED SPOTS

LINES AND WRINKLES APPEAR

DECREASE OF HAIR FOLLICLES AND SEBACEOUS GLANDS

INTRINSIC AGING: GENES AND INHERITANCE

Genes carry the coded information that allows characteristics to be inherited from one generation to the next. The sequence of the chemical base pairs in DNA creates a code that defines the way the gene expresses itself in its human owner. Tiny changes in genes between generations provide the mechanism for biological genetic evolution, and variations in genes form the basis of differences between individuals. Even before the discovery of chromosomes and genes and DNA, humans were debating whether, how, and to what extent human characteristics might be hereditary or caused by upbringing. Nature or nurture? Or as we describe it today, genes or environment?

So, what determines our intelligence, opinions, health, longevity and desires? Why do some people grow older faster than others? Why do some people suffer lots of illnesses while others lead lives that are mostly healthy? Is it genetics? Are we more influenced by what happens to us as we grow and learn? Or is it a mix of these two? Armed with the answers to these questions, we can begin to make changes in our lives that will allow us to maintain (and even improve) our health and live longer.

You may have heard a variation of this sentiment when it comes to aging: "It's all in our genes. Sure, modern medicine can ease the pain a little as we grow older, but our fate is clear." This is a common attitude—but it's a mistake. Genes can influence many aspects of our lives, including our health, but we now know for certain that genes do not pre-determine everything.

Genetic researchers try to identify the DNA coding differences among different individuals and populations; they look for correlations between coding patterns and differences observed. For example, gene patterns can be linked to physical attributes, like whether you have dimples in your cheeks, your hair color or your eye color. Susceptibility to certain diseases also can be identified in the gene patterns.

But it's not straightforward. There are relatively few genes simply and directly related to physical attributes. For example, if you have the gene for cheek dimples, you'll have cheek dimples. If you have the gene for a cleft chin, you'll have a cleft chin. For the most part, however, genes don't work like that. Often, our genes only create a pre-disposition to a certain attribute—and other external factors interact with genes to influence the outcome.

Most human genetic markers that have been linked to specific age-related illness do not behave deterministically, in the sense that having a specific set of gene markers definitely causes the disease. Certain gene patterns can increase the risk, some patterns can reduce it, but few patterns cause it for sure. In these cases, we need to be careful to describe the gene pattern not as causing the disease but as being a "genetic risk factor."

For example, there are several different gene forms that can affect the likelihood of developing Alzheimer's disease. With the most common gene combination, Alzheimer's afflicts some people, but not others. A different variant has been linked to a reduced risk of late-onset Alzheimer's compared to the most common form, and yet another variant may increase the risk. There is still another gene that influences early-onset Alzheimer's. If present, it makes early-onset highly likely; if absent, highly unlikely. In every case, it's all about degrees of risk, not inevitability.[24]

That's just one example. Consistently, we find that genes mostly affect probabilities and less often operate in a deterministic way. We can combat illnesses and rapid aging that is linked to such probabilistic gene patterns by understanding the environmental factors that allow or encourage those genes to be expressed.

Our improved knowledge of gene structure detail (thanks in large part to the efforts of researchers contributing to the Human Genome Project[25]) has enabled researchers to be more definite about the actual impact of genes on the likelihood of incurring specific diseases. Such research projects also have given us a basis for more accurate insights into links between genes, illness and age-related deterioration. Researchers can assess with greater confidence whether a condition is the inevitable result of a certain genetic marker—or not significantly influenced by genes at all.

For everything in between, we now can make more informed risk assessments. It seems that there are not many diseases or conditions that are genetically inevitable; in most diseases, genes provide a greater or smaller predisposition to a specific illness. Even with a genetic marker that suggests a strong predisposition to a disease, it's often possible to decrease the odds of getting that illness with a combination of healthy living choices and preventive medical measures.

Our knowledge today has reached a point where we can say with confidence that, although there's a genetic component to aging and illness, environmental factors matter a lot more. [26]That means we have a huge opportunity to reduce the risks from genetic inheritance by controlling our own environment. In other words, we can impact how those genes come into play by choosing how to care for and nourish our own bodies.

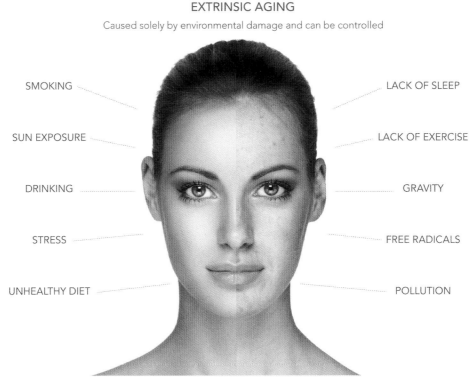

EXTRINSIC AGING
Caused solely by environmental damage and can be controlled

SMOKING

SUN EXPOSURE

DRINKING

STRESS

UNHEALTHY DIET

LACK OF SLEEP

LACK OF EXERCISE

GRAVITY

FREE RADICALS

POLLUTION

EXTRINSIC AGING: WE ARE IN CONTROL

Extrinsic aging is caused by factors other than the genetic dispositions to aging and illness described in the previous section. Extrinsic aging is driven by the environment we live in, the food we choose to eat, how we look after our physical bodies, how mentally resilient we are to stress and anxiety, and much more. The outside world affects our body every day, through our skin, lungs and what we choose to eat and drink. These extrinsic factors can lead directly to cell deterioration, which results in what we call aging. Furthermore, they can cause illness, and illness accelerates aging.

Let's take a deeper dive into extrinsic factors:

- Your body cells need good nutrition and hydration, so choose food and beverages that nourish, and avoid those that damage. Your food needs to contain adequate cell-building materials, provide energy and nutrients, and deliver dietary fiber so that your internal digestive system can keep its microbial flora in peak condition.

- There are many ways to inflict damage on the body's cells. Smoking cigarettes causes inflammation throughout the body and can cause or increase the risk of diseases in the lungs and other major organs. Too much alcohol can compromise the immune system, cause inflammation and lead to cardiovascular disease, liver problems and other health problems. Same with excessive drug use. All of these vices accelerate cell aging.

- Physical activity plays an important role in body health. Exercise increases blood circulation and oxygen supply to the muscles, internal organs and skin, all of which assists cell formation and health. Exercise improves your sleep quality, which, in turn, enhances the condition of cells throughout your body. Exercise also protects against multiple diseases associated with aging. Bottom line: If you don't get enough physical exercise, you are more prone to illness—and you'll age faster.

- Sunlight damages our skin, and skin damage can have repercussions for the rest of the body. Our skin has to fight off damage-causing chemicals in the air and in the water.

- Mental stress can alter the way your nervous system operates, and that can have an impact on the way your skin works. In particular, it can result in a weakening of your skin's barriers against microbes and other bugs, making you more susceptible to illnesses. This is why unpredictable rashes and skin eruptions can accompany exposure to stressful situations.

We now know that around 70 percent to 80 percent of aging is due to extrinsic factors. That gives us window after window of opportunity to challenge the aging process by making healthy living choices about food, exercise, skin care and mental balance.

Extrinsic aging affects more than just the skin on our face and body. Environmental factors coupled with a subpar lifestyle can force the hair growth cycle to experience a major shift. About 50 percent of American men and women suffer from, what I would call, environmental hair loss—thinning hair and hair loss caused by stress, a poor diet and a lack of exercise. Sure, it is natural for the hair cycle to slow and the size of the hair follicle to miniaturize as we age, but a change in the way you take care of your body can make a dramatic change to the hair on your head.

If thinning hair and hair loss are of concern, I highly recommend consulting with a board-certified dermatologist, and making a change to your diet, monitoring your stress levels, getting enough sleep, exercising regularly and adding a hair specific nutraceutical, like Hush & Hush DeeplyRooted, to the mix. Supplements that focus on regrowing healthy hair and improving hair and scalp health contain botanicals, vitamins and other ingredients to help normalize growth patterns, decrease oil production and inflammation.

WHEN THINGS GO WRONG

CELL DAMAGE AND REPLICATION ERRORS

Earlier, I explained how the process of mitosis (cell division) continues throughout our lives to create new cells. Mitosis preserves genetic information and results in the body having two cells that both should be the same as the original cell. More often than not, the replication process works just fine, but occasionally a mistake can happen. When it does, DNA replication will not result in an exact copy. Sometimes there's an obvious cause for faults occurring: A cell's DNA could be damaged before the splitting process starts, perhaps by excessive sunlight, chemicals, tobacco or other drugs. Other times, faulty replication is (as far as we know) completely random.

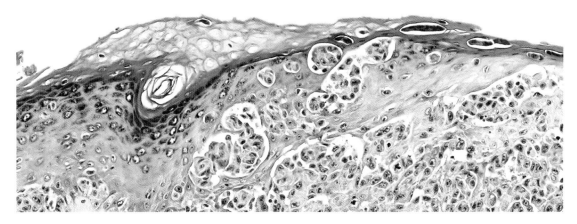

Whenever a cell is damaged either by physical factors or by a random event, the immune system usually will identify what's happening and send out appropriate chemical signals to the mitochondria within the affected cells. The mitochondria will then quietly and efficiently shut that cell down, which is the process of apoptosis mentioned earlier.[27]

Sometimes, apoptosis doesn't happen. If for some reason the immune system slips up, or the mitochondria don't do their job, the damaged cell will be replicated. If it replicates once it can replicate many times; this unrestricted growth can result in a mass of unwanted cells—aka, a tumor—that continues to grow and potentially do damage.

The good news is that you can help prevent this from happening. By minimizing your exposure to damaging events and nourishing your cells, each cell will live longer. Mitosis will take place at longer intervals, thus reducing the chances of defects in cell replication.

DNA damage is not the only hazard the human body encounters during mitosis. Something else happens to the chromosomes that contain our DNA.

DNA's End Game

Chromosomes consist of long strands of DNA, and each strand has loose ends.[28] Every time a chromosome splits during cell division, the ends become shortened in the process. If those chromosome ends contained vital genetic information, we'd be in trouble after just one or two generations of cell replication.

But we survive. This is because the ends of our chromosome strands are not loaded with important data; they consist of a short length of apparently meaningless DNA called a telomere. Instead of losing necessary DNA, we just lose a bit off the end of that telomere.

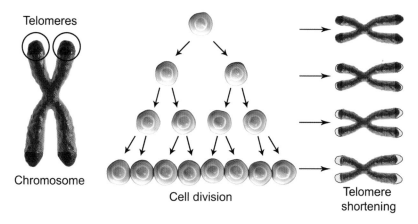

Telomeres

Chromosome

Cell division

Telomere shortening

Unfortunately, telomeres don't last forever. Every time a chromosome is divided, you lose another section of telomere on each strand. Eventually, the telomeres become so short that cell division cannot take place without damaging the DNA.[29] At this stage either too many cells die, leading to atrophy, or else the damaged cells survive and thrive, with a high probability of becoming cancer cells. Neither outcome is something you want.

Healthy cells live longer and divide less often. To extend the number of years that our telomeres stay in business protecting our DNA, we need to keep our cells healthy. And that depends on making the right living choices.

To Express or Not to Express

Having specific genes does not guarantee that you will or will not contract a given illness, or age more or less quickly. Sometimes genes are expressed, which means that they are switched on and have an impact. Sometimes they are not expressed, and so they do nothing.

There are several ways in which events in your body can control the way your genes are expressed through a process called DNA methylation.[30]

The ability of the body to turn gene expression on and off at the right times and under the appropriate conditions is an essential part of healthy embryonic development, cell differentiation and chromosome stability.[31] When this process is working correctly, methylation turns on or turns off the expression of genes as needed to ensure that cell differentiation functions properly and that chromosomes are maintained in a stable, healthy condition.

It doesn't always work that way. Sometimes genes that should be switched off are switched on, and vice versa. When that happens your body is failing in one of its most important functions. Inappropriate methylation, consisting of an absence of methylation where it is needed (hypomethylation) or the presence of methylation where it is unwanted (hypermethylation) has been linked in adults to certain types of cancer, lupus and muscular dystrophy.[32]

As research gradually illuminates the exact mechanisms of methylation, the various causes, including dietary, are becoming clearer. There are several dietary components that have been shown to fight de-methylation and support appropriate methylation by, for example, inhibiting hypermethylation of cancer-causing genes.[33]

All fruits and vegetables support appropriate methylation. Folate and other B-vitamin components, as well as phenolic compounds in plant foods all fight de-methylation. Selenium deficiency is associated with hypomethylation, so we need to maintain a reasonable level of selenium by eating nuts and seeds and other selenium-rich foods.

On the other hand, there are substances we should avoid in order to keep our DNA methylation process working for us, not against us. Two danger factors already are well known.

Smoking tobacco is known to trigger abnormal methylation in more than 7,000 genes, which represents around one-third of your gene population.[34] Smoking affects methylation in genes that are associated with cardiovascular illnesses and cancers. Stopping smoking will repair some of the damage over time, but some residual damage probably will last for decades. So, if you smoke, stop now before you do more irreparable damage.

Consumption of alcohol is strongly associated with hypomethylation.[35] In fact, the connection is so strong that methylation levels can be used as an indicator to measure alcohol consumption. The more alcohol you consume, the more you affect DNA methylation in your genes.

LINES OF DEFENSE

The human body naturally tries to prevent harmful substances from entering it. Keeping the bad stuff out starts with the skin, which works tirelessly to keep damaging substances and pathogens outside our delicate bodies. The skin has a partner in the skin microbiome (your own personal army of friendly microorganisms that live in and on your skin). If healthy, the microbiome will neutralize certain pathogens before they invade. If it becomes unbalanced, the microbiome is less able to destroy invading forces. Skin microorganisms are an integral part of your border patrol team.

Salivary glands, tear glands, gut, kidneys and a variety of mucus sources also play a role in neutralizing pathogens—or capturing them and expelling them from the body. Our brave mito-chondria will, if necessary, signal the cell they inhabit to commit suicide if that is the best thing for an invaded body.

Inflammation is part of the defensive process too. It's a natural reaction to some kind of body invasion or cell damage. Inflammation can be a response to an infection by bacteria, fungus or physical damage, as the immune system deploys forces to combat pathogens or other intruders. It's triggered by the release of certain chemicals from injured cells, which produces a rush of blood to the site of the problem. This delivers an army of lymphocytes (white blood cells), including different types—each type with its own specialized capability to zap intruders.

Inflammation often causes pain. Pain, unpleasant as it usually is, sometimes serves a useful purpose. It's telling your brain that something is going on that might not be good. Usually, but not infallibly, it's suggesting you should do something to help your body reduce the pain. If mending the pain involves something simple like resting a sore muscle for a short time, ev-erything is fine. If we focus more on treating the pain than identifying its cause—and treating that—then that can lead to problems.

Your body has a terrific array of tools to resist invasion and repair damage. Yet the immune system itself can be damaged. If the immune system is consistently pushed to its limits, that can result in excess inflammation, which may become chronic. That causes increased blood pressure, damage to the arteries and cell damage. At that stage, body cells can succumb to any number of inflammatory diseases: arthritis, joint pain and stiffness, heart disease, diabetes, bowel disease and more. None of this is good if you want to lead a long and healthy life.

To understand the link between the immune system and excessive inflammation, we also need to look at the closely related topics of oxidation and the formation of free radicals.

Radical Approach

Oxidation happens throughout the natural world, not just in the human body. It's a simple chemical reaction in which one atom or molecule loses one or more electrons to another atom or molecule. This usually results in the creation of a new molecule of a different kind[36]. A classic example of oxidation is the formation of rust from iron and atmospheric oxygen. The iron is said to be oxidized by the oxygen. Oxygen grabs electrons from iron, or, to put it another way, iron loses electrons to the oxygen. This type of reaction is called a reduction-oxidation reaction (or redox). The result is rust.

In a sense, what goes on in our bodies is a bit like rusting; as you age, you oxidize. Cells re-sponsible for creating energy process the nutrients we eat and the oxygen in the air we breathe. In our internal cellular power station, the oxygen aggressively steals electrons from some molecules: These molecules have been oxidized, so they lack an electron—meaning they are pos-itively charged. A charged molecule is called a radical, and radicals usually are eager to bond with any other molecule that's in the neighborhood. If there isn't anything available nearby, they float around, chemically reactive and ready to bond. An unattached radical is called a "free radical." Not all free radicals are bad. After all, they're an essential part of the power production process, and in moderate amounts they are needed for some biological signaling functions that can protect against diseases. However, an abundance of free radicals can be dangerous.

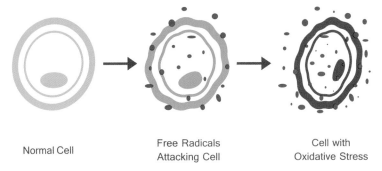

Normal Cell | Free Radicals Attacking Cell | Cell with Oxidative Stress

A host of things contribute to the production of excess free radicals: too much blood sugar, ingested chemicals, drugs, smoke, foods that have been heavily processed and other foreign substances. Stress, lack of sleep and physical damage also may play a role. When there are too many free radicals (sometimes described as oxidative stress), those charged particles seize electrons wherever they can, resulting in actual damage to body cells, proteins and even genes. The result is inflammation as the body's immune system tries, unsuccessfully, to combat the unknown cause of the damage.

Your power generation system always produces free radicals, but fortunately the body has a natural way of zapping excessive amounts of free radicals about as soon as they are formed. Antioxidants are substances that donate electrons freely to any nearby radicals that need them. That is, they restore free radicals to their original molecular form, thus reducing oxidative stress.

The oxidation-inflammation theory of cell aging has been around for a long time. Research seems to confirm that this process (described here in a simplified way) plays a role in human aging, and that inflammation contributes to a variety of diseases that shorten the lives of humans.

The good news is that natural human foods contain lots of antioxidants; foods that contain antioxidants fight inflammation and can help regulate the immune system (regular exercise also reduces oxidative stress). The bad news is that many of us have stopped eating natural human food, specifically fresh fruit and vegetables (many humans also don't get enough exercise). Without a healthy intake of antioxidants, the body can't match the excess free radicals in its normal energy creation system—nor can it combat the extra oxidative stress from chemicals, smoke and other oxidizing agents in our food and air.

Foods that contain antioxidants fight inflammation and can help regulate the immune system. Antioxidants can be found in some nuts, and in all fruits and vegetables (the darker and more intense the coloration, the better). Blueberries, blackberries and grapes are all great antioxidants. Lots of spices and herbs are good too—like cinnamon, turmeric, oregano and just about anything else in your spice drawer.

The kind of antioxidants that are added to meat products during processing (or fed to animals before slaughter) are mostly there to extend product shelf life, but don't do much for human longevity; so stick to plants.

Antioxidants also come in supplement form, which can be useful if your day-to-day diet is lacking. In my opinion, supplements like Hush & Hush's TimeCapsule (hushandhush.com) not only can be useful, but are essential in order to boost the antioxidant capacity in your body. Many of the recommended daily intake dosages aren't enough to combat free radical damage in the body. Just be careful. Overdoing antioxidant supplements can cause problems,[37] and most are not FDA regulated. I recommend that you have blood work done to check your antioxidant levels.

Eating antioxidant-rich foods that can help reduce inflammation is essential. At the same time, it's important to avoid enemy foods that boost the oxidizing process and trigger inflammation. Foods that stimulate your body to produce more energy than it needs also create excess free radicals that can't always be scooped up by antioxidants. The culprits are well-known, starting with refined sugar and refined starches. Processed vegetable oils, fried foods and many food additives also boost free radicals, leading to oxidative stress.

WHY THIS AGE MATTERS

In recent years, cellular health and inflammation researchers have been paying a lot of attention to a body process called glycation—and to the molecules created by that process, which are advanced glycation end products (AGEs). The formation and presence of AGEs appear to be closely correlated to a range of body dysfunctions, including excessive inflammation, protein degradation and cell aging.

Glycation occurs when sugar (in the bloodstream) combines with certain proteins to produce AGE molecules, which are essentially degraded versions of normal proteins.

The glycation process was first studied in diabetic patients with exceptionally high levels of glucose in their blood. High blood sugar levels drive high levels of glycation. That results in diabetics having AGEs spread throughout the body.[38] In diabetics, the relationship between AGE, protein degradation and inflammation has been firmly established. One of the proteins damaged by AGE is collagen, which is widely present in our joints, connective tissues and skin.

Further research[39] found that non-diabetics can be affected by AGEs, especially as our skin ages and the health of our collagen becomes even more important. AGEs (specifically certain AGEs now recognized as "Toxic AGEs") are implicated in aging and illness for everyone (not just diabetics).[40] There is now evidence that toxic AGEs also are implicated in the formation of neurological diseases.[41]

You have control over many factors that affect, in one way or another, the amount of AGEs that are in your body. For example:

Smoking tobacco is linked to the creation of AGEs throughout your skin and body.[42]

The ultraviolet component of sunlight causes oxidative stress and this increases the formation of AGEs in the skin.[43]

Many food products contain AGEs, especially meat products, processed foods and foods cooked at high temperatures. Although it's difficult to eliminate AGEs from your food intake completely, sensible healthy food choices can reduce the AGEs you ingest.

We can improve our body's ability to fight AGE formation by exercising[44] and eating foods high in AGE-fighting agents.

A Maintenance Plan for Humans

Our efforts to understand how the human body works have led to many insights into ways we can take care of our bodies to slow aging and improve our health. An encouraging feature of this research is that some common factors emerge over and over. Whether we are trying to fight inflammation and oxidation, maintain neurological health, reduce the toxic advance of glycation, or nourish and care for the building blocks of our bodies (our cells), the reasoning leads to the same conclusions about the choices that are good for us—and the choices that are damaging.

Those insights are reflected throughout the *Age Later* program in specific recommendations. If you make healthy living choices to defend your body against illness and aging, you will experience better health and age more gracefully. If your body provides an environment that welcomes illness and aging, you won't.

Which will you choose?

Now, let's move on to what you need to do to look younger and live longer.

Chapter 3

GET MOTIVATED, GET STARTED

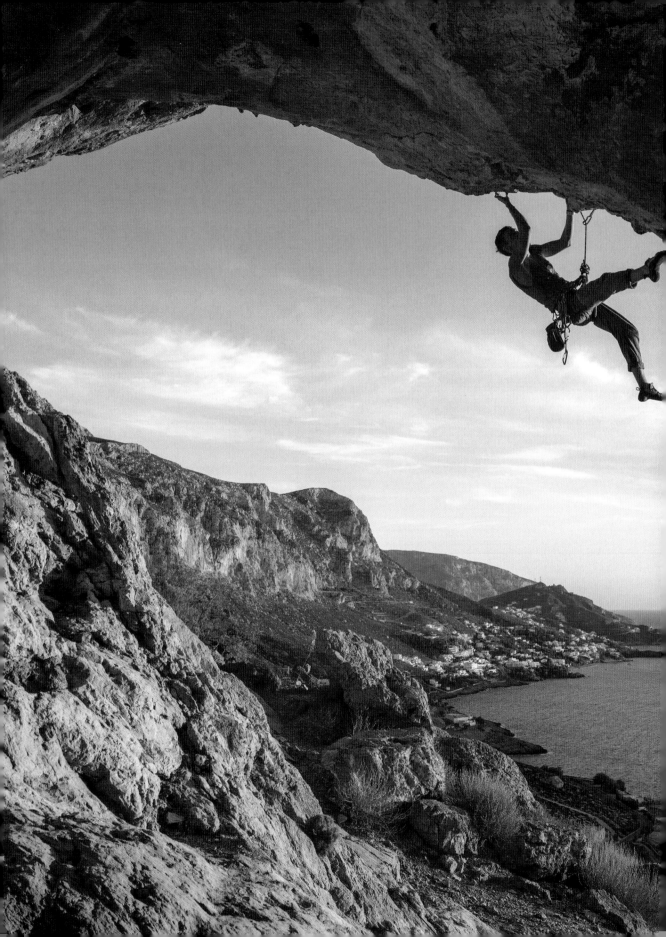

GET MOTIVATED, GET STARTED

For those of you who aren't already living a lifestyle based on the choices I describe in *Age Later*, this is the moment of truth. A journey of a thousand miles begins with a single step.

Are you ready to take the step—one that leads toward improved health, increased stamina and strength, and a more youthful appearance?

These are the life-changing benefits that are within your reach. If you follow the *Age Later* program for seven weeks, and give it serious attention, you will notice significant improvements. Your skin will feel smoother and hydrated, you'll have more energy, you'll think more clearly, your posture will improve—you'll feel more alive.

As always, results will depend on your degree of aging and state of health at the start of the program, not to mention how enthusiastic and diligent you are about following through on the program.

Although anyone of any age can benefit from the healthy living choices suggested in the *Age Later* program, those who benefit most and with least effort are those who start the transformation before they've caused too much damage to their bodies. So, the sooner you start the better.

Are you ready?

Let's take the leap.

TRANSFORMATION

My *Age Later* program recommends a range of healthy living choices that will change your life in multiple ways. However, the program is flexible.

The more elements you build into your life, the more improvements you'll see. Even one small change will bring benefits; as you begin to recognize these enhancements, you'll be motivated to do more and more. But those who go all in—who adopt the program in all its breadth—stand to benefit the most.

The *Age Later* program can be fun and fulfilling for those who approach it with the right frame of mind. This is not about forcing a new lifestyle. This is about you choosing to adopt new habits, ones that will benefit you in the short term as well as in the long run. To that end, the first seven weeks are crucial. You must work hard to build your foundation. You're making good habits an everlasting part of your new lifestyle. Expect some of these changes to be challenging at first. I promise you, they'll get easier; that's how good habits work.

Ultimately, this book is about a permanent lifestyle change. You are about to reprogram your body.

You'll start with your conscious mind, the mind that is reading this book now and absorbing its messages. To acquire a new habit, you not only need to be convinced at the level of your conscious mind, but you need to reprogram your subconscious so that new habits and skills are embedded. It's like being on autopilot. This is how people learn skills that need to operate reliably when the conscious mind is otherwise occupied, or when events happen too quickly for the conscious mind to keep up. This is how people become skilled at baseball, tennis, golf, skiing, playing piano or driving a car. You do this with practice, multiple repetitions over a long period of time.

New persistent habits will change the sort of person you are. The way you change is completely under your control. You are free to choose habits that are good for your appearance, physical health and mental strength. You can choose a lifestyle that will extend your life and make it more productive and enjoyable. Or you can choose to do none of these things.

If you really want to transform your life, this book is here to help.

Why Seven Weeks?

You may have heard that it takes just 21 days to form a new habit. If only that were true, but it's not![45]

A few minutes contemplating your own habit-forming characteristics can demonstrate this. How long does it take you to form a new (good) habit? You might say that it all depends—and you would be right. It depends on how simple or complex your new habit is, how enjoyable or irksome it feels, how motivated you are to achieve the benefits of the new habit. It depends on how frequently you repeat the action during the training period; if you repeat the action six times a day, you'll likely learn sooner than if you repeat it just once a month.

Other factors can delay or accelerate habit acquisition. For example, if your friends and family are all supportive and encouraging when they observe you trying to change your life, then your new good habits are more likely to stick sooner—and more likely to last. On the other hand, if your friends and family are not supportive, transformation could take a long time.

The amount of time needed to initiate the transformation and see results will vary from person to person, especially if you're changing several things all at once. In those cases, a few days definitely will not be enough.

That's why I suggest seven weeks of serious effort to make a good start on these fundamental changes to your lifestyle. By the end of that time, the new ways of caring for yourself will have become natural and almost automatic. At that point, you'll want to continue adding to your good habits, naturally and almost effortlessly. That's when the benefits of your new healthy living choices will become readily apparent.

At the end of the seven weeks, you will have acquired a new set of good habits and eliminated a number of bad habits. You will have established the foundation for your new lifestyle, one that you will need to maintain in order to achieve long-term benefits.

But seven weeks is only the beginning. It's the first chapter in a story that will redefine the way you live, the way you feel and the way you look.

MEASURING PROGRESS

The mirror never lies. For some, that will be the easiest way to chart progress as the lifestyle changes in *Age Later* begin to take root.

For others, a more organized, detailed approach will work best—especially given the progress in multiple areas that *Age Later* has the potential to deliver. I find that those who keep track of progress, even in a simple way, discover that they not only become more motivated, but they stay motivated.

Use a spiral notebook, a computer spreadsheet, a tracking app like Fitness & Health Habit Tracker or Lifesum—or a big chart on the wall. Whatever works best for you. Keeping some sort of a visible record helps to maintain your motivation, especially when you see progress every week.

What's important to you? Here are some ideas:

- Measure improvements to your overall appearance, skin condition and posture by taking a sequence of photographs.

- Chart your blood pressure or heart rate variability (HRV) as a measure of your cardio-vascular health (and also as an indication of your mental stress levels).

- Weigh yourself once a day.

- Count the number of repetitions you achieve in strength exercises.

- Measure your achievement in a selected long-duration exercise (walking, biking, running) every session.

- Measure the general fitness of your heart and lungs by timing how long it takes for your pulse to return to normal after vigorous exercise.

Everything in the program contributes to these measurements. For example, your blood pressure will be influenced by the food you eat, your exercise regimen, your ability to control or curtail your smoking and/or alcohol habits, your success at stress reduction and achieving inner peace. Your skin condition is influenced not just by skin care but also by food and exercise (as well as smoking and alcohol consumption). Everything is connected.

When you measure any of these parameters, you are measuring progress in all aspects of the *Age Later* program.

A couple of quick suggestions: 1) Measure your progress regularly; once a week works for most people; 2) Whatever measurements you take, record them on the same day and around the same time, so that you're measuring in consistent conditions; 3) Wait at least 30 minutes after exercise before measuring blood pressure, HRV or pulse rate; 4) If you have an activity tracker it will do much of the work for you when it comes to charting progress—some even measure pulse rate and HVR for you; 5) If you load data into a spreadsheet, consider printing out graphs that illustrate your progress—and then post them someplace you regularly look (like the refrigerator door) for added encouragement.

YOUR FIRST CHOICE

Age Later presents one of those challenges that looks daunting at the outset. However, once you've immersed yourself in the changes, you'll wonder why you even hesitated.

Remember when you learned to ride a bike? When you learned to swim? How about when you first learned to drive a car, to ski, to ride a horse, to play guitar or piano? I'm assuming that you've done at least one of those things in your life. Remember how difficult it looked before you started? And how great it was to find you were able to do it? And how, after some time, you looked back and thought that the challenge hadn't been such a big deal after all?

Making and taking action involving healthy living choices is the same. It's about learning to do something new. There are a few different things you have to learn, but that's OK—you're more than capable of spinning these plates at once.

Developing positive, life-altering habits is accomplished in steps. First, you have to have the courage and determination to start. Early in the process, you have to recognize that this new way of doing things might be awkward and uncomfortable until you've mastered it. And, later, you have to allow yourself to revel in what you've learned and how it makes you feel—so much so that you can't live without this new lifestyle.

This is what I want for you, and that is what you should want for yourself.

Your first healthy living choice is to decide to be healthy.

WHAT COULD STOP YOU (IF YOU LET IT)?

Everyone can benefit from making healthy living choices, but some may feel that they can't get started on this journey because of some aspect of their current life or condition of health.

Don't go down that road. What's the problem? Say it out loud, then tackle it.

Anything that makes you feel like you can't lead a healthier life is a roadblock—and we need to eliminate them.

HEALTH PROBLEMS

Perhaps you have a health issue that requires professional care and that limits you physically. It might be something that, say, prohibits you from running 5 miles every day—but it shouldn't stop you from reforming your eating habits, improving your mental well-being and taking care of your skin. Depending on the condition, perhaps you can still do some form of physical exercise—although, to be safe, consult your medical adviser before doing something you've never done before.

Clearly, for people with such medical issues, it's vitally important to take your physical condition into account. But it's also possible to maneuver around that roadblock and make progress toward a healthier future.

OLD INJURIES

The most common reason for feeling cautious about increasing your level of exercise is fear of pain. You might be worried about an old injury or condition and how a new exercise routine might trigger dormant aches or, worse, lead to additional problems. Maybe, you have an issue with persistent pain that has no obvious single cause. Or, perhaps you nicked your finger yesterday cutting cabbage. Sorry, that one is no excuse.

Let's go back to the "old injury" roadblock.

Many people manage to adapt to old injuries and live with them for a long time, working around the residual pain. Sometimes old injuries cause further damage, such as bone spurs, or leave some muscles in a weakened condition. So, it's conceivable that a change to your routine, like increased and consistent exercise, could wreak havoc on an old injury. If the pain is tolerable most of the time, it may seem to you that it isn't worth the trouble to fix it. But if you become more active, the pain could become a real barrier to success.

The good news is that the same condition you decided to live with a decade ago may be treatable now. Injuries that challenged surgeons years ago often can be fixed today with a relatively simple operation.

Don't let apprehension regarding longtime ailments trip you up. There may be a modern-day solution for your old injury.

CHRONIC PAIN

On the other hand, perhaps you suffer from generalized pain with no obvious cause, including joint pains and headaches.

According to a 2012 survey,[46] around 11 percent of people in the United States reported experiencing pain every day for more than three months (which is defined as chronic pain). Pain is a real problem if it persistently prohibits you from doing what you want to do or need to do. It's even worse if you don't know what's causing it. At that point, you may be thinking more about pain management than pain elimination.

Different people have different levels of sensitivity to pain. Some people have an abnormally high pain threshold. On the other end of the spectrum, other people experience pain all the time, and mostly for no apparent reason. Between these two extremes, there is a spectrum of sensitivity to pain. Because of this, it's not likely that there is one simple remedy for chronic pain that will work for everyone.

Too many people are treated with the blunt instrument of never-ending doses of pain-killing drugs. Some of these drugs can be addictive; many of them will damage your health if taken over long periods.

The science of addressing pain without the use of pain-killing medication has advanced significantly in recent years. Before asking your doctor for more painkillers, consider whether you might benefit from an approach that involves less-potent drugs—or even no drugs. These approaches are based on the understanding that pain is more than a sensory issue. The way the nervous system and brain process pain can make a difference in the way that pain is perceived.

Every person is different, and I would not attempt to prescribe one course of drug-free pain relief for everyone. Nor is it easy to attempt drug-free pain management all alone without appropriate support. Your first step should be to discuss the topic frankly with your doctor, who may refer you to a multidisciplinary pain management center that offers a customized program to meet your specific needs.

A pain management program may involve drugs at some point, but the aim often will be to move to a non-drug regimen that lowers the level of pain to a point at which you can function well.

Here are examples [47] [48] of treatments that have proven to be successful for many people:

Acupuncture	Massage
Bioelectronics	Meditation Therapy
Biofeedback	Mindfulness Based Stress Reduction
Cognitive-Behavioral Therapy	Psychotherapy
	Physical Therapy
Deep Breathing	Relaxation Therapy
Electrical stimulation	Yoga

Tell the professional responsible for your pain treatment about your plans regarding the *Age Later* program; he or she may suggest some modifications until you're better able to fully immerse yourself in your healthier lifestyle.

Once you get started, you may find that the multifaceted approach of the *Age Later* program actually helps with your pain. Caring for your skin properly, changing the balance of the food you eat, adding moderate amounts of exercise to your routine, and focusing on your own peace of mind and mental well-being, all work together to improve the general health of your body. Healthy bodies usually experience less pain.

Don't allow concerns about pain to be a permanent roadblock in the way of becoming healthier and looking younger.

YOU'RE OVERWEIGHT?

If you're overweight, you're not alone. Maybe you've tried for years to reduce your weight and nothing has worked: diet after diet, gym memberships, pills, expensive exercise machines that are now collecting dust in the garage.

Do not despair. I can't promise to eliminate your excess weight overnight, but I'm confident that healthy living choices will lead you in the right direction.

Most weight loss regimens are narrowly focused and designed for the short term. My program is broad in its approach and built for the long run. That means that it is not a quick or easy fix. But it is a fix.

What causes people to pack on more pounds than they would like? Overeating is one reason, of course, as is lack of exercise. We all know that. But it's not just the amount of food you eat. What you eat matters just as much.

There are other factors that make a difference, such as the condition and balance of your stomach's microbial population, the way we move around in our daily lives, and even our mental attitude about ourselves and the world around us. In this book, I outline ways to eat more sensibly and get enough exercise. The program also helps address many other factors that, taken together, may help with your weight-management plans.

Being overweight should not prevent you from embracing the lessons in *Age Later*. No matter how much you weigh today, you can benefit from the program. Follow *Age Later* for seven weeks, and you'll establish the life patterns that will lead to a fitter, leaner and healthier future.

You Have Recurring Allergies?

Allergies are a nuisance. Why are so many people suffering with so many allergies today? One reason is that modern life is assaulting us with chemicals, vapors and other substances. Our bodies can't cope well with all these new dangers, but they react anyway, and that causes sniffling and discomfort. Our bodies sometimes also react badly to substances that have been in our environment and food for thousands of years, such as cedar pollen, dust, shellfish and nuts.

If you suffer from recurring and serious allergies, you may be worried about embarking on a program, like *Age Later*, that requires changes to your lifestyle. What if it makes your allergies worse?

Talk to people. Ask your friends. Who is miserable all summer, and who gets through life with just the occasional sniffle? Compare their diets, their exercise routines, and their attitude toward life.

Many people are living with an immune system that is out of balance, or a stomach that's populated with the wrong balance of microbes. Or they're living with too much mental stress. Any of these factors can affect your response to allergens in the environment. Perhaps you should tackle your allergies by following a multifaceted program that boosts your general health. No matter what, don't shrink from the *Age Later* program because of allergies. They're not roadblocks.

Chronic Procrastination

Sometimes, when it comes to making lifestyle changes, the most daunting obstacle has nothing to do with external forces. It's the battle within. Why do so many people fail to do things that are in their own interest? Why do they put off until tomorrow what they should start today?

Everyone procrastinates occasionally. It's not uncommon, especially in this tech-savvy age of cell phones and social media, to become distracted and waste time. For the average person, whose real problem is a lack of personal organization or the ability to prioritize, there are hundreds of helpful books out there.

Chronic procrastinators are different. They slip into procrastination mode almost every time there is something important to be done. For them, failing to get things started (and finished) is a way of life.

For chronic procrastinators, the problem has less to do with being unorganized or having poor time management skills. It's psychological, and it's emotional[49]. Some psychologists estimate that around 20 percent of adults fit the description of chronic procrastinator.

- Have you read more than a couple of books and articles on how to organize and prioritize—and still can't seem to stop procrastinating?

- Do you avoid doing things because you feel you have to be in the mood before you start, or you'll be wasting time?

- Do you sometimes feel that you can't do something because you're not in the right frame of mind, so it probably won't go well?

- Do you sometimes take a break or even a nap before doing something because you feel you need to build energy for the task?

- Do you sometimes persuade yourself to put off a chore because you feel like you'll probably mess it up?

- Do you sometimes feel fearful of starting a task because you don't think it will be successful?

- Have you ever really wanted to do something—but found that there was something inside you that just wouldn't let you do it?

I can't offer a formal diagnosis, of course, but if you answered yes to most of those questions, there's a chance you may fit the definition of a chronic procrastinator.

Procrastinators give all sorts of reasons for constantly putting off important tasks. Yet people who habitually procrastinate do so knowingly, and they end up feeling guilty and unhappy because they've failed to do something important. That leads to lack of enthusiasm for anything, resulting in further procrastination and a mental aversion to anything involving a commitment. Chronic procrastinators believe that if they hide that exercise plan in the back of the mind, then it won't cause as much guilt. They're usually wrong about that.

To-do lists don't help chronic procrastinators much. Lists just make them more unhappy. (Or, they don't get around to preparing a list.)

In this book, I invite you to take actions to change the way you live. It will be interesting and fun, and you don't need to push yourself further than makes you comfortable.

Yet some people reading this book won't be able take that first step. If you are a chronic procrastinator, and you fail to recognize that about yourself, chances are you will not make the necessary progress to improve your health. Every change you need to attempt will be a struggle.

Psychologist Timothy Pychyl puts it this way. "I think the basic notion of procrastination as self-regulation failure is pretty clear ... You know what you ought to do, and you're not able to bring yourself to do it. It's that gap between intention and action."[50]

If you understand that you are, or you're close to being, a chronic procrastinator, what can you do? It's possible that psychological therapy can help, but before that, try some of these suggestions as you take action to start, and continue, the *Age Later* program.

Don't get hung up if you stall one time. Forgive yourself and try again.

No one is judging you by your success or failure in your attempt to become healthier. Just try it. You probably will find that just starting gives you more momentum than you ever thought possible.

After you have read this book, you might feel that the number of things you need to do is overwhelming. Take a deep breath. Choose one topic that appeals most to you, and do that first. Then add one little thing at a time, every day.

Remember that this is not work, and it's not a duty to anyone except you. It's a gift to yourself, just like a visit to the movies or a great vacation overseas. Do it and enjoy it without overthinking it.

Here is another quote from the psychologist Timothy Pychyl: "It's an existentially relevant problem, because it's not getting on with life itself. You only get a certain number of years. What are you doing?"

ANYTHING ELSE?

Addictions? Relatives? Marital issues? Work problems?

There always will be roadblocks. The question is whether you're going to turn them into excuses. Don't. You may not be able to do everything I recommend in this book, but you certainly can do something. So, do what you can, then do a little more. In seven weeks, you'll wonder why you ever doubted your ability to *Age Later*.

Chapter 4

LOSING YOUR DANGEROUS HABITS

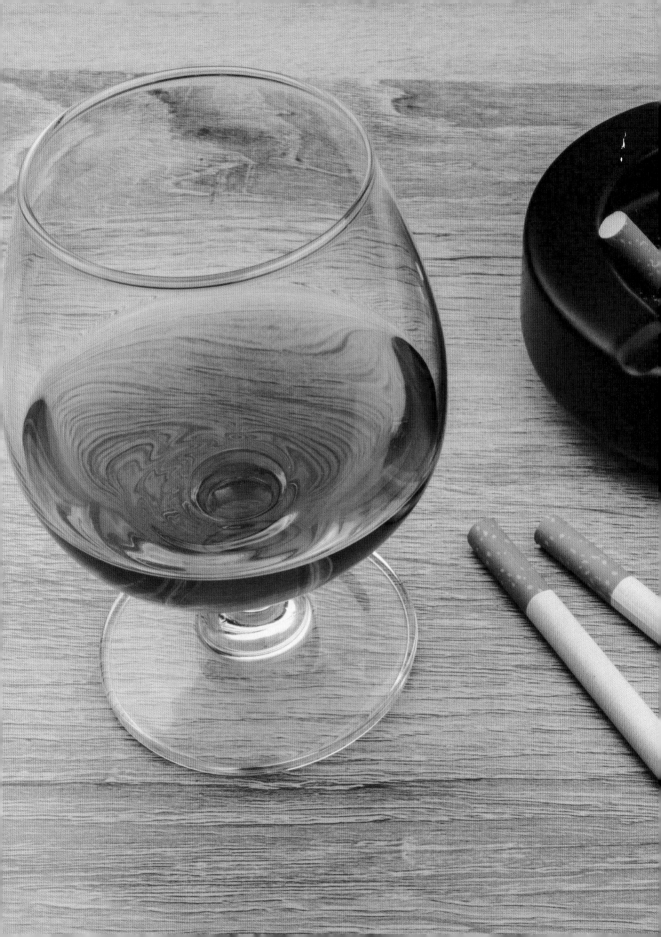

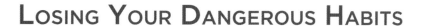

LOSING YOUR DANGEROUS HABITS

Earlier, we touched on some of the obstacles that can prevent people, at least in their minds, from taking a life-changing leap—like the healthy choices outlined in *Age Later*. I saved two of those roadblocks to address separately because they involve products that are widely consumed, marketed to the masses and easy to obtain.

They also will shorten your life.

Of course, placing tobacco and alcohol in the "bad habit" category is hardly revolutionary. Still, I bring both up early in *Age Later* because their debilitating effects impact so many people around the world. Even if you do make healthy choices in other parts of your life—like those recommended later in the book—smoking and/or excessive drinking will limit or negate the progress you're capable of making, and you will always be at higher risk for a range of diseases.

To some people, these habits may not seem like a big deal. After all, we're not that far removed from eras where people routinely smoked cigarettes on television and where the three-martini lunch was socially acceptable.

But why roll those dice? These habits are responsible for millions of premature deaths. Smokers die, on average, at least 10 years earlier than non-smokers.[51] People with an alcohol dependency die, on average, more than seven years earlier than those who consume little or no alcohol.[52]

QUIT SMOKING

It's easy to identify longtime smokers. They look old, because smoking accelerates aging. And many of them know it. But, still, they keep smoking.

Why? Like any addiction, it's not easy to quit. But to receive the full benefits of *Age Later*, you have no choice. You must avoid inhaling any type of smoke, but especially tobacco smoke. No cigarettes, no cigars, no pipes, no hookahs.

Perhaps some knowledge about the deadly effects of smoking on the human body can help.

Although many other substances we inhale can be harmful,[53] tobacco is unique in that so many people smoke in damaging amounts every day. Smoking is an efficient way to populate your body with poisons that work together to damage your body cells and DNA, dramatically affect your skin quality, increase your blood pressure and cause life-ending diseases.

Cigarette smoke contains a vicious cocktail of thousands of different substances, including hundreds of known toxic substances and at least 60 known cancer-causing substances.[54]

People who smoke take longer to recover from illness and from injuries. I and other surgeons have noted for years that our patients who smoke have more post-surgical skin infections and heal more slowly.

Tobacco also contains nicotine. Apart from being an essential ingredient in tobacco products (essential because it's addictive), it's also used widely as an insecticide. Think about that. Smokers are inhaling a chemical used to kill insects. Nicotine ingestion is harmful, even without the smoke.

If you're still a smoker, you probably already feel like a bit of a social outcast—and you may not welcome more advice from me. I know it's not easy to give up if you've been a slave to the habit for years. If it were easy, you would have done it already—because the statistics about smoking are startling. In the United States alone, around 1,700 people die every day from smoking-related illnesses. That's more than one person every minute.

For many of us, that would be enough incentive to stop, yet for some habitual smokers, there seem to be no facts or statistics powerful enough to curb the desire. Perhaps this is because some smokers feel the damage is done, and there's no way back, so they might as well enjoy a few more smokes before their inevitable early death. It's true that some damage is lasting, and it's possible that residual harm in the form of DNA methylation can hang around for a long time.[55] Your body will do its best to counteract the impact, but some risk may still be present decades after you quit smoking.

That said, there are measurable benefits to quitting, no matter how long you've been smoking. That means you should stop smoking now before you do more damage. Give your body the best chance possible of repairing the destruction already done. If you quit smoking now, chances are that you will experience immediate and longer-term health benefits.[56] Among them:

- The same day you stop smoking, your heart rate drops and your blood pressure drops to less dangerous levels. Within about 12 hours, the carbon monoxide level in your blood drops to a normal level.

- Within a few weeks, your blood circulation improves and your lungs become more effective.

- It takes from a few weeks up to several months, but gradually your coughing decreases and you can breathe more easily.

- At the end of a year after quitting completely you will have reduced your risk of coronary heart disease by about half.

- After 10 years, your risk of lung cancer falls to about half; there also are reductions in the risk of all other cancers caused by smoking (mouth, throat, esophagus, bladder, cervix and pancreas).

- After 15 years, your risk of stroke and your risk of coronary heart disease could be around the same or not much higher than that of a lifetime non-smoker.

Smokers who try to quit just to please others tend to have low success rates. Smokers who are seriously motivated to quit because they want to look better and live longer have more chance of success, but if they do it without support their chances of quitting permanently are still low. When people are motivated to find support, by joining a local or online group, or working with a friend, the success rate rises. If a smoker is motivated, has support, and also consults with a family doctor for advice and coaching, then the quit rate goes up to more than 80 percent.

It's worth noting that by not smoking you're also benefiting the people around you who may have suffered coughing, lung irritation, stinging eyes or worse from second-hand smoke. Moreover, your smoking puts their health at risk.

One more thing: By not smoking, you'll be in much better shape to follow the *Age Later* program, and your bad habit no longer will undermine its benefits.

SENSIBLE ALCOHOL USE

Should we all eliminate alcohol from our lives? Some people think so, pointing to the health risks, social damage and time lost resulting from overindulgence. Others can hardly imagine a life without the taste of fine wine, or a sophisticated single malt, or the social lubrication that comes with a moderate amount of alcohol.

There are strong health arguments against heavy alcohol consumption, and the damage caused by this is well documented. Chronic alcohol abuse falls into the same category as smoking—it's harmful and life-shortening.

Among other things, excessive alcohol use can: lead to liver damage and cancers, diminish brain functioning, cause weight gain and high blood pressure, increase risk of heart disease and type 2 diabetes, and pave the way for depressive tendencies. For more details involving the long list of problems caused by heavy alcohol consumption, see Appendix A.

There are some indications that light alcohol consumption may bring some benefits.[57] More details about how small amounts of alcohol can bring benefits are listed in Appendix A.

My advice regarding alcohol in your lifestyle is that if you do not consume alcohol now, there is no good reason to start. If you do consume alcohol, and you can comfortably keep within the moderate consumption limits, there's no strong scientific reason to stop.

According to the National Institute on Alcohol Abuse & Alcoholism (NIAAA), moderate alcohol consumption is defined as follows:

- For an adult woman: consuming no more than seven alcoholic drinks a week, with no more than two on any one day, and at least one day per week with no alcohol.

- For an adult male: consuming no more than 14 drinks a week, with no more than three on any one day, and one day per week at least with no alcohol.

- Even if you are a moderate consumer, you may be tempted to binge once in a while. You shouldn't, even if it's your birthday. But if you do, abstain for a few days (just to prove to yourself that you can do it) and then go back to moderate consumption.

These guidelines for moderate drinking assume that each drink contains about 14 grams of alcohol.[58] That's about right for most standard bar drinks, but you should be aware that some drinks contain more alcohol than a standard drink (craft beers, cocktails, cask-strength whiskeys and so on). Drinks you pour at home, or that your friends make for you, likely will exceed standard alcohol pours, so take that into account.

While it's possible that red wine has more health benefits than any other alcoholic drink, bear in mind that it's still subject to the same limits—so if you have a glass of red wine that still counts against your daily total. Finally, try to avoid sweet cocktails completely; on top of the alcohol, you're consuming lots of sugar. Not a good combination.

For the purposes of the *Age Later* program, I would limit the "moderate" drinking standards even more. I suggest no more than five drinks per week (one glass of wine or cocktail per day, with two days of no alcohol) for both men and women.

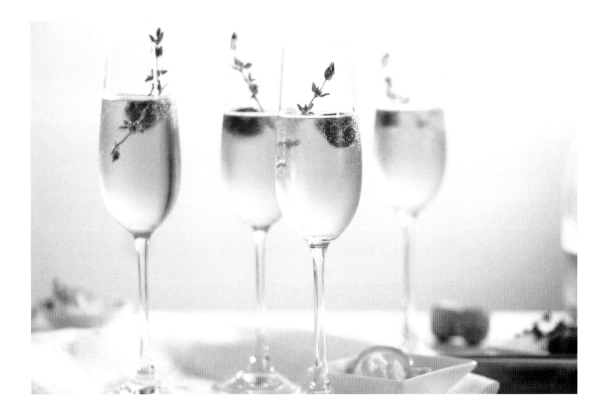

If you do follow the NIAAA standard for moderate drinking, avoid consuming more than 14 drinks (for men; seven for women) in a week. Anything beyond those levels is considered heavy drinking, and that's dangerous to your health. Reduce your consumption to moderate levels or lower as quickly as possible.

If you find you are unable to make the change from "heavy" to "moderate," you're harming your body. Your aim should be to stop drinking alcohol altogether. If you have a problem quitting, speak to a medical professional about getting help.

How to Gain Control

Kicking bad habits means taking control of your own choices.

A method of kicking bad habits that is used in some professional therapy approaches is a form of Behavioral Modification Therapy. For example, Habit Reversal Therapy[59] involves keeping track of the cues that cause you to think of doing something—and then replacing the bad habit with something else (a competing, less troublesome action, possibly something that's good for you).

Another approach used in therapy is Motivational Interviewing[60], in which the therapist works with the client to reposition the habit.

You may find that just understanding these psychological approaches can help, but the most effective way of quitting is to work with a therapist.

Your family doctor can help. For some people there are non-addictive prescription medications that can help,[61] and your family doctor should be able to advise on other therapies that are appropriate for you.[62]

It always helps to get the support and cooperation of friends and family. Tell them what you are doing and ask them to commit to helping and supporting you.

For some people, kicking the worst of their bad habits will be, perhaps, the most difficult step. For others, the timing might be perfect. Perhaps, they've been psychologically ready to make the change, but they just needed the push. Either way, it's possible to close this chapter in your life on a positive note. You can make the healthy living choice you know you need to make. Whether you achieve it alone or with professional help, you'll feel a sense of pride and accomplishment for leaving behind a seriously damaging bad habit.

Better still, you'll find the remaining *Age Later* challenges a breeze.

Whatever you do, press on with other healthy living choices. You may find they help build motivation to help you kick your bad habits.

CARE FOR YOUR SKIN

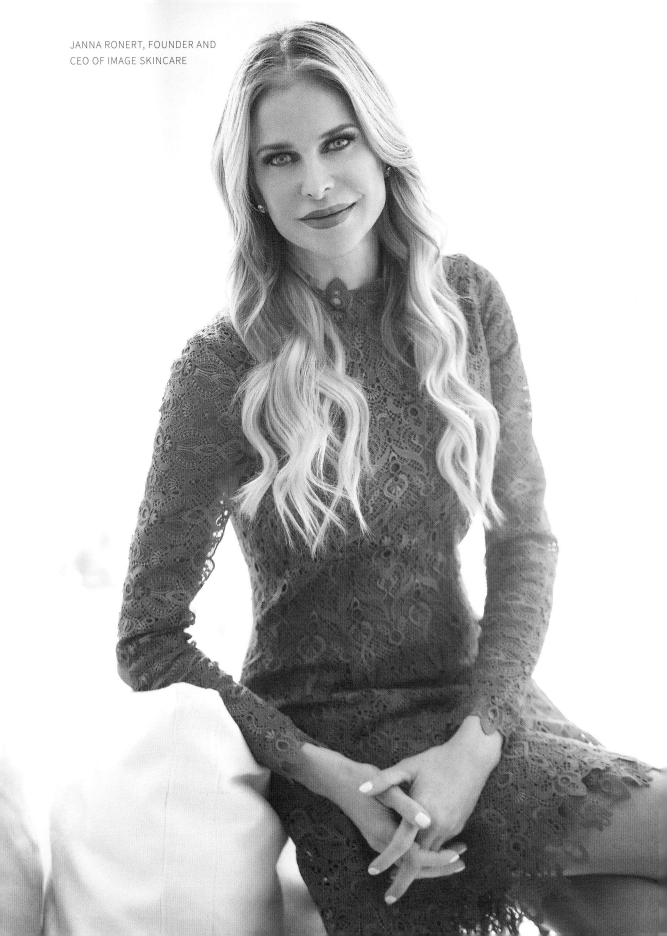

"THE NEW PERSPECTIVE ON SKIN"

They say that beauty is in the eyes of the beholder, but, for me, beauty is skin deep—figuratively and physically. Healthy, beautiful skin reflects light just right that it possesses a lit-from-within appearance, a look that we are all constantly chasing and trying to achieve. Skin that looks years younger than it genuinely is, is the true testament to looking and feeling good. And if you have ever been complimented on your skin, you know that there is no greater feeling. Taking care of your skin and body is rule number one in attaining a beautiful complexion, and skincare takes center stage here.

As we age, the skin ages, too. It's a natural, inevitable progression that can't totally be stopped but it can be limited. And that's where great skin-care products come in. Sure, the tactile sensation of applying a luxurious cream or delectably scented serum to your skin is, for some, a ritualistic act and the only way to start the day; for others, it serves a functional means to treat a bothersome issue. No matter the motive a common thread exists: we all use products as an attempt to stave off the aging process and make ourselves look that much better, regardless of how extreme our individual anti-aging plan may be.

As the Founder and CEO of Image Skincare, a prominent and successful skin-care company, I can never stress enough the importance of good skincare. Since starting Image Skincare 15 years ago with an intention to create products powered by smart botanicals and high percentages of safe, proven active ingredients—something I personally could not find on the market—I have witnessed a major pendulum swing in the skincare industry. Women (and men for that fact) are embracing the necessary efforts that come with maintaining beautiful, ageless skin. And that means taking a holistic approach and nurturing your skin from the inside out and the outside in. The industry, as a whole, is adopting these philosophies, too, with the advent of new products and technologies. No longer one-sided, skincare works more symbiotically than ever before with wellness, diet and exercise—each piece of the puzzle is as important as the next, and heavily influences the functionality and image of your skin.

With the convergence of skincare and wellness, nutraceuticals are an essential part of the puzzle that can't be ignored. They're like a little well-known secret that bridges the gap between great skin and living longer and aging better. I see what a great nutraceutical supplement can do for the mind, body and soul, which is why I am so excited to be a part of our newest venture, Hush & Hush, a line of scientifically-backed luxury nutraceuticals.

The multi-billion-dollar world of skincare is more comprehensive and inclusive than ever, yet some people still find it daunting to navigate. Skincare should not be passed over just because new brands emerge on a daily basis and unique ingredients and formulations constantly come to the forefront.

To those women and men that say they don't have time to use skincare or avoid wearing sunscreen every single day (this is non-negotiable) because they can't find one that, "doesn't sting", or "won't leave a white cast," I say keep searching; don't give up because that perfect product does exist. Yes, taking care of your skin requires time and due diligence, but you can tailor your routine to fit your morning and nighttime schedule so that proper skin care does not seem like a chore or burden, but more like self-care because it is. And, I'll let you in on a little secret: great skincare doesn't have to break the bank.

I always recognize the impact that good skincare has on one's self-esteem, self-confidence and overall appearance. And nothing looks and feels as good as young, healthy, ageless skin.

- Janna Ronert, Founder and CEO of Image Skincare

Age later.

• • • • • • • • • •

CARE FOR YOUR SKIN

For over 15 years, my team at Image Skincare has developed skin-care products with one primary aim: to delay the aging process as it affects our skin. Keeping skin healthier and more youthful looking for longer has played such a vital role within our company, that our tagline for Image Skincare is *"Age Later."* Many ingredients and healthy living choices are, in fact, also healthy for our skin. Many of the ideas and suggestions we've developed through the years at Image Skincare can be found in the following chapter.

The skin is the largest body organ you possess. It's a tough, flexible and sophisticated envelope for your entire inner body, providing protection, thermal regulation and much more. It's the first line of defense against the outside world, your protection against daily assaults from natural elements (sun, wind, etc.) and a physical defense against chemicals and pathogens in the environment. Millions of friendly microorganisms that crowd out bad bacteria and fungi assist in this defense, helping to keep your skin in good condition.[63]

Your skin also is part of the system of organs that detect what's going on in the outside world. Cells in the skin act as sensors that relay information to your brain and nervous system. Different types of sensors in the skin enable you to feel pain and avoid injury, and sense heat and cold as part of a complex system of whole body heat regulation. In addition, your skin contains sweat glands, thermal insulation, pigmentation and other essential equipment.

That's a lot of responsibility for the skin to shoulder. Though it does its best to look after itself naturally, the skin deserves your help.

Over the last 15 years, I've worked to develop skin-care solutions that delay aging. We've created a range of products that are easy to use—and that really work. My advice is based on those years of research and development. I now know that great skin-care products are essential—but that other lifestyle changes also can make a profound difference.

Healthy skin is a psychological booster. Skin that is smooth, supple and resilient is immediately more attractive to others, so people with glowing, healthy skin feel good about themselves. Feeling good creates reactions in the body that fight depression, reduce stress and motivate people to work for further self-improvement, adding momentum to the process of resisting aging and looking younger.

Good feelings can extend your life.

This chapter introduces you to a collection of healthy living choices related to caring for your skin. Making the right decisions in the short term will lead to adopting new habits, day-to-day actions that can transform you in more ways than you can imagine.

THE STRUCTURE OF THE SKIN

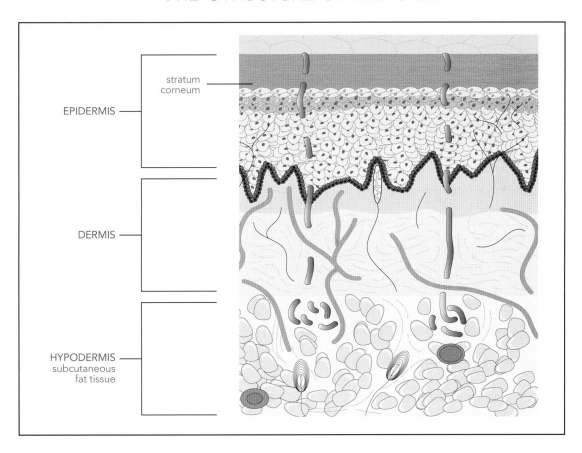

Let's take a brief look at the structure of the skin. If you know how it's built, then you will better understand how and why to care for it.

Skin comes in layers. Each layer is slightly different in its structure, ingredients and function. The layers aren't physically distinct with sharp boundaries; they are firmly unified with connective tissue, with one layer gradually blending into the next. Let's start from the outside and work in.

There are three layers that all perform vital roles to ensure skin health:

- The **stratum corneum** is the surface layer, consisting mainly of dead skin cells; it provides a protective cover for the living cells below.

- The **epidermis** consists of layers of living tissue and includes the stratum basale, the deepest layer of the epidermis and one with an array of duties.

- The **dermis** is the layer than connects the skin to the underlying body tissues, such as muscle and fat.

THE OUTER SKIN: STRATUM CORNEUM

The outermost layer of your skin is called the stratum corneum, which means "horn-like layer." This layer is made of dead skin cells (corneocytes) that accumulate as the lower layers of skin create new cells, pushing the dead cells up toward the surface. The stratum corneum varies in thickness and toughness depending on where it is on your body, but it's usually comprised of 20 or so layers of dead cells, squashed flat and tightly bound together.

The stratum corneum mainly consists of keratin, a strong and fibrous protein, bound together with proteins and lipids. This layer does the hard work when it comes to separating your inside from the outside world. It's a deceptively tough layer, considering how flexible it needs to be. The stratum corneum resists the flow of fluids from inside to outside, helping to ensure that the living cells in lower layers of the skin remain hydrated.

These dead surface cells are tightly arrayed to form a strong outside surface that prevents entry of potentially damaging microbes, fungi, chemicals and other unwanted substances. In areas of the body where the skin needs to be thicker (the palms of the hands and soles of the feet), the stratum corneum is reinforced by additional layers of dead cells, the stratum lucidum.

EPIDERMIS

The epidermis layer itself consists of several layers, but to keep things simple let's focus on one that is fundamental to skin health, the stratum basale or basal layer.[64] The basal layer is the innermost layer of the epidermis. Cell division takes place in the stratum basale, providing a continuing source of cells that pass through successively higher layers until they reach the stratum corneum. This progression through the epidermal layers takes from 14 to 40 days, depending on the location of the skin and your age.

The skin stem cells in the basal layer regulate all healing and regenerative processes and therefore play a vital role in maintaining skin health and integrity. Also in the basal layer, there are specialist cells that play roles in sensing (touch receptors), pigmentation of the skin and immunity.

Dermis

Underneath the epidermis is a layer called the dermis, containing some of the skin's nerve endings, capillaries carrying blood, hair roots, sweat glands and pigmentation. It's where a lot of action takes place.

There are two layers within the dermis.[65]

The elastin and collagen in the dermis are essential for healthy functioning of the skin—and also important in terms of your appearance. Elastin and collagen enable skin elasticity, allowing the skin to smoothly stretch and contract back into place. Collagen in the skin also performs a host of other services, such as moisture retention, cushioning and resilience. Healthy collagen means fewer wrinkles and less sagging. That's another good reason for looking after your collagen. Collagen plays a role not just in the skin but in all the body's moving parts. That's why people with stiff joints sometimes find that their skin lacks elasticity and is tired-looking.

Subcutaneous Fat

Immediately below the dermis is a layer that is sometimes called the hypodermis. It's not strictly part of your skin, but it's an important component of your body covering. This is where your subcutaneous fat lives, in cells called adipocytes.

The upper layer has folds and creases of collagen and elastin where it meets the layer above, the dermis. Then there's the fat. Having the right amount of fat is important, and aiming for zero fat is a not a good idea.

Your subcutaneous fat protects your inner tissues and organs from cold and heat in the environment outside. Fat is a thermal insulator, so it slows down the transfer of heat in both directions. When the air is colder than your body, it prevents your body heat from escaping too fast. When the air is warmer than your body, your fat slows the movement of thermal energy from the outside to the inside, thus helping to keep your internal organs at a stable temperature.

Along with being an essential layer of insulation, subcutaneous fat is one of the sources of stored energy available to the body to meet extra energy needs, for example during strenuous exercise.

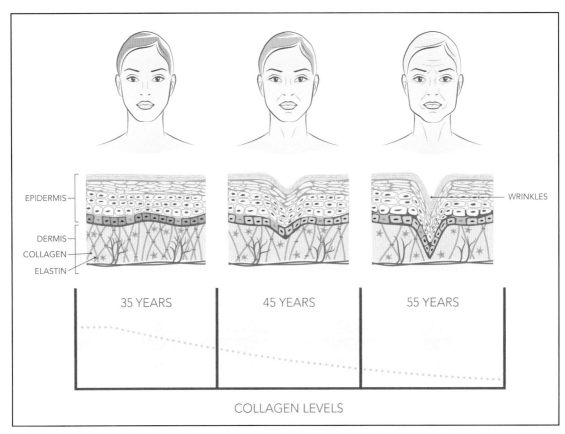

EPIDERMIS
DERMIS
COLLAGEN
ELASTIN
WRINKLES

35 YEARS　　45 YEARS　　55 YEARS

COLLAGEN LEVELS

AGING OF THE SKIN

Your skin is a mirror that reveals the state of health of your entire body. The same genetic mechanisms and the same exposures to an aggressive environment that cause damage and aging inside our bodies also drive the deterioration of skin cells.

Genes do have an impact. Your inner biological clock ticks on, no matter what you do. This is largely determined by the biological coding in your DNA. Your cells cannot replicate forever, and eventually cell damage leads to apoptosis, or cell death. Your DNA also determines your susceptibility to certain illnesses, and those illnesses can accelerate cell aging. Still, most of the visible signs of aging are caused by years of damage to our skin, at all levels, simply by living in the world.

Aging of the skin, by whatever mechanism, reduces our resistance to outside assaults, so aged skin becomes less of a barrier to disease, toxins and allergens. If our skin isn't healthy, we're more likely to get sick. At the same time, an unhealthy body leads to skin deterioration.

However, the opposite also is true. Healthy skin reflects a healthy body.

SMILING AND FROWNING

Your face is the great communicator. You express emotions by smiling, frowning, looking alarmed, looking puzzled. Our facial skin is tightly connected to the underlying muscle system and to the superficial muscular aponeurotic system (SMAS), which is a distinct fiber-muscular layer that ages with use. When we smile or frown, the skin follows the muscle movement, as does the SMAS.

If you frown once, it does not have a noticeable impact, and the wrinkle created disappears once you stop frowning. When you smile and frown thousands of times, year after year, the wrinkles get engraved into your skin and into the SMAS, leaving permanent lines behind. At the same time, gravity exerts a constant downward pull on the skin and your muscles, eventually causing sagging.

Up to a point, these facial changes as we grow older might be described as "showing character." Eventually, it's best described as "looking old."

Skin care can address the quality of skin layers and reduce the appearance of wrinkles and sagging, but surface skin care has very little impact on the SMAS underneath. Tightening and rejuvenating the SMAS may require surgical intervention.

SUNLIGHT

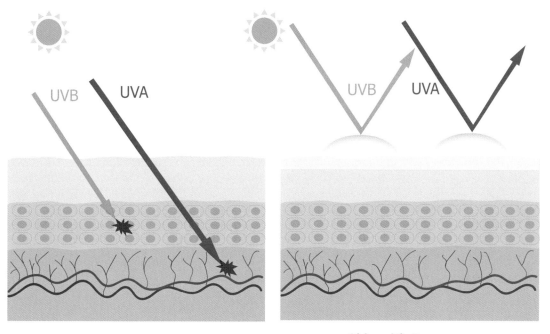

Normal skin   **Skin with Sunscreen**

Of the many factors that cause extrinsic aging of the skin, the everyday assault by sunlight is the number one danger.

Being out in the fresh air and daylight is psychologically uplifting, even therapeutic. Sunlight is instrumental in enabling our bodies to make vitamin D, which in turn is needed to make use of calcium to build healthy teeth and bones. So is sunlight good for us? To some extent, yes.

But there's a downside. Sunlight is damaging; it's the biggest single cause of skin aging. The visible part of sunlight has some impact,[66] but the most severe skin damage is caused by rays of invisible ultraviolet light (UV) that impact our skin every day. It damages the cells in your eyes too.

UV is the component of sunlight that causes skin to darken as it tans, redden as it burns and peel when it's burned too much. Too much UV exposure causes skin cell damage that can evolve into a variety of problems, including forms of skin cancer. In the U.S., Americans who live into their 60s have at least a 40 percent chance of having skin cancer at some point in their lives.[67] If you live in Australia, and you make the most of the outdoor life, your chances rise to more than 60 percent according to the Australian Cancer Council.[68]

Just as visible light is defined in terms of wavelengths, invisible UV light is categorized in the same way. There are three different subgroups within the UV spectrum: UVA, UVB and UVC.[69]

UVA is the group with the longest wavelength and represents around 95 percent of the UV radiation that reaches Earth. UVA is the radiation that causes tanning, which is an attempt by the body to protect the skin from damage. It penetrates the skin deeply and damages skin cells in the dermis and epidermis, causing wrinkles and other signs of aging. UVA has been shown to contribute to DNA damage in skin cells,[70] which can lead to melanoma. It passes right through clouds and ozone; even on a dull and cloudy day, you're still receiving a heavy dose of UVA (and thus need skin protection).

UVB, unlike UVA is blocked somewhat by ozone and clouds, so UVB represents (on average) only around 5 percent of the UV radiation at the Earth's surface (more on a clear sunny day). Nevertheless, UVB is more energetic than UVA and is absorbed in high concentrations in the epidermis (the top outer layer), where it causes a lot of damage. UVB has a shorter wavelength than UVA and so UVB cannot penetrate so deeply into the skin's layers. That means all of its energy is absorbed in just a small layer of surface skin. It's UVB that causes most of the reddening of skin exposed to sunlight. If your skin goes red, your skin has been damaged by UVB. Overexposure to UVB is a significant risk factor for skin cancers.

UVC is even more energetic—and more dangerous—than UVB, but because of its short wavelength it's almost entirely blocked by the ozone layer. (There are some industrial sources of UVC, welding equipment for example, and people close to such equipment must wear protection for the skin and the eyes to avoid serious damage.)

THE SKIN DISCONNECT

You might have met some older people who are slim, fit and full of vigor. They are alert and move around like someone 20 years younger. Yet, their skin doesn't look like the skin of a young person. It doesn't look like the skin of an elderly person either, but there's no doubt the skin is older than the body. This is what I call the "skin disconnect"—a young body with older skin.

People like this come from a generation that understood about health-giving foods, they valued exercise and they kept their brains active. They took great care of everything, except their skin. Back then, it was cool to have an outdoors life—and a sexy tan to go with it. They spent lots of time at the beach, or on the golf course, or playing tennis, with little or no protection from the sun's UV rays.

The result is a young body with older skin. Modern methods of skin care and rejuvenation can go a long way toward correcting sun damage caused years ago, but some signs always will remain. So, while we can help people look seven years younger than they look today, it's not always possible to completely reverse the clock.

People from that generation would look quite different today had they protected and cared for their skin as enthusiastically as they nourished and exercised their bodies and brains. They'd still behave younger than their age in years—and they would have skin to match that inner youthfulness, with no disconnect.

EXPOSURE TO THE ELEMENTS

In addition to the ravages of sunlight, just being in the atmosphere causes stress to our skin. Dry air outside and inside damages skin cells by dehydrating them. Polluted air, polluted water, and wind all attack your skin. Tobacco smoke and other pollutants lead to a decrease in oxygen levels in your skin and accelerate aging by reducing the skin's regenerative capabilities.

Your skin also can be damaged by what is taking place inside your body. Damage at the cellular level can be caused by poor food choices, consuming damaging substances, lack of exercise and too much mental stress.

THE VITAMIN D CONTROVERSY

Your skin helps your body make vitamin D. You benefit from having adequate levels of vitamin D in the body; it's a great antioxidant and can help with cell growth and repair. The benefits of vitamin D apply to skin cells themselves, so there's a two-way relationship here: Healthy skin provides vitamin D to the body, and the presence of vitamin D in skin is associated with healthy skin cells.[71]

Ultraviolet radiation from the sun is needed by the body to create vitamin D. The amount of UVB reaching the Earth's surface varies because it's partially blocked or reflected (more than visible light) by the ozone layer, atmosphere and clouds. The amount of outdoor exposure required for people to manufacture their daily needs of vitamin D varies according to weather, conditions in the upper atmosphere, altitude and time of year. Also, not every person can synthesize vitamin D at the same rate. In ideal conditions, it might take 10 or 15 minutes to synthesize enough vitamin D. In the worst case, you might never reach your daily quota.

There's another problem. Although vitamin D is vital for health, and UVB is required for you to create vitamin D, UVB itself is harmful. Many people assume they must spend lots of time in the sun to make their vitamin D, but that will accelerate aging and can be dangerous. Extended exposure to UVB causes sunburn in the outer skin layer. This is the type of sunburn that doesn't appear immediately but causes redness after you've been exposed. Excess UVB exposure, to the extent that burning occurs, is definitely linked to skin aging as well as to skin cancers.

What to do? Once again, as in so many issues related to health, it's all about balance. When you're outside, you should use a moisturizer with sun protection factor 30 (preferably containing zinc oxide), such as Image Skincare Prevention + Daily Ultimate Protection Moisturizer (imageskincare.com), to reduce the intensity of UV interacting with your skin cells. Avoid direct exposure to the sun by seeking shade whenever possible—and, please, don't sunbathe.

You can obtain some vitamin D from sunlight and some from foods. Yet vitamin D deficiency is becoming more prevalent; some estimates suggest the deficiency exists in upward of 50 percent of the population worldwide.[72] I recommend that you have your vitamin D content measured in a blood test. If the test reveals that your lifestyle, location, metabolism and skin sensitivity conspire to keep your vitamin D levels low, then take a raw-sourced vitamin D3 supplement every day, 2,000 IU. Do not try to address low vitamin D levels by spending more time in the sun.

Also, take a vitamin D supplement that includes vitamin K2 to help absorption.

Healthy Living Choices for Your Skin

Specialists in Skin Care

We all understand the need to now and again consult professionals: family doctor, dentist, lawyer, optometrist, interior designer, car mechanic. But skin care seems to be perceived differently. Some believe that skin takes care of itself. People (especially men) who never miss a single dental checkup will avoid visiting a dermatologist until there is a real problem. I strongly recommend that everyone—no matter your age, sex and current skin condition—visit a skin-care specialist at least once a year. Even seemingly healthy skin can have conditions that lead to problems; a specialist can identify problems early, when they're easy to fix.

There are three levels of skin specialists that you should know about.

A **certified aesthetician** has received formal full-time training in care and protection of the entire integumentary system: skin, hair and nails. Aestheticians' skills include assessment of skin condition, styling and cosmetics, the application of skin-care techniques such as facial treatments, peels, microdermabrasion, facial hair removal, manicures and pedicures, and treatments for skin conditions such as acne and pigmentation problems. Aestheticians can provide consultations that enable you to provide effective daily home care using a selection of products specific to your skin type and condition. In most cases, they offer professional, clinical skin-care products not found in drugstores and department stores; these professional products contain higher concentrations of active ingredients and are made to a higher quality standard than mass-produced products.

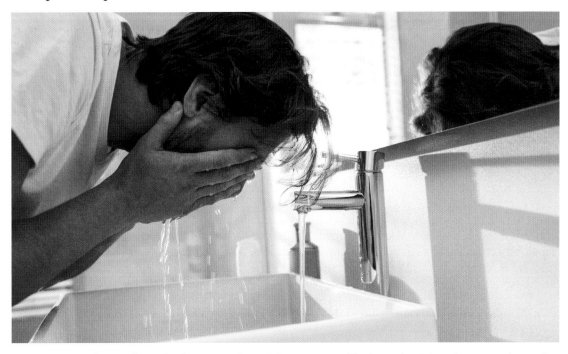

Many people can benefit from regular visits to a certified aesthetician for more intensive treatments than are possible at home. (It's like the relationship with your dental hygienist; you know you need to brush and floss every day, but you still visit a hygienist every six months for a deep clean and checkup.) Not only will the aesthetician provide the necessary corrective and restorative treatment, he or she also will provide advice on adjustments to your daily routine. If signs of skin damage are evident, a certified aesthetician can refer you to a board-certified dermatologist or a board-certified plastic surgeon.

A **board-certified dermatologist** is a registered medical practitioner who specializes in the diagnosis and treatment of more severe skin problems—like sun damage, chronic acne, eczema and psoriasis. This physician also can provide a range of cosmetic skin treatments, such as peels, Botox Cosmetic injections, fillers and laser treatments, as well as effective treatment for some skin cancer conditions. Since dermatologists are licensed medical doctors, they can prescribe drugs and lotions not available over the counter. If you have a previous history of skin damage (such as skin cancers) then you should visit a board-certified dermatologist regularly.

A **board-certified plastic surgeon** is a registered medical practitioner who specializes in more invasive treatments involving cosmetic or reconstructive surgery. Examples of cosmetic treatments are facelifts, liposuction and tummy tucks. Reconstructive surgery can restore appearance and function following accidents or surgery, or fix congenital defects such as a cleft palate.

From the *Age Later* perspective, each of these board-certified professionals has a role to play.

Make an appointment first to visit a certified aesthetician or a board-certified dermatologist for advice on tackling signs of aging. If you don't already have a specialist, ask friends and your primary care physician for recommendations. You need to find a specialist who makes you feel confident and at ease.

A professional can assess your condition and make recommendations for appropriate products to revitalize and maintain your skin, taking into account your specific skin type, skin condition and other factors related to your overall health.

Skin Care Self-Assessment

Inspect your skin at least once a month. Look for signs of potential trouble and check on general skin health and signs of aging. If you find problems or large changes, make an appointment to see a certified aesthetician, your family doctor or a board-certified dermatologist as soon as you can.

Here are some of those troubling signs:

- Rough, raised or darkened areas that stay around more than a few weeks

- Moles or other marks that start to grow or become irregular in shape

- Small areas that bleed, become flaky, become itchy or painful

- Substantial changes over a short period of time

Signs of skin aging include:

- Lack of elasticity and resilience: Aging skin does not spring back into place as quickly as young skin; this eventually results in visible sags and wrinkles.

- Dryness: Aging skin retains less moisture, resulting sometimes in flakiness and itching.

- Textural changes: Aging skin sometimes becomes crepey and resembles orange peel in texture.

- Fragility: Aging skin becomes thinner and less resilient, so it bruises and tears more easily, and takes longer to heal.

- Lumps, rough patches, age spots.

Some people take photographs (selfies) during their regular inspections. This helps to identify anything new that has appeared. Also, you will have an ongoing record to see how you've changed for the better as a result of your healthy living choices.

TAKE ACTION WHEN YOU NOTICE A SKIN PROBLEM

If you identify damage during a skin inspection—lumps, rough patches, age spots, moles that are itchy or infected—then do something about it. These are signs of potentially serious problems, and it makes sense to visit your doctor or a board-certified dermatologist without delay. Similarly, persistent conditions such as eczema, psoriasis, acne and dermatitis may need professional attention. There are numerous skin treatments available these days (too many to list in this book) for specific conditions.

Early treatment is simpler, easier and more likely to be effective. Dealing with troubling issues straight away establishes a foundation for enhancements to your skin that further healthy living choices can provide.

REVERSING SKIN AGING

Make a resolution to fix those general signs of age-related damage, which may include wrinkles, dryness and lack of elasticity.

Your skin-care specialist will be happy to work with you to create a program that reverses signs of aging. Suggestions may include the following:

- An upgrade to some or all of the skin-care products and methods used in your daily cleansing routine. This routine is outlined in the next section and may need to be adjusted from time to time as your skin changes.

- Regular (two or three times a week) use of masks—like Image Skincare's AGELESS Total Resurfacing Masque and I MASK Biomolecular Hydrating Recovery Mask (imageskincare.com)—for resurfacing and rejuvenation, hydration, increasing firmness, and reducing lines and wrinkles. Different masks are available for different skin conditions. Masks typically contain enzymes, hydroxy acids or retinol, vitamins and natural nutrients such as green tea and aloe vera.

- The use of peels, either at home or under the supervision of a certified aesthetician (the Image Skincare I-Peel is a great professional treatment), for a deeper removal of dead cells than can be achieved with daily exfoliants. A peel also can provide nutrition, smoothing and wrinkle reduction. There are a variety of peels designed for different skin conditions.

- A course of lotions and treatments to adjust pigmentation for more uniform skin tones, such as the Image Skincare Iluma Collection (imageskincare.com).

- Additional hydration to reduce wrinkles around the eyes and mouth. You'll find it in Image Skincare Vital C Hydrating Eye Recovery Gel (imagesksincare.com).

- Oral shots of collagen, like Image Skincare YANA Daily Collagen Shots (imageskincare.com) are ingestible products containing collagen peptides and other substances that help the body gradually create its own collagen. Since collagen loss is one of the by-products of aging, oral consumption of the substances the body needs to create more collagen can produce visible improvements in just two or three weeks.

Some damage cannot be reversed easily, or at all, by skin treatments and non-invasive techniques. The fact is that most permanent skin damage happens when people are under the age of 16. Damage done in childhood often is not apparent until well into maturity, and people don't associate their aging skin condition, deep wrinkles, lack of tone and lack of elasticity with childhood damage. When skin treatments and non-invasive techniques fail to address the damage, your skin-care provider may suggest more assertive approaches periodically.

These may include:

- Dermal filler injections to plump your skin and restore volume

- Botox Cosmetic injections

- Various laser treatments, such as cellulite removal, removal of scars, sun spots and age spots, skin firming, skin rejuvenation and wrinkle reduction

- More aggressive peels that need to be used under supervision

- Photodynamic therapy for pre-cancerous and cancerous conditions

Some skin problems may need invasive techniques, specifically surgery. For example, when a mature person has been overweight, significant weight loss will result in sagging skin in the upper arms, in the face and neck, and around the waist. Some of these results can be psychologically damaging and impede the mindset necessary to maintain a healthy lifestyle. In such cases, surgical intervention may be the only way to address the condition. Well-chosen and well-implemented surgery can restore that person's ability to improve health through diet, exercise and continued skin care. Almost any part of the body can be treated surgically for cosmetic improvement, but the usual targets for these procedures are:

- Face, chin and neck

- Upper arms

- Thighs

- Hips

- Waist ("tummy tuck," which may be used following substantial weight loss or liposuction)

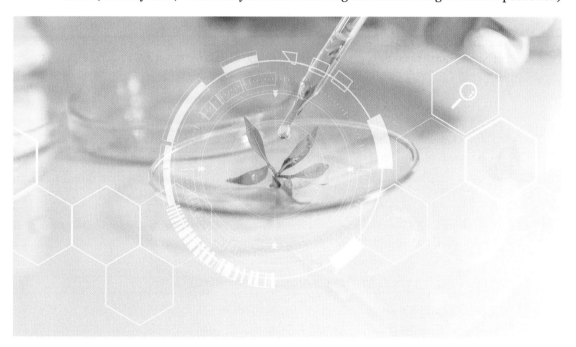

SKIN CARE PRODUCT INGREDIENTS

Today's skin-care industry offers a wide and sometimes perplexing range of products, containing a vast inventory of ingredients—some traditional, many relatively new as research continues into how the skin grows and protects itself. Choosing a product based on its ingredients is more useful than relying on advertising claims. To help you select skin-care products, I have provided a list on my website (agelaterbook.com) of many of the ingredients commonly found in topical products.

SURGICAL INTERVENTIONS

Our facial skin is interlinked with our so-called superficial muscular aponeurotic system (SMAS). As I mentioned earlier, everyday facial movements, such as smiling, frowning and expressing surprise, lead to wrinkling, and the constant pull of gravity eventually can result in noticeable sagging. The skin not only sags over the years, but it also loses volume, which contributes to loose skin.

Daily skin care will improve the quality of the skin and minimize surface wrinkles, but it has limited impact on the SMAS beneath. In order to tighten and rejuvenate sagging skin, tightening of the SMAS is crucial for effective, long-lasting results.

This can be achieved through plastic surgery.

Surgical procedures that address sagging and loose skin include: upper and lower blepharoplasty (eyelids); forehead lifts; upper, mid and lower facelifts; and neck lifts. Volume loss can be corrected with autologous tissue, like fat, which is harvested from other body parts of the same patient. Tissue fillers like hyaluronic acid also are effective, but they are shorter term solutions since the body absorbs these foreign substances over time. Foreign permanent fillers (tissue from other people) are less popular because they can increase the risk of complications, like inflammation, bumps and irregularities.

Carefully selected and planned procedures using these techniques mean that we can correct sagging and loose skin, and restore volume in almost every part of the face, including the lips, cheeks, chin and nose. I've found that, for some people, the results provide a motivating boost that prompts them to address extrinsic causes of aging; they'll start eating more healthy, exercising regularly and taking better care of their skin.

Choose your board-certified plastic surgeon carefully. In the U.S., it's important to select a board-certified surgeon. To find a qualified surgeon in your area, visit plasticsurgery.org, where only board-certified plastic surgeons are listed.

This chapter outlined ways in which you can improve the health and appearance of your skin by following simple routines of correction, protection and nutrition.

So far, so good: By caring for your skin as described, you can go a long way toward achieving a youthful appearance.

But as you understand by now, the secrets of *Age Later* aren't just skin-deep. The next few chapters provide more healthy living choices—additional keys to unlock a way of life that will drive your mental and physical wellness to new heights.

CARE FOR YOUR SKIN EVERY DAY

Everyday care of the skin is vitally important for children, adolescents and adults, no matter where you live. Those who spend a lot of time in harsh environments need to pay extra attention to their skin. Some examples of harsh environments include:

- Anywhere the climate reaches extremes—very hot or cold, very humid or dry. That probably covers much of the planet.

- Some office workplaces have inadequate air circulation leading to over-dry air.

- Industrial and agricultural environments, whether you work there or live nearby, add dust and chemicals to the air, which stress your skin's defensive mechanisms.

- Being outside in strong or persistent winds can have a drying effect.

- Outside activities can be harsh. Skiing, for example, typically takes place in a cold, bright, windy and dry environment. That's a challenging combination for your skin, even if you only expose tiny areas when you're on the slopes.

- Sunbathing of any kind—without skin protection—is terrible for the skin, no matter how good it makes you feel.

Even with preventive measures, we inevitably experience some small amount of environmental damage every day. It's important to take daily steps to restore the skin as best as possible, so that it's ready for the next round of assaults.

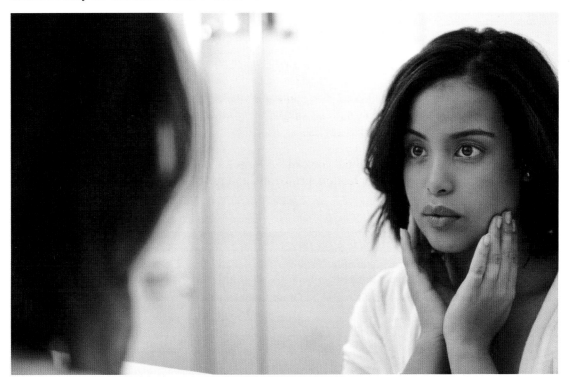

Caring for skin every day requires an investment in skin-care products. Some people (especially men) become so overwhelmed by the number of available products that the investment doesn't seem worth it. But, trust me, it is.

A few factors to consider during your research: 1) Along with quality ingredients, products must be right for your skin type; 2) New products should be compatible with other cleansing and skin-care items you use (your skin will tell you if it's sensitive to a product or new combination);

3) If your choice is not clear after a bit of research, your skin-care specialist can advise you.

You probably will start your new skin-care routine by using a mix of products that you already have. However, at some point you should sit down with a professional and get some advice on products that are right for you in terms of capability and affordability. It's worth noting, by the way, that the most expensive products aren't necessarily the best.

Your daily regimen for facial care should include three simple steps each morning and three simple steps each night:

- Morning: cleanser, serum, then moisturizer with sun protection

- Evening: cleanser, serum and a repair cream

For the rest of your body, use a cleanser (other than soap) and apply a quality body moisturizer, twice daily, that contains antioxidants and nutrients.

Consult your certified aesthetician or go to imageskincare.com for more professional skin-care advice.

Daily Cleansing

Careful daily cleansing is the starting point for skin health. Routine washing of the body removes debris and deposits that can clog pores and provide hiding places for unwanted visitors, microbes and fungi. Cleansing also provides an environment for additional skin-care products (used for exfoliation, moisturizing, protection, rejuvenation and more) to work with full effectiveness.

Both for face and body, you should use cleansers that are hypoallergenic and hydrating. I recommend a cleanser that is glycolic-acid-based, like Image Skincare Ageless Total Facial Cleanser, which combines mild exfoliation with deep cleansing. These products will maintain your skin's pH, hydration and microbial balance while preserving your natural oils (unlike regular soap which strip off surface oils). Some cleansers that work well for most of your body can be too harsh for sensitive facial skin, so you should use a facial cleanser that is formulated specifically for your face.

You don't need antibacterial soaps. Regular cleansers can remove the daily surface dirt and debris, allowing your skin to retain natural oils and a good balance of friendly microbes.

When choosing a cleanser, take into account the characteristics and condition of your skin. Some cleansers are better for dry skin, which usually needs something creamier and more moisturizing. Other cleansers are better at removing excess oils, and trapped dust and debris, without eliminating all the natural oils. Those that include an exfoliant (such as alpha hydroxy acids or microexfoliating beads) help remove dead skin cells and allow the cleanser (and other skin-care products) to reach the new skin where it can do most good.

DAILY EXFOLIATION

Some of your skin cells die every day and are replaced. A mild daily exfoliation helps the skin to shed those dead skin cells leaving the surface of the skin clear of debris, smoother and ready to receive further skin-care treatment. Exfoliation increases blood circulation to the skin, allows more oxygen and nutrients to reach the skin cells, and improves skin tone. Some cleansers contain a mild exfoliant along with the cleaning agents. These combined products make daily exfoliation less of a chore.

A daily exfoliation makes sense, providing it is gentle, since all it has to do is remove the accumulated debris from the previous 24 hours. For everyday exfoliation, avoid exfoliating multiple times with different products during one session; this can cause irritation and sensitivity. Also, never use an aggressive traditional exfoliant on a daily basis; many of these are designed to be used once a week or even once a month. (Not sure? Read the label.)

There is a range of abrasive and acid-based exfoliants suitable for daily use, so choosing the right one can be complicated. The exfoliating component itself has to be chosen carefully according to your skin type. If the exfoliation is too severe, it can damage new living skin cells as it removes the old ones. You wouldn't use sandpaper on your skin, would you? On the other hand, if the exfoliation is too mild, it will not sufficiently clear the surface debris.

Some exfoliants use fine particles of natural products as the abrasion material: tiny beads made from substances including apricot kernels, walnut shells, almond shells, salt and more. Other exfoliants include a carefully calculated mix of acids (for example, alpha-hydroxy acids, glycolic, lactic, citric or salicylic acids). In the correct quantity and concentration, these acids are skin-friendly and loosen clumps of dead cells on the skin's surface. All exfoliant products, whether acid-based or abrasive usually contain moisturizers, pH-balancing components and nutrients.

For a more intensive exfoliation on occasion, use a peel recommended by your aesthetician or book a professional treatment every month or two.

DAILY REGENERATION, REPAIR AND NUTRITION

Everyday life damages your skin, whether you notice it immediately or not. Rather than wait for the damage to become obvious, it makes sense to aim for daily regeneration and repair, in order to catch minor damage as soon as it happens. Repairing damage also requires building new skin cells that need nourishment.

Today, all of those objectives—regeneration, repair and nourishment—can be achieved using a serum designed for those purposes. I recommend a lightweight, water-based serum that contains high concentrations of vitamin C, peptides for collagen and elastin regeneration, and botanicals and other antioxidants. Some serums also contain one or more plant stem cell ingredients. Plant stem cells are produced from a variety of plant sources, each one with its own special capabilities to improve skin functioning and longevity.

Some natural products, used for thousands of years to maintain skin health, continue to provide benefits today. Examples are aloe vera, which assists in healing and also acts as a moisturizer; and green tea, which provides lots of antioxidants to fight free radical damage. Vitamin C from berries and other plants is highly effective when applied to the skin; it stimulates production of collagen and protects cells from free radicals.

Choosing the correct serum should not be left to chance; the most effective products in this category are generally only available from certified aestheticians and board-certified dermatologists. That's another reason to seek professional advice as you design and evolve your daily skin-care routine. If you need to build up collagen levels, consider including daily collagen shots.

At the end of each day, it's imperative to address the skin damage that has taken place. There are overnight creams designed for that purpose. I recommend a repair cream high in alpha hydroxy acids, a percentage of retinol, and antioxidants. The strength of the repair cream recommended by your aesthetician depends on your age, the severity of your skin damage and signs of aging. Some overnight products also contain a mixture of plant stem cell ingredients designed to protect skin stem cells and DNA against oxidative stress.

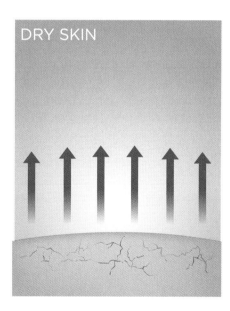 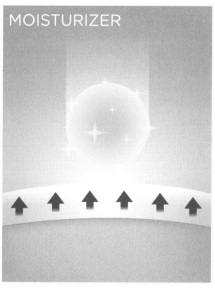

Daily Hydration

Even the best cleansers reduce skin hydration a little, so replacing the moisture is essential. Some serums, including Image Skincare Ageless Total Pure Hyaluronic Filler, are based on hyaluronic acid, a natural ingredient that locks in moisture. For extra hydration, use moisturizer before applying sunscreen, or use a combination product that contains both a moisturizer and SPF. You also need to hydrate your skin from inside, so drink sufficient fluids throughout the day.

SPF SELECTION GUIDE

Outdoor Hours	Skin Tone				
	VERY FAIR Never tans, always burns	**FAIR** Tans slowly, burns easily	**LIGHT** Usually burns first	**MEDIUM** Burns minimally	**DARK** Rarely burns
1	SPF 30	SPF 15	SPF 15	SPF 8-14	SPF 8-14
2	SPF 30	SPF 30	SPF 30	SPF 15	SPF 8-14
3	SPF 50+	SPF 50+	SPF 30	SPF 15	SPF 15
4	SPF 50-100	SPF 50+	SPF 30	SPF 30	SPF 15
5	SPF 50-100	SPF 50-100	SPF 50-100	SPF 50+	SPF 30

Reapply at least every 2 hours or as directed on package to help ensure adequate protection.

DAILY PROTECTION

If you really want to *Age Later*, stick to a daily routine of protecting your skin in order to prevent damage, every day of every year, no matter where you live. Daily skin protection is not an option. It's another healthy living choice you must make.

If you're going to be outside for extended periods, cover all exposed skin with a quality professional sunscreen of at least SPF30, like the Image Skincare Prevention collection (imageskincare.com). I strongly recommend a sunscreen that contains a strong physical blocker (such as titanium dioxide or zinc oxide) that prevents the UV rays from reaching the surface of the skin. Avoid sunscreen lotions that contain only UV-absorbing chemicals as their active ingredient— and especially avoid sunscreens that use retinyl palmitate, which accelerates cell aging when exposed to sunlight.[73] The best sunscreen products also include antioxidants, vitamins and an effective moisturizer. These will nourish the skin, protect against free radical damage, and make your skin cells more resilient to the attacks of sunlight, wind and air-conditioned interiors.

Clothing also is something to consider when talking about skin care. Normal light clothing, for example a thin shirt or blouse, will not block UV effectively. The more tightly woven and heavy the fabric, the better the protection—so don't spend hours in the sun wearing mesh finishes or other loose weaves. In general, if you can see light through the clothing, then it won't provide ample UV protection. If you must spend extended periods in the sun for work or travel, look for specialized clothing that claims to block UV and carries a UV SPF rating.

A hat with a brim provides extra protection for the face, neck, eyes and ears, and the top of your head. The hair on your head does not provide enough protection on a bright day. In fact, hair follicles can be damaged by sunlight, just like the skin cells around them.

Your eye cells are specially adapted cells that are sensitive to visible light, but they are made of the same basic materials as your skin cells, so your eyes need protection too. Sunglasses should be rated for 99 percent or 100 percent UVA and UVB blocking. Wear eye protection during the summer, even on cloudy days.

Even if you're using sunscreen lotion and wearing sun-resistant clothing, restrict your exposure to direct sunlight to less than a couple of hours in any day. Do not sunbathe. Do not sit for long periods in the sun. When you feel burning, no matter how slight, or if you see any part of your skin turning red, that's a warning sign. Pay attention to the message from your skin, and take cover.

Food for Your Skin

My *Age Later* food plan will ensure that you are receiving everything you need to keep your body and skin healthy. There are some foods and food components that are especially good for your skin, so to drive home the point about the importance of skin nutrition from within, here are some nutrients that should appear often in your meal plans. The chapter on Food will explain more; it lists the foods that include these skin-friendly nutrients.

Nutrient	Sources	Benefits for the skin
Glucosinolates	Broccoli, cauliflower, cabbage	Collagen protectors
Lycopene	Tomatoes and tomato products, watermelon, pink grapefruit and guavas	Prevents collagen degradation and may help reduce the damage caused by UVB. Foods that contain lycopene include tomatoes and tomato products, watermelon, pink grapefruit and guava.

Nutrient	Sources	Benefits for the skin
Omega-3	Olives and olive oil, nuts, seeds, avocado, fruits and vegetables, avocado, kidney beans, oily fish	Strengthens skin cell membranes, helping them resist cell damage and hold more water. Enables efficient uptake of nutrients. Fights inflammation in skin layers, making skin more healthy and resilient.
Omega-6	Olives and olive oil, nuts, seeds, avocado, fruits and vegetables, avocado, kidney beans, oily fish, palm oil, whole grains, poultry and eggs	Strengthens skin cell membranes, helping them resist cell damage and hold more water. Enables efficient uptake of nutrients. Fights inflammation in skin layers, making skin more healthy and resilient.
Omega-9	Olives, nuts, seeds, and oils cold-pressed from those foods. Olive oil is very high in oleic acid, and also is a good source of omega-3 and omega-6	Maintains skin health and manages cholesterol levels.
Vitamin A	Vegetables, eggs, dairy	Helps prevent UV damage, stimulates skin cell renewal and encourages fibroblast production, which helps make your skin firm and resilient.
Vitamin B group	Fruits, vegetables, seafood, beans, eggs, dairy, meat	Helps maintain the health of skin, hair and nails. Niacin (B3) helps to maintain hydration, B5 works alongside vitamin C to repair skin damage.

Nutrient	Sources	Benefits for the skin
Vitamin C, and other anti-oxidants.	All fruits and vegetables	Vitamin C helps prevent cell degeneration and fights inflammation. Also helps build collagen throughout the body: skin, tendons, ligaments and more, making skin smooth, youthful and glowing.
Water	Water and all water-based drinks	Hydrates skin from inside.

Chapter 6

EXERCISE AND ACTIVITY

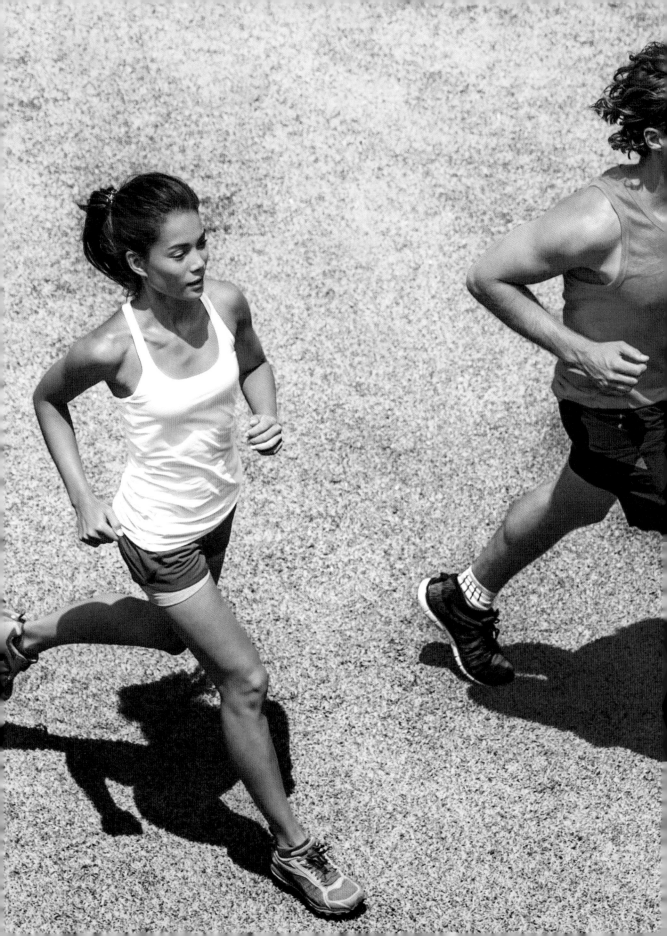

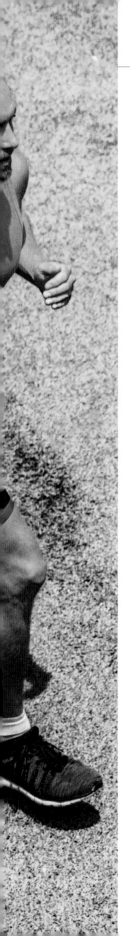

EXERCISE AND ACTIVITY

A SLUGGISH NATION

In the developed world today, and in the United States especially, people generally are overweight and unfit. Centers for Disease Control and Prevention (CDC) estimates that almost half the U.S. adult population does not get enough aerobic exercise; less than 22 percent of adults ages 18 and over meet the CDC's guidelines for physical activity levels.[74]

The U.S. is not alone. Where America leads, other countries follow. As countries become richer, the general level of physical activity in the population becomes lower and lower. High-income countries average around 55 percent of adults who get enough activity; low-income countries average around 80 percent.

Insufficient exercise leads to illness and a shorter life. People who don't exercise regularly are at greater risk of suffering from heart disease, diabetes and cancer.[75] Without regular exercise, your body accumulates higher levels of advanced glycation end products (AGEs),[76] which are linked to inflammation in the body. Exercise, along with control of food intake, is essential for weight control, so when we learn that around two-thirds of the adult population is either overweight or obese, we should take notice.

We use technology to make life easier and assume that makes life better at the same time. Yet simple activities like walking to the store, doing housework and mowing the lawn used to boost our health levels. Today, we don't even have to leave the house to shop; we can go online and order goods for delivery. We've made many physical tasks easier with tools and technology, but we've failed to recognize how that was our affecting our physical health.

This is not just laziness, although that's part of the problem for some people. When we're preoccupied or exhausted or just busy with day-to-day life, it's easy to slip into convenient habits, like choosing to drive the car instead of walking, taking the elevator instead of the stairs—or sleeping an extra 30 minutes instead of going on that morning jog.

The problem is that we can't set daily exercise on a back burner. A life without activity and exercise, inevitably, will lead to health issues.

But it doesn't have to be like that. Activity levels are driven by habits. You can choose to take the easy road and not exercise. Or you can make healthy living choices, adopt better habits, and increase your strength, stamina and overall well-being.

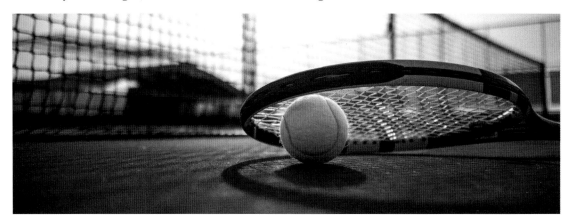

THE BENEFITS OF EXERCISE

Your body is good at sending nutrients to the places where those nutrients are most needed. If you don't use parts of your body, the nutrients will go somewhere else, notably to build your energy reserves in the form of fat deposit. This is why if you don't employ your muscles, they will start to waste away, and if you don't stress your bones, they will become less dense and more fragile. Your brain needs plenty of blood to function, but if your circulation is always slow, the blood your brain craves may not be there when it needs to be.

Moving your limbs strengthens your muscles, increases bone density and improves the flexibility of your joints. Fit people look better; they have better posture, improved muscle tone and smoother skin.

Physical exercise also increases blood circulation. The extra blood flow delivers more oxygen and nutrients to all your cells, and flushes out unwanted free radicals and toxins. This diminishes inflammation throughout the body, which reduces cell damage and extends cell life.

Making your body work hard benefits your heart and lungs, because those organs are driven by muscle power. Exercise converts reserves of fat to muscle and energy, helping you maintain a healthy weight. This all goes to improve the performance of your cardiovascular and respiratory systems, reducing the risk of heart disease and diabetes. Exercise also reduces the risk of suffering from internal organ cancers and neuro-deficiency diseases, including Alzheimer's and Parkinson's.

Exercise boosts the health of all body cells, even your skin cells.[77] Exercise can slow down the aging process and even reverse some effects of skin aging,[78] improving your skin's health and appearance.

Regular exercise not only reduces levels of stress, anxiety and depression,[79] but it contributes toward maintaining cognition and brain functioning. Exercise results in better sleep patterns; adequate sleep is essential for the health of your nervous system, your skin—your whole body.

The right kinds of exercise build every part of the body—but it's not the kind of bodybuilding that results in extreme bulk and curvature. My version of bodybuilding is about healthy and sustained strength, balance, posture, poise and flexibility, and for that you don't need giant muscles.

Put simply, if you don't exercise, your health will deteriorate. If you do exercise, especially if you're committed to a consistent regimen, you will be more healthy—in mind and in body. So, move your body!

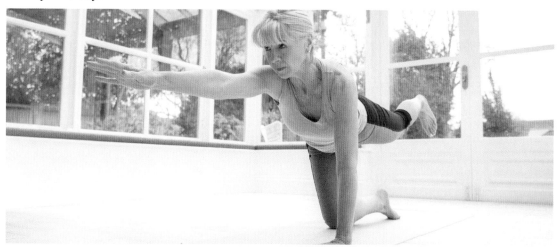

FIGHTING AGING WITH EXERCISE

You don't necessarily have to go to the gym to exercise, although, if you can, you'll likely make faster progress. I recommend a morning jog or a morning warm-up, or both, first thing every day.

Beyond formal workouts, opportunities to exercise arise during a normal day of walking about, shopping, working, gardening and so on. If you can boost the amount of "incidental physical activity" you do, it's an easy and painless way of getting the exercise you need. Most of us don't take those daily opportunities, so that is something you can probably change. Simple stretching and balancing exercises also are good for your muscles and joints, and help improve posture.

Strengthening exercises maintain muscle tone. Muscle decay often is the first sign of advancing age, and regular strength exercises will fight off the natural weakening of muscles that occurs if they aren't regularly used.

Your heart and lung muscles also need exercise. Strengthening them is crucial for cardiovascular health; this is the aim of moderate and vigorous aerobic exercise.

How Much Exercise Does a Body Need?

You don't need to train like a professional athlete or a bodybuilder to benefit from exercise. It only takes a few minutes of purposeful exercise every day to make a difference—but the more you exercise, the more you will benefit. The official line is that for a healthy adult to remain healthy, the minimum amount of exercise needed is about 150 minutes a week of moderate aerobic physical activity (or 75 minutes per week of vigorous aerobic activity), plus two short sessions of weight training per week.[80]

Still, a small amount of daily regular exercise is better than none, especially if it includes some sessions that are vigorous enough for you to be out of breath.

Try starting with whatever level of exercise you can manage, and ramp up as rapidly as you can to something close to those targets. Regular exercise is more useful than infrequent long sessions: 20 minutes each day for five days a week is more valuable than 100 minutes in one day.

In the detailed descriptions for each type of exercise, I make suggestions for how much time to devote in order to achieve results.

Exercise and Nutrition

Exercise and nutrition are tightly linked. You can eat all the right foods, but unless you exercise you won't be able to take full advantage of those foods—and that still leaves you susceptible to age-related illnesses. Conversely, you might be an exercise fanatic, but if you don't provide your body with the nutrients it needs to build healthy cells and muscle, then your exercise won't be as effective as it could be.

Your food plan and your exercise plan go hand in hand. Making healthy living choices in both areas will be more effective than focusing on just one or the other.

Exercise and Weight Loss

Exercise improves your health, and exercise is an essential component of a weight-loss program, but don't count on exercise alone to lose weight. You still need to manage your food intake. Exercise can help with weight management by simply burning fat; exercise dissipates energy that is stored in fat—some of that energy is used to build muscle, some is dissipated as heat.

Muscles use more energy than fat, even when resting. So, exercise boosts your resting metabolic rate, which means you will consume more energy even when you're sitting on the couch. Once again, the source of that energy is stored fat.

However, the relationship between exercise and weight loss is quite complex because of the ways in which the body prioritizes use of the calories it consumes.[81] That's why exercise works for some people who are trying to lose weight but not others. Some overweight people work hard; they exercise regularly and are perplexed that their efforts are not paying off. They might feel better, have more energy and breathe more easily, but their weight stays much the same.

To lose weight you almost certainly need to exercise even more than you might think. The calories you spend during exercise, although important, may not totally add up to calories lost in fat, because the body efficiently reduces energy expenditure in other departments while you're exercising.

The more intense your daily exercise routine, the more calories you use during exercise. Very intense exercise forces your body to keep demanding calories even after the exercise period is finished, which accelerates fat-burning. For this reason using the exercises described as part of High Intensity Interval Training (HIIT) program will yield even more benefits.

To achieve a boost to your resting metabolic rate, occasional gentle exercise is not enough. You need exercise that is regular, sustained and vigorous enough to result in conversion of fat to muscle.[82]

Even if you successfully increase resting metabolic rate, that improvement may be offset by an increase in the efficiency of your metabolism, which allows you to extract more energy from your food intake. So, you still need to manage food intake carefully.

If you need to lose weight, make sure that exercise is a part of your weight management program. Just don't expect it to achieve the results you want all by itself. Food intake, both the quantity and the quality, remain crucial. Your fitter body and increased metabolic rate do not give you an excuse to eat more food.

WHEN IS THE BEST TIME TO EXERCISE?

Your muscles, joints and body organs will benefit no matter what time of day you choose to exercise. The best time of day is what works best for you, based on your mood and your schedule.

Some people are naturally morning people, alert and enthusiastic as soon as they wake up. Others really don't get energized until later in the day. There are some advantages to exercising first thing in the morning. I already have mentioned the value of warm-up exercises immediately after waking up to boost circulation and get the muscles moving. It's a seamless progression to move from there to other exercise routines, have a shower and get on with the day.

For many people this approach is more reliable than leaving the exercise until later in the day. Things happen, schedules change and real life sometimes just gets in the way. For this reason, late morning or afternoon sessions require more self-organization and self-discipline than early morning exercises.

On the flip side, one benefit of late-afternoon or early-evening exercise, right after a long day of work, is that it's a great way of counteracting the stresses of the day. Even if you do most of your exercise in the morning, some stretches or aerobics after work can be a great benefit.

Late-evening exercise has become popular, with some people out at the gym until midnight. Especially in metropolitan areas, some gyms are open 24 hours. This works well for certain people, but don't expect to be able to drop off to sleep immediately after finishing strenuous exercise or a lengthy aerobic workout. Allow yourself a good hour or so to wind down.

If you exercise in the early evening (that is, before your evening meal) you stand less chance of having sleep disruption.[83]

Another consideration is the impact of exercise on your eating habits. If you eat before a workout, you will almost always feel like eating again afterward. If you are at all concerned about weight management, avoid this. The best time to exercise is just before breakfast, lunch or dinner. That means you can satisfy your post-workout desire for food with a scheduled meal, not with an extra snack.

Whatever time of day you prefer, try to get into some sort of routine. You should have predictable slots in your schedule for planned exercise; follow that routine every week. People who rely on just "finding some time" for exercise, often don't.

But there can't be excuses when it comes to the exercise necessary to your overall well-being. Everyone claims to be busy, and we mostly are, but it's possible to create space by limiting the time you spend on other activities. For starters, put down your phone, close your laptop or turn off your television. Stop and think about how much time you spend online without real purpose, immersed in social media or watching mindless TV programs. By scheduling time for a purposeful workout, you're making exercise a high priority. Other, less important activities are the ones you should allow to slip.

You have 168 hours available to you every week. Assuming you spend 60 of them sleeping or getting ready for bed, around 48 in some kind of committed activity (work), and, say 40 eating, socializing, driving, entertaining yourself, etc., there are still 20 hours left. Devote a small slice of your weekly hours to boosting your health with regular exercise—and see what a difference it makes in your life.

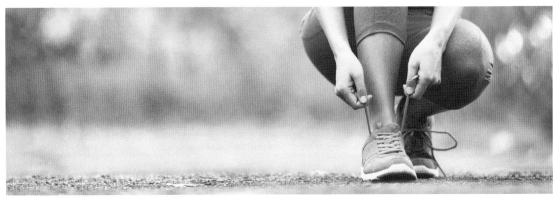

GETTING READY TO EXERCISE

Most healthy people can increase the amount of moderate exercise they do without danger. However, if you consider yourself to be something of a couch potato, or if you have respiratory problems, suffer from chest pains, experience dizziness—or have any history of heart problems or medical conditions that might interfere with effective exercise—then it's imperative that you check with your primary care physician to determine whether the workout program can present problems.

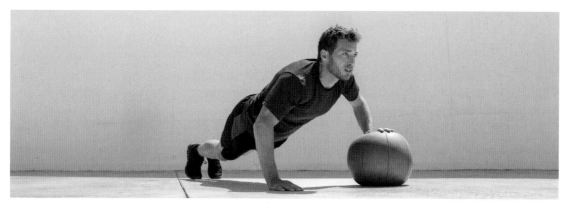

For anyone concerned that they are too old to do serious exercise, don't be. It's just not true. Older people who haven't exercised for a long time do need to be careful, especially if they also have health-related conditions, but moderate exercise is good for you at any age.[84] The usual reservations apply: If you intend to make a dramatic change in your level of exercise, consult with your doctor first.

If you already are fairly active, and you make an effort to get at least some weekly exercise, then it's time to ramp up your exercise level. Even for this group, it's worth visiting your doctor to see just how far you can go, and how quickly.

YOUR HEART

One of the tests you should request from your physician is a cardiac stress test. This will give you a measured figure for your "maximum heart rate," which is the safe limit for you to reach during exercise. Knowing your maximum heart rate is the way to set safe limits on your exercise and to gauge how intensive each type of exercise is for you.

If you haven't had a cardiac stress test, you can refer to a chart provided by the American Heart Association, which provides typical maximum and resting heart rates for different age groups. I have adapted that chart to provide some simple beats-per-minute guidance, this way you can check that you are raising your heart rate adequately, while also staying within safe limits for your age, especially during vigorous exercise. (The chart also is available on my website, agelaterbook.com).

The maximum heart rate for exercising in the ensuing table (Heart Rate Exercise Zones) is based on chronological age. Some people are physically younger than others of the same age, as we know. Nevertheless the maximum heart rate for your age is a reasonable guide to setting yourself limits and targets for exercise.

If a trainer or medical advisor suggests different limits for you, no problem: Everyone is a bit different.

Heart Rate Exercise Zones

Age	During moderate aerobic exercise, aim to exceed this heart rate bpm during the session	During moderate aerobic exercise, to keep below this heart rate bpm	During vigorous aerobic exercise, aim to exceed this heart rate bpm during the session	During vigorous aerobic exercise, to keep below this heart rate bpm	Typically the maximum heart rate bpm for the age group
Age	**50%**	**65%**	**70%**	**85%**	**100%**
20	100	130	140	170	200
25	98	127	137	166	195
30	95	124	133	162	190
35	93	120	130	157	185
40	90	117	126	153	180
45	88	114	123	149	175
50	85	111	119	145	170
55	83	107	116	140	165
60	80	104	112	136	160
65	78	101	109	132	155
70	75	98	105	128	150
75	73	94	102	123	145
80	70	91	98	119	140
85	68	88	95	115	135
90	65	85	91	111	130
95	63	81	88	106	125
100	60	78	84	102	120

This Heart Rate chart, as mentioned, is adapted from data provided by the American Heart Association.[85] Be aware that some medications can reduce the Maximum Heart Rate. If you are on any medications, speak to your doctor. You may have to base your targets and limits on a lower Maximum Heart Rate number while you are using those drugs.

Moderate aerobic exercise is intended to increase your circulation and move your muscles and joints without causing excessive breathlessness. The target zone for heart rate during moderate exercise is between 50 percent and 65 percent of the Maximum Heart Rate for the age group.

Vigorous aerobic exercise is intended to increase your circulation and give all your muscles a strenuous workout, including the muscles of the heart. You should breathe heavily during these exercises, or you're not working hard enough. The target zone for heart rate during vigorous aerobic exercise is between 70 percent and 85 percent of the Maximum Heart Rate for your age group.

To avoid exceeding your maximum heart rate, you need to know exactly what your heart rate is at any time. You can measure your heart rate the old-fashioned way by counting your pulse beats for a measured minute; but you may find it more convenient and more accurate to use a device that constantly monitors your heart rate. You can buy a device that is just a heart monitor, or you can buy an activity tracker that includes heart monitor capability. These are now widely available, and there are plenty from which to choose, depending on how much you want to spend. This is a worthwhile and cost-effective investment if you're serious about fighting the aging process with exercise.

Start by measuring your normal resting heart rate. This will allow you to time how long it takes for your heart rate to return to normal after exercise. To work out a benchmark for your resting heart rate, measure your pulse (or check your heart rate monitor) two or three times at different times of the day, each time at least 15 minutes after you have stopped exercising (or wait longer if you still feel out of breath), and after lying down in a quiet place for at least 10 minutes. Average the results and write it down.

As you go through the exercise program you should measure your average resting heart rate again, say every four weeks. You may find that it goes down slightly. That means your exercise routine is having some benefit.

EXERCISE AND YOUR SKIN

Exercise generally improves skin health and condition. For example, improved circulation often helps reduce acne or eczema.

For a few people the combination of greater blood flow to the skin, higher skin temperature and more perspiration may at times cause more irritation. People with conditions such as acne, eczema, rosacea or psoriasis should be aware that this could occur.[86]

Nevertheless, the benefits of exercise are so great that you should not allow these conditions to get in the way. You may have to ramp up your exercise level gradually, staying with light to moderate activities and increasing as your skin quality improves. You should moisturize before vigorous activities, as well-hydrated skin is more resistant to the salt in perspiration, which is sometimes the cause of irritation. Avoid exercising in overheated places.

Activities like tai chi and yoga can provide many health benefits and may be less likely to trigger skin inflammation in those with pre-existing skin conditions. Yoga and other moderate types of exercise are shown to reduce stress, which has been linked to certain skin conditions.

Finally, please note that there's no rule saying that you have to wear tight clothing for exercise. If you are more comfortable wearing looser natural fiber clothing, do so.

YOUR JOINTS

Your joints will benefit from exercise, but only if you ensure the exercise doesn't damage them first. If you have pre-existing joint conditions, and are just embarking on a workout program, start by engaging in low-impact exercises.

Elliptical machines, and cycling or walking on level ground might be good ways to get started if you have knee or hip problems. People in this category should avoid the following: stair-climbing (as an exercise), running and jumping. Exercises involving stretching may be helpful, as long as you start gently and gradually increase as you discover what your body is capable of doing.

People who stress their joints aggressively on a regular basis, such as football players, competitive skiers and tennis players, need well-developed muscular systems (and sometimes joint braces) to help protect their joints from serious injury. Learn from those professionals. Before engaging in activity that has a high impact on any joint, first build up the muscles that support that joint and hold it in position. If you have a serious joint problem, consider working with a therapist or trainer until you've built up both your muscles and the integrity of your joint.

HEALTHY LIVING CHOICE: MOVE YOUR BODY

FROM ZERO TO ACTIVE

One way to kick-start a new fitness routine, especially for those going from zero activity to light exercise, is to start the morning with a moderate run. It doesn't require a gym membership or a trainer. And it's an invigorating way to begin your day.

Need help getting motivated? Try this. Keep your running shoes next to your bed, as a daily reminder. Set your alarm 30 minutes earlier than normal. Start by jogging for just 10 minutes, then gradually extend the time you spend running. Push to 30 minutes, or even 45 minutes.

Jogging 30 minutes or more feeds extra oxygen to the brain, which improves mood and brain health; plus, it can protect against Alzheimer's. Carrying light weights as you jog will increase the benefit to your arms and upper body.

The modest pace of jogging serves as a perfect warm-up. As you advance in your training, add some other light exercises before or after your jog—or, after finishing your run, go straight to a more vigorous workout to further improve your strength and balance.

In the meantime, just a simple morning jog will create noticeable improvements to your overall health.

Warm Up

The purpose of warming up is to move your muscles enough to (literally) increase their temperature, making them looser and more flexible. Because you're starting from cold, you must do this gradually and gently. Along the way, you'll increase your heart rate and respiration, but only a little. At the end of a warm-up, you should feel ready for action—not ready for a break.

Warming up before more strenuous exercise is essential to avoid muscle strain, but the components of a warm-up depend on your level of fitness and the activities you are going to do. A warm-up routine that's appropriate for a professional athlete may resemble a full-blown workout to someone who does minimal exercise.

Your day is going to contain physical activity: walking, taking out the trash, moving furniture, carrying boxes, etc. Doesn't it make sense to warm up before starting the day? It's a painless way to get going and makes sure you are awake, especially if you include jogging or running-on-the-spot in your routine. Early morning wake-up exercises used to be a tradition in many countries, and we would all be healthier if it became widespread again.

You will benefit from warming up before any moderate or vigorous activity, such as aerobic exercises, golf or tennis, going for a morning jog, a hike, or even a shopping expedition. Build your own warm-up routine using a mix of moderate aerobic (without weights) and dynamic stretches[87] that you enjoy, with the aim of targeting all of your muscles. Choose two to four different warm-up activities and build a routine that lasts 5 to 10 minutes. The regimen might consist of two or three different dynamic stretching exercises, followed by one or two aerobic activities. If you have another exercise session later in the day, warm up again before starting that workout.

Here are a few warm-up suggestions:

- Dynamic stretching exercises: forward lunges, walking lunges, arm swings, leg swings.

- Rope jumps: If you haven't done rope jumps since junior high, you've been missing out on a great warm-up exercise that also improves coordination and balance.

- Jumping jacks: Another exercise from your grade-school physical education class that still works. If you can't quite remember how to do it, check out a video on the Internet.[88]

- Exercise machine: For a warm-up, a few minutes at an easy pace on a cycling machine, rowing machine, elliptical or treadmill will do the trick.

- Jogging, or jogging on the spot: I always include jogging in my morning warm-up. It's an easy way to get the circulation moving.

Whatever combination of warm-up exercises you choose, don't force any movements, don't overwork painful joints or muscles, and don't overexert to the point of being out of breath. That comes later.

Change your routine now and again by including different exercises and by changing the sequence. Sticking to one fixed routine runs the risk of overlooking certain muscles and joints. Also change your sequence of exercises every week.

When warming up before participating in a specific sport or activity (cycling, rowing, skiing, tennis), some coaches suggest you start limbering up by practicing that activity. If that appeals to you, do it slowly and gently for five to 10 minutes. That way, you'll loosen the exact muscles you need to loosen.

Like other elements of *Age Later* that we've discussed, building a foundation—in this case, as part of your new fitness routine—is important. The warm-up is your jumping-off point, one that leads to more involved workouts, and to greater enthusiasm and appreciation for the way exercise makes you feel.

EVERYDAY ACTIVITY: EXERCISE THAT COMES NATURALLY

You can decide to upgrade the level of physical activity in your everyday life. That is a healthy living choice that brings significant benefits without a lot of extra time expenditure.

Morning runs around the block are great, but you'll get even more benefit if you don't spend the rest of the day sitting at a desk and all evening sitting on a couch. Think of your everyday physical behavior as an exercise opportunity—and make the most of it.

Unscheduled exercise is activity that takes place every day. Some researchers call this activity "Incidental Physical Activity" (IPA), and the benefits of this type of activity are now receiving some attention.[89] Most of us don't consciously think of everyday activity as an exercise, but if it involves moving, bending or stretching your body, it's exercise.

Once you recognize that everyday movements potentially are making you healthier, they take on new value. One study found that simply being aware that everyday movement is exercise somehow makes that exercise more effective.[90] If you recognize its value, even loading and emptying the dishwasher can be exercise, especially if you arrange to keep your dinnerware on some high and some low shelves.

You do need scheduled purposeful exercise, but if you adopt good everyday activity habits, then you win yourself an exercise bonus. Everyday activity in the form of IPA has value, so consider any situation that requires body movements as an extra investment in your body's health.

The Path of More Resistance

Ordinary activities all help: Climbing stairs instead of using the elevator, doing housework, being active at work, tending to your herbs and vegetables. Even passionate behavior makes a contribution; anything that raises your heart rate and makes you slightly out of breath is useful exercise.[91]

However, our natural inclination is to be efficient. If you forget your keys, the extra walk back to the house makes you frustrated. On the other hand, it's not necessarily bad to walk a bit more. A change in attitude about any inconvenience that involves extra walking—an understanding that such movement is good for your health—not only can reduce stress-inducing annoyances, it can lead to a lifestyle change.

Instead of always looking for the shortest path when at home or at work or at the department store, select different routes. Don't move the coffee machine that's on the other side of the office; enjoy the walk. Take the stairs from the second floor of the mall instead of the elevator. Don't stress out searching for the closest parking spot; just park the car. Choose movement.

Walk More, Drive Less

The invention of the motorcar was responsible for a massive decline in human physical activity, perhaps even more than the invention of the cushioned sofa.

If you can find ways of using your legs instead of sitting in a car, you can add significantly to your quota of Incidental Physical Activity.

Do you live close to shops, supermarkets, bars and restaurants? If so, what is your decision point for driving rather than taking the car? A 10-minute walk? A 30-minute walk? Think about it. Many people take the car to avoid even a short walk. It's understandable if weather is an issue, if you have children, if you're making a grocery run or another legitimate reason. But for the rest of you, there's no excuse. So, try this: Instead of driving, say to a nearby restaurant, try parking five minutes away. You can walk off some of the meal afterward—and you'll take advantage of an IPA opportunity at the same time.

If you have a gym membership, it's probably not far from where you live given all the fitness locations that abound. Consider walking, running or biking to the gym and back home again. If you have a 10-minute jog to the gym and 10 minutes back again, that's 20 minutes of cardio work and a bonus toward that day's IPA achievement.

If you can walk or cycle to work, consider doing it—even if it's only on occasion. Some of you have opportunities to combine walking or cycling with the use of public transport. Public transport can be an exercise enabler that fits right in to your everyday life. Bring a change of clothes and some toiletries in your backpack; even if there's no shower at work, you can still clean up before clocking in. Too many people simply make the obvious choice: driving. Get past the obvious and examine your commuting options with an open mind.

Pick Up the Pace

Little children, once they learn to walk, seem to want to run everywhere. Older children are not good at sitting still or standing in one place; they fidget and move around. Most adolescents and young adults still fidget and walk briskly, sometimes they run and walk alternately if they are in a hurry, which is a highly effective way of covering a distance without getting too breathless.

At some point as humans mature, they start to stroll instead of walk. There's nothing wrong with strolling sometimes. But all the time?

I suppose that if someone has everything in their life so well-organized that they're never late, then there's no sense of urgency. But some people drive their cars at outrageous and illegal speeds, then meander slowly across the parking lot upon arriving at their destination.

Whether you think of yourself as a slow or fast person, decide to kick it up a notch from time to time. In addition to taking every opportunity to walk more, aim to walk just a little faster without running out of breath. Be brisk!

Stand More, Sit Less

While it's difficult to separate out the health risk of sitting from other factors, we still know for sure that more exercise is better than less exercise. Your joints and muscles are more active when you're standing or walking, compared to sitting down for long periods. So it makes sense to avoid sitting if you don't have to.[92]

If you have to wait for a bus or a train or a plane, spend as much time as possible standing or strolling around. Even if you're waiting to see a doctor, walk around the waiting room or outside the office if there's some delay. Ask reception to ping you on your cellphone; they'll be happy to do it, because it's all for the good of your health.

In a confined space, like a plane, it's not easy to find IPA opportunities. Still, you can walk the aisle and stretch during a flight. On some airlines, the cabin crew will remind passengers of the dangers of sitting in one position too long, including the potential for deep vein thrombosis. Walking the aisle might annoy a few of the passengers, but the benefits outweigh their issues. Sitting still in a cramped space is bad for your circulation, muscles and lungs—so get up and move around.

If you work at a desk, and you have a say over your working environment, ask for a sit-stand desk—and aim to move between standing, sitting and walking around several times each day.

Your boss isn't cooperating? Remind her or him that requiring you to sit for extended periods will damage your health. Additionally, being unable to control aspects of your working environment adds to your stress. We all know that employees who are happy do better work,[93] so an uncooperative boss is deliberately damaging productivity. You might not want to put it to your boss that way—then again, no one can fault you for advocating for your well-being.

How do you spend your evenings? If it involves more sitting, remember to stand up and walk twice an hour, at least. Ever tried watching a movie standing up? Reading a book? It's possible. You can buy a couple of high-top tables, the type you see in many bars. Using one of those makes the act of standing up feel obvious and natural. A martini is not required for this exercise.

Our modern culture is predominantly sedentary. So much of our daily routine involves sitting down. Fight the norm. A thousand or more years before chairs were invented,[94] our ancestors were naturally inclined to stand, squat or lie down instead of sit. There is evidence that their knees were in better condition than ours are today, even with all that running around chasing their meals.[95]

STRETCHING, FLEXIBILITY, POSTURE AND BALANCE

Generally speaking, stretching is an underrated activity. Most fitness programs tend to emphasize contraction of the muscles; muscles contract when they are used to exert pressure, which is fundamental to strength training and a lot of aerobic exercise. Stretching is the opposite approach.

Stretching the muscles increases blood flow to the muscle and provides a healthy balance to the stresses of contraction, as well as improving joint flexibility and mobility. As stretching releases locked-in pressures in your body, you may find it also alleviates mental stress. In addition, stretching exercises help to improve balance and posture.

There are many modern and traditional ways of stretching your body, and I suggest incorporating at least one of these regularly. At a minimum, learn a few basic stretching exercises to use when you are fully warmed up, after moderate or vigorous aerobic exercise.

Some basic stretching exercises that you can do at any time are listed on my website (agelaterbook.com), where I provide information about two different types of stretching exercises.

Static stretching is where the muscles are gradually stretched and held in a stretched position for around 10 seconds. Dynamic stretching involves more movement, and the positions are held for much shorter times; the movement is an important part of dynamic stretching.

Perform a selection of these basic static and dynamic stretching exercises at least once a week (twice a week is better).

Basic stretching is fine to get started, but at some point you may wish to add variety. To that end, there are other ways—modern and traditional—to stretch your muscles. You can achieve great results from disciplines such as tai-chi, yoga, calisthenics and even ballet practice. I recommend that you start by taking a class in order to receive expert instruction on how to perform the moves correctly. You may also enjoy the companionship of working on these moves in a group.

These traditional forms of exercise bring another benefit: The disciplines generally recognize the synergistic relationship between mind and body, and thus emphasize tranquility and inner peace as part of the process of learning and participating.

Some massage techniques (for example Thai massage) emphasize the extension of muscles and joints by stretching. Although it can be argued that the person giving the massage gets more exercise than the person receiving it, there are real benefits to massage—especially when the body has been stressed (via sporting activities, overdoing it in the gym, a long airplane flight, work-related issues, etc.). A form of do-it-yourself massage involves the use of a sports medicine foam roller[96] that, used according to instructions, can help release knotted muscle tissue and reduce feelings of tension in the body.

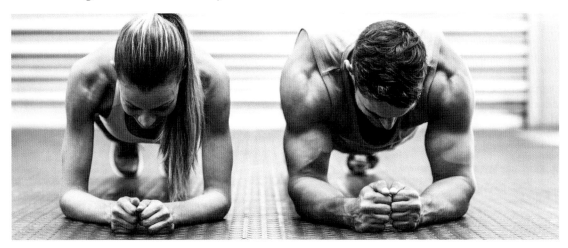

STRENGTH TRAINING

Some people believe that as we grow older, our muscles naturally become weaker. The reality is that, as people grow older, most reduce their level of physical activity—and without daily activity, the muscles weaken. If you don't regularly use every muscle in your body, the body will decide that those muscles aren't necessary—and it will stop feeding them. In the same way, stressing your bones makes them stronger too.

Strength training is a type of anaerobic training involving intensive and short duration exercise that aims to build reserves of energy and muscle power. My recommendation is to do strength training two days a week, with rest days in between. These exercises are designed to stress your muscles; you'll obtain the most benefit by allowing two or three days between sessions for your muscles to self-repair and adjust. If possible, do your vigorous aerobics and strength exercises on different days of the week.

Listed below are a number of strength exercises that can be done at home with no equipment, or, in a couple of cases, with some simple weights. These specific examples come from the CDC website, where you also can find detailed instructions and videos.[97] These exercises are a great place to start. They are all known to work and have been used successfully for decades.

- Squat: Strengthens lower legs, upper legs and hips. Also provides exercise for thigh muscles and helps improve balance.

- Superman: Strengthens back muscles.

- Sit-ups: Strengthens abdominal muscles.

- Push-ups: Strengthens chest, shoulders and arms.

- Bicep curls (with weights): Strengthens arm muscles.

- Overhead press (with weights): Strengthens arms, shoulders and upper back.

Instructions for performing these exercises are on my website (agelaterbook.com), which also includes links to videos. You should be able to perform all of these exercises in one session in less than 20 minutes. If you stress your muscles sufficiently in that time frame, there's no real benefit to working out longer than 20 minutes—in fact, it might be counterproductive. You may choose to start with just two or three exercises, and then add new exercises until you're tackling the full set of seven.

Start by repeating each activity until you reach the initial target or feel you are too tired to continue. Make a note of what you have achieved. At the next session, adjust the exercise as suggested to increase the effort. Also, aim to increase the repetitions.

As you gain fitness and muscle tone, the exercises will become easier. If you decide to stop increasing repetitions, at least stay at the maintenance level—between two and three minutes on each exercise, twice a week.

If possible, keep strength exercises and your vigorous aerobic exercises (or HIIT) separate by scheduling them on different days.

All yoga provides muscle strengthening, as well as low-impact joint exercise and muscle extension. If you already incorporate yoga into your exercise program, consider putting together a set of yoga-based strength exercises to do at home in addition to (or instead of) the basic strength exercises on my website.[98] Do this in consultation with your yoga instructor (if you have one).

You can also use weights and other gym equipment to achieve the necessary amount of muscle strength training. Modern gym equipment can produce even faster and more impressive results. CDC also provides details and videos of selected exercises using gym equipment [99] either in a gym or at home (if you have the equipment). If you use heavy-duty gym equipment and serious weights, I recommend working with a professional trainer or coach to ensure that you don't damage muscle tissue and joints.

Once you establish a routine, think about combining your weightlifting with dynamic exercises. The advantage of this approach, which is called full-body strength training, is that all the body's muscles are exercised together, ensuring that muscle development takes place everywhere you need it. Work with a trainer on this type of exercising, at least initially, and discuss which types of full-body strength training are appropriate for you.

Aerobic Exercise

Moderate Aerobic Exercise

Moderate aerobic exercise is activity that is typically prolonged and steady. During moderate aerobic exercise your heart rate and breathing rate will increase somewhat, but not enough to prohibit you from continuing for an extended period (say, at least 30 minutes). Examples are walking and hiking, and steady-paced slow running. Gentle and sustained exercise on an elliptical machine or stationary exercise bike, or walking on a treadmill, also should be regarded as moderate aerobic exercise. Moderate exercise in the *Age Later* program should raise your heart rate to a level of around 50 percent of your heart rate maximum—but should not exceed 65 percent of the maximum heart rate for your age group, as given in the table "Heart Rate Exercise Zones," which appears earlier in the book and on my website (agelaterbook.com).

Here are some moderate aerobic exercises to include in your program:

- Walking (briskly): fairly level ground, faster and more purposeful than a stroll.

- Jogging: moderate steady pace, no sprinting; carry light weights to give your arms more exercise.

- Hiking on trails: steady pace, even surface, with some inclines uphill and downhill.

- Road cycling: steady cadence with some hills.

- Tennis, squash, badminton, basketball, indoor soccer and volleyball: friendly and relaxed games, not highly competitive.

- Swimming: Easy pace, depending on your level of proficiency; the sort of pace you can maintain for a long time.

- Water aerobics, gentle.

- Running in place

- Dancing

- Treadmill: brisk walking pace, gentle to moderate incline.

- Elliptical machine or stationary bike: moderate pace.

- Jumping rope, jumping jacks and similar exercises.

The amount of time to spend on moderate aerobic exercise depends on your level of fitness and what you want to achieve, as described later in this chapter. You can do planned moderate aerobic exercise more than once in a day, but try to make each session at least 10 minutes, otherwise the effort has limited value. I suggest spreading your moderate aerobic exercise over at least two days, and up to five days per week, with each session lasting at least 10 minutes (preferably, 15).

If you're on a tight schedule, replace some of your moderate aerobic exercise with vigorous aerobic exercise. For every 10 minutes of moderate exercise substitute five minutes of vigorous exercise; you'll cut that chunk of exercise time in half—and gain a similar or even greater benefit.

VIGOROUS AEROBIC EXERCISE

Vigorous aerobic exercise is activity that raises your heart rate substantially further than moderate exercise, and so it makes you breathe more heavily. Vigorous aerobic exercise should raise your heart rate to about 65 percent of the suggested maximum heart rate for your age as given in the aforementioned "Heart Rate Exercise Zones" table. Above that level, you may start to feel burning in your muscles; that's a sign that you're crossing the boundary into anaerobic exercise. Some slight muscle pain is indicative of progress in breaking down and rebuilding muscle tissue, but don't take this too far and don't stress sore muscles for too long. If you want to go further and build significant muscle, see my notes below on strength training.

- Running or fast jogging: fairly level ground, some inclines; faster than a gentle jog.

- Treadmill: running pace, gentle to severe incline.

- Hiking on trails: Steady brisk pace, mixed surfaces, some steep inclines uphill and downhill.

- Swimming: Fast pace, depending on your level of proficiency; the sort of pace that will tire you in less than 10 minutes.

- Road and trail cycling: Steady fast cadence with steep hills, up and down.

- Elliptical machine, stationary bike or rowing machine: set to a high resistance to get the lungs going.

- Tennis, squash, badminton, basketball, indoor soccer, outdoor soccer or volleyball: competitive matches.

The minimum amount of time you spend on vigorous aerobic exercise depends on the level of exercise you choose. To be of most value, each vigorous aerobic session should be at least 15 minutes. Try to space out your vigorous aerobic sessions. Don't do two sets on the same day, or on two days in a row. This allows your muscles to repair and recover between sessions. If possible, do your vigorous aerobics and your strength exercises on different days of the week.

HIGH INTENSITY INTERVAL TRAINING

A step up from vigorous aerobic exercise is High Intensity Interval Training (HIIT), which is an approach to exercise that may have some advantages compared to moderate or aerobic exercise. In HIIT, you exercise to an extreme degree (that is, as hard and fast as you can) for a short time, and then you coast at a moderate level for a period. Then you repeat.

HIIT can be used with almost any type of exercise listed in the Vigorous Aerobic Exercise section. The periods of intense activity can be as short as a few seconds, up to five minutes or more. The relaxation periods in between usually run about the same length but can be much longer. Because there are many variants of HIIT, each with its own benefits, I recommend waiting until you've been exercising for a few weeks before considering HIIT; this will ensure that you've reached a reasonable level of fitness. When you're ready, consider first discussing HIIT options with a trainer.

As with all exercises, HIIT will improve the condition of your muscles and cardiovascular system, but HIIT may deliver results more quickly and with a smaller investment of time than other exercise patterns. HIIT may also help you to burn more fat. HIIT should be seen primarily as a replacement for vigorous aerobic activity. Continue to include other exercises—such as stretching and strength exercises—in your program.

For more information on HIIT, download the short brochure provided by the American College of Sports Medicine.[100] Visit the website at acsm.org.

CHOOSING TO EXERCISE

Making an effort to exercise is a lifestyle decision, one of the more important choices you will make when it comes to your health. You can try any or all of the exercises suggested in this chapter, but the important thing is to move your body, and do it regularly. And if you exercise hard enough to run out of breath from time to time, trust me, that's a good thing.

Just breaking a sweat will encourage you to do more. After a couple of weeks of regular workouts, you'll feel inspired to take it a step further, and then a little more. At a certain point, you'll find that a weekly exercise routine is not only second nature, but it's a habit you can't live without.

Do it. You'll feel the benefit sooner than you might think.

Chapter 7

FOOD CHOICES FOR HEALTH AND YOUTHFULNESS

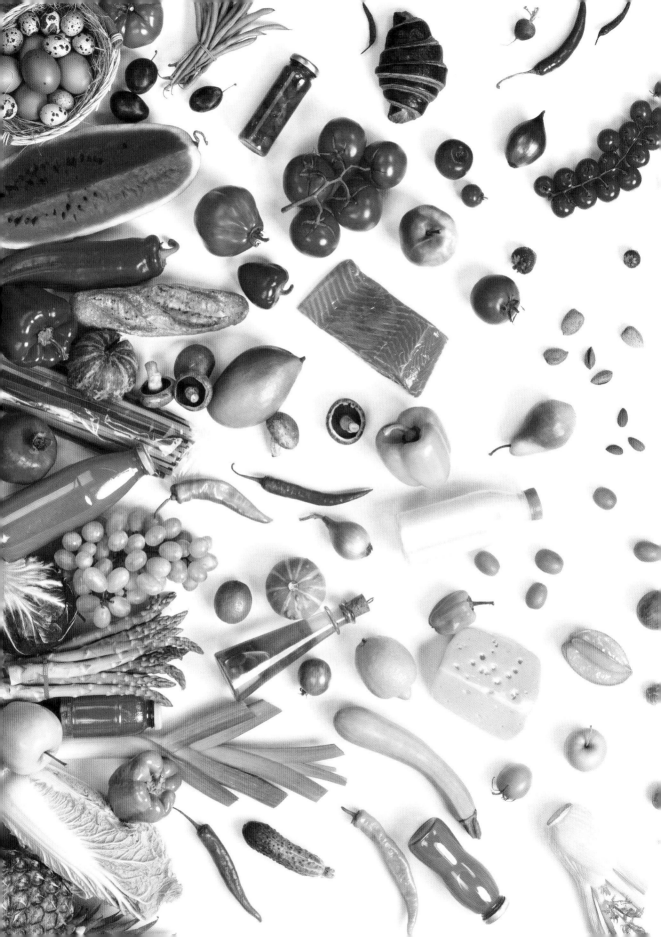

FOOD CHOICES FOR HEALTH AND YOUTHFULNESS

Statistics show that people in the United States make their share of life-shortening decisions when it comes to nutrition, often opting for food that makes them unhealthy, and overweight or obese.[101] If you think it's unfair to single out America, think again. Overall, the percentage of the world's population that qualifies as obese has nearly tripled since 1975. However, of the 35 nations in the Organisation for Economic Co-operation and Development (OECD), the U.S. tops the chart for obesity. In fact, it's done so for many years.[102] According to global statistics for 2015, more than 38 percent of the U.S. population is obese. Compare this to Southeast Asia (3 percent), Japan (3.7 percent), Italy (9.8 percent) and Germany (23.6 percent).

When the figures for being overweight and obese are combined, it accounts for some 70 percent of the U.S. adult population. Think about it: Fewer than one-third of adults living in the United States are at a weight considered healthy.

The international statistics quoted above are based on Body Mass Index. This provides a rough guide to healthy weights, but it doesn't take into account body fat levels, which, ideally, should be below 10 percent. In addition to BMI, you should monitor your Waist to Hip ratio (WHR), which is your waist measurement divided by your hip measurement. That provides an indication of the amount of excess fat you are carrying. WHR targets are 0.9 for men and 0.85 for women. A WHR over 1.0 is cause for concern.[103]

The typical American eats too much food and, more often than not, the wrong types of food. This, coupled with low levels of physical activity, is a formula for illness, disease and a shortened life expectancy. If that's not enough to sound the alarm, consider this: Obese people have 8 percent less brain tissue than people of the same age with normal weight.[104]

The *Age Later* plan is designed to change your poor eating habits—for the good of your body and your mind.

Recent nutrition research has focused on foods implicated in cell aging and inflammation, which, as noted earlier, make our bodies more susceptible to diseases. On the positive side, research also has generated information about foods that lead to health and youthfulness. We probably are the first generation in human history that has access to a reliable and scientifically tested list of foods that are definitely good for us—and a list of those we should avoid if we want to live longer.

Some of this research has resulted in interesting changes regarding what nutritionists recommend. Foods regarded as bad for you only a few decades ago—think red wine, butter and coffee—are now viewed differently (when used in moderation). Other foods that were long considered healthy are now on the unhealthy list—red meat, processed vegetable oils and refined sugar.

I've based the food recommendations in *Age Later* on decades of research, as well as on my own experiences. The result is a food plan that I can confidently recommend for everyone, with priority given to a rich mixture of vegetables, fruits and a variety of vegan protein sources. I also make suggestions for supplementing your daily food with certain vitamins, minerals and antioxidants to ensure that you reap all the benefits of the *Age Later* program.

This chapter is all about bringing healthy living choices to the forefront in your food selection and eating habits. These choices apply to everyone, not just those who are overweight or obese. In fact, this is not a typical weight-loss diet: It's a plan for permanently changing your attitude toward food and the way you eat.[105] As a result, you'll have more energy, your weight will gradually stabilize at a level that's right for you, and you'll look and feel better than ever.

Some of my *Age Later* recommendations align with common factors in well-known diets: less refined sugar, less highly processed flour, less meat, more fiber and avoiding processed foods. For example, the Mediterranean diet lines up well with the *Age Later* recommendations.

On the other hand, I don't agree with the limited range of nourishment that many modern diets advocate by focusing solely on eliminating certain foods, or on eating just a narrow range of foods (the zero carb diet, the pineapple diet, the cookie diet, the meat-only diet, and so on). Limiting the range and balance of nutrients and essential elements may lead to short-term weight loss, but it does not lead to a healthier life.

Age Later has bigger-picture aspirations; it's not just about losing weight. That said, most overweight people who change the balance of their food intake (and exercise regularly) according to my plan eventually will lose unwanted pounds. This gradual and steady weight reduction comes with an important benefit: Once you reach your appropriate weight level, you'll find it much easier to maintain it thanks to your new and improved lifestyle.

FOOD AND NUTRITION

Every molecule the human body needs enters the body in the form of food and drink (which includes supplements). Not everything we eat is useful to the body, but some things are. The components of foods that humans need to consume routinely to survive and flourish are generally called nutrients. Nutrients come in various forms. Some are pure elements or simple molecules. Others are much more complex molecules. Every chemical element in the structure of a normal healthy body must be available in one form or another in our food.

Five groups of nutrients are commonly recognized: amino acids and proteins, carbohydrates, fats, vitamins and minerals. I like to take this a little further and add two more essentials: fiber (which is a type of carbohydrate) and water.

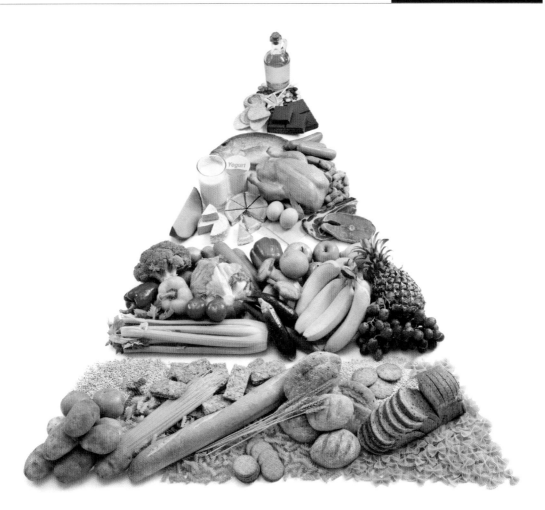

- Proteins (and amino acids, which are used to build proteins); the soft-tissue parts of your body (skin, brain, muscles, nervous system are mostly made of proteins.

- Carbohydrates, a source of energy for the body and the brain.

- Fiber, which is commonly considered a subset of carbohydrates.

- Fats provide energy and also help the body to absorb vitamins, which are fat-soluble.

- Vitamins perform a range of duties in our bodies, from assisting in building and maintaining healthy tissue to fighting inflammation and more.

- Minerals are elemental chemicals that work with the body's organs and nervous system in several ways. Some minerals are part of our body's structure; our bones and teeth, for example, consist largely of the mineral calcium.

- Water is essential to life on Earth, and your body contains lots of it. We use that water every day, so it's imperative to replenish every drop.

The body needs all of these nutrients to maintain its health. We're capable of manufacturing some based on other nutrients in foods we eat. Others can't be made inside the body, so we have to consume enough to meet the body's needs. These are called essential nutrients.

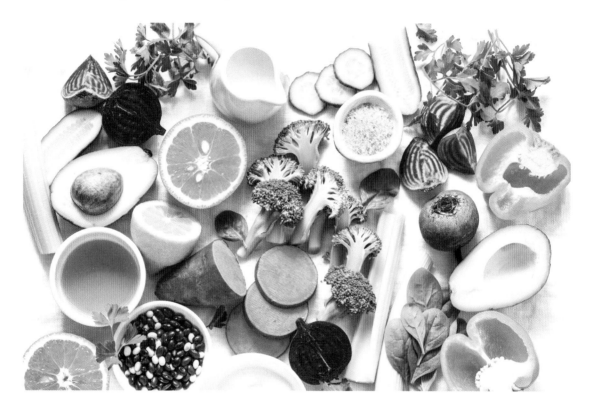

Proteins and Amino Acids

Our cells contain proteins. Proteins are assembled according to instructions encoded in DNA, mainly from amino acids. Proteins and amino acids are therefore fundamental to human life: The cells in our muscles, skin, brain, organs and nervous system could not exist without proteins and the amino acids from which they are made.

There are many different types of proteins in your body. Collagen and elastin are structural proteins essential to proper functioning of skin, joints and connective tissue. Fibronectin plays a part in cell growth, development and healing. Other proteins play a role in nervous system and brain functioning. Some hormones are proteins; others are amino acids or derivatives. Most enzymes are proteins. Enzymes operate to support and accelerate chemical reactions throughout the body. Most of our life-supporting processes depend on the existence and effective behavior of enzymes.

Our foods must provide the raw materials for cell-building. The plant- or animal-based foods we ingest supply most of our whole proteins, which our digestive system dismantles into the constituent amino acids. In turn, those are used to build the range of proteins needed in the human body.

"Essential" amino acids cannot be synthesized inside our bodies, so we need to obtain them from our food.

"Complete" proteins include all the essential amino acids. Meat and dairy products and a few plants (quinoa, soybeans and buckwheat) contain complete proteins. The complete set of amino acids also can be obtained from plant foods by incorporating different groups (grains, beans, leafy vegetables).

Appendix B contains a list of all amino acids important to human growth and health.

CARBOHYDRATES

Carbohydrates are compounds that consist mainly of carbon, hydrogen and oxygen; they're produced naturally and in varying quantities by an array of plants. Your body uses carbohydrates to make glucose, which is converted into energy to run the systems of your body, including your brain. If your carbohydrate intake exceeds your immediate energy needs, then your body will send the extra energy into storage. Your body's short-term storage is in the form of glycogen in the muscles and liver, where it's readily available for action. Longer-term storage is in the form of fats.

If your energy needs exceed the energy immediately available from your food, then the body will extract it from stored fat. If you are overweight, the best approach is two-fold—consume less energy-containing foods and increase your energy usage by being more physically active.

If body fat is used up, you'll start to burn protein—that can lead to muscle atrophy. Always having some fats in reserve will prevent that.

Ideally, our intake of energy-giving foods should result in enough fuel to meet our daily needs and maintain a sufficient level of fats for emergencies. We need to balance energy in and energy out to maintain a stable weight. In the modern world, most adults consume too much fuel; they carry the excess all day, every day, in the form of fat. An overweight person is like a small car with the gas tank of a truck—and the tank is always full.

Carbohydrates are not the only source of energy for our bodies, but they are the quickest to take effect. Your body can convert carbs to glucose quickly and with less energy loss. Fats contain around twice as much energy as carbs, but it takes longer for your body to extract that energy. Protein contains about the same amount of energy by weight as carbs, but it takes even more processing. Rapid conversion sounds like a good thing, and it can be if you are an Olympic sprinter. But for most of us, too much energy in too short a time is both unnecessary and unhealthy.

When you ingest an abundance of easily convertible carbohydrates—even if you balance your energy input and output over the entire day—it quickly overloads your blood with glucose. This triggers body responses that can lead to excess weight, diabetes and cardiovascular problems.

The most easily convertible carbs are refined sugars and refined starches. Sweets and candies, sweetened drinks, white bread and pastries are all products that will spike your blood glucose level.

Some rise in blood glucose after eating a meal is normal and natural. Glucose in the blood directs the energy to where it's needed. It's sudden and severe spiking that does the damage.

Some diet programs demonize carbohydrates. I don't think that is necessary, but I do recognize the dangers of refined sugar and starches. You do need some carbs, but probably not as much as you think. You take in carbohydrates when you eat any fruit or vegetable, so a genuinely zero-carb diet is not, strictly speaking, possible.

When bundled inside natural plant foods, sugars and starches are accompanied by substances (fibers, proteins and enzymes) that work to buffer their impact on the body. The result is a gradual rise and fall of glucose levels, not a dangerous spike. Also, the accompanying fiber bulk makes it more difficult to consume enough sugar to cause damage. Once the food has been processed, the chemical structure of the sugars released into your body is about the same as if you consumed that amount of sugar in refined form. The difference is in the delivery rate—a steady drip feed over an extended period, not a rapid and damaging flood.

Even if you cut out all refined sugar and white flour products, you can easily secure enough energy for the day from vegetables, fruits, whole grains and plant-derived oils and fats.

While I don't advocate a zero-carb diet, we need to think about the balance between fats and carbs. Plant-based oils provide a host of health advantages, but they do contain more calories than carbohydrates. To balance an increase in fat intake, we need to reduce carb intake. The body will store fat no matter which foods provide the excess calories. A moderate reduction of foods that are highest in carbs—such as starchy plants and bread products (even whole grain bread)—allows room for the addition of olive oil and other nutritious oils.

Fats

Between 1950 and 1970, deaths across the U.S. from heart disease increased steadily.[106] By 1970, there was a growing belief that consumption of fats was the main culprit; that prompted a government effort to persuade people to reduce or eliminate fat from their diets. Unfortunately, the blanket condemnation of all fats not only was unnecessary but probably damaging. At the time, many researchers contested the decision as being over-simplistic. It already was clear back then that refined carbohydrates were part of the problem too—or even most of the problem.[107]

A particularly harmful result of the all-fats-are-bad approach was that fats in the diet rapidly became replaced by refined carbohydrates (sugar and white flour). The absence of fat in food made it feel less satisfying to many people, and that satisfaction deficit was filled with sugar and starch—exactly the opposite of what was needed.[108]

Today, it's clear that some fats are necessary in our diets and that lowering the level of those needed fats causes health problems. Some fats and oils in our food are good for us. These include omega-3, omega-6 and omega-9 groups of fats, and others, including butyrates. Dangerous fats are industrial trans-fats. Fats that lie somewhere in between are certain saturated fats, once thought to be dangerous. Now, the experts aren't so sure: Some may be beneficial, some probably are not good.

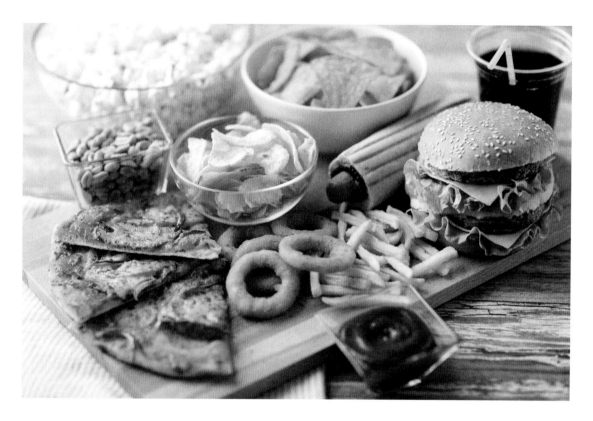

BENEFICIAL FATS

Fatty acids are critical for cell health and renewal throughout the body. These fats strengthen your cells and help them to hold moisture.

Omega group fatty acids are involved in supporting important body functions, including circulation, cell-building, skin renewal and brain functioning. They are critical for skin health and joint health, and they can fight heart disease, depression and Alzheimer's.

Two omega fatty acids are defined as essential because they cannot be synthesized within the body: alpha-linolenic acid (ALA, an omega-3 fatty acid) and linoleic acid (LA, an omega-6 fatty acid). Another, oleic acid (an omega-9 fatty acid), can be synthesized within the body from omega-3 and omega-6 fatty acids but only in limited quantities, so the body also needs a food source of omega-9.

Other important omega-3 fatty acids are eicosapentaenoic acid (EPA) and docosahexaenoic acid (DHA). EPA helps control inflammation throughout the body and may reduce symptoms of depression. DHA is important for brain development and maintenance. If we consume enough ALA from dietary sources, then the body can convert some of it to EPA and DHA. But if our intake of ALA is insufficient, we can't make it ourselves.

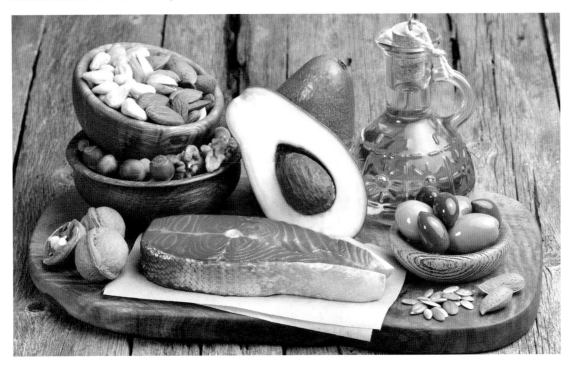

We can obtain ALA and other omega-3 fatty acids from many vegetables, beans, nuts, seeds and fruits. Especially good sources are flax seeds, chia seeds, walnuts, kidney beans and black beans. Olive oil and oils made from flax seeds, canola seeds, sunflower seeds and soybeans all contain omega-3. Marine algae and phytoplankton are good omega-3 sources, which is why oily fresh fish (that eat algae and plankton) also are a valued source of the EPA and DHA omega-3 fatty acids (but not necessarily of ALA).

Most sources of omega-3 are also sources of omega-6. However, omega-6 can be obtained from other products, like cold-pressed olive oil, palm oil, whole grains, poultry and eggs. Because of the wider range of sources, humans generally ingest more omega-6 than omega-3 (and easily obtain sufficient omega-6 from a normal healthy diet). Ideally, intake of omega-3 and omega-6 should be in balance, but typical food choices today provide around 10 times as much omega-6 fatty acids as omega-3. That's why it's important to supplement omega-3.

Oleic acid, one of the most common fats in the body, plays a role in skin health and in managing cholesterol levels. Good sources of oleic acid and other omega-9 acids include: olives, nuts, seeds and oils cold-pressed from those foods. Olive oil is very high in oleic acid (and also is a good source of omega-3 and omega-6).

Butyrates are compounds formed from butyric acid (a fatty acid). They are essential for stomach health as they provide food for good bacteria, a strong population of which is vital for a healthy body. Some stomach microbes can consume dietary fiber and convert that fiber to butyrates—so dietary fiber is not just a source of bulk in the gut; it's a source of useful butyrates. All fruits and vegetables contain useful fiber, but among those that provide food for butyrate production are asparagus, chicory, garlic, Jerusalem artichoke, unripe bananas, leeks and onions.

Alpha lipoic acid is a powerful antioxidant fatty acid. It plays a role in supporting the health and function of the cardiovascular system, brain, nervous system, skin and muscles. It's present in many foods (nuts and seeds, green vegetables) and in animal tissues. The body also can synthesize alpha lipoid acid from octanoic acid (caprylic acid), a constituent of mammal milk and some vegetable oils.

Lecithin, a fatty substance found in a variety of plants and animals, is a source of several valuable micronutrients, including choline, inositol and other glycerophospholipids and various lipids. It occurs naturally in almost all plant and animal food sources. Foods especially rich in lecithin include eggs, beans, fruit, grains, nuts, milk and seafood. It acts as a natural emulsifier in traditional recipes and is widely used in manufactured products.

DANGEROUS FATS

The fats that should have been banned many years ago are trans fats (or industrial trans-unsaturated fatty acids). Industrial trans fats cause inflammation throughout the body, especially in heart tissue. Consumption of industrial trans fats, even in small quantities, is known to increase the risk of coronary heart disease. It has no known health benefits. That's why there is an effort, worldwide, to eliminate them from food products.

Industrial trans fats are manufactured. Starting usually with normal (healthy) vegetable oil, a process called hydrogenation changes the molecules to make them more stable and enduring. The benefits are entirely in the form of extended shelf life, which is why trans fats were used widely in processed and packaged food products. Margarine, vegetable shortening, processed vegetable oils and anything containing partially hydrogenated vegetable oil, contain industrial trans fats. Many processed foods and fried foods also contain some trans fats.

FATS THAT MIGHT BE OK

There are two broad categories of fats that may be less damaging (overall) than previously thought: some saturated fats and natural trans fats.

Saturated fats are plentiful in many common foods, including all meats, whole milk, cheese, yogurt, butter and cream. They're also present in coconut oil, palm oil and cocoa butter. Although most vegetable-based oils contain monounsaturated or polyunsaturated fats, many do contain a small amount of saturated oils. Human breast milk contains a high proportion of saturated fats,[109] and for infants these saturated fatty acids provide energy and components vital to the efficient development of healthy brains and healthy bodies. So, it's unreasonable to suggest that all saturated fats are harmful. Adult human beings have been consuming saturated fatty acids for tens of thousands of years, at least. However, our ancient ancestors probably consumed small quantities—along with large quantities of fruits and vegetables, providing lots of antioxidants and fiber. It's difficult to avoid all saturated fats—nor should we. Even the healthy Mediterranean diet contains some saturated fats.

We do know that saturated fat isn't a unique substance; in fact, there are numerous saturated fatty acids. As researchers identify the pathways in the body that these different substances follow, they find that some saturated fatty acids may be harmful, especially when consumed in large quantities. Other may be more or less neutral, and others may even be beneficial. The picture is further complicated by the fact that foods that contain fatty acids also contain a cocktail of many other substances, so the net impact on the body is not easily predictable.

There is a debate in progress, with people lining up on both sides. Research results are conflicting.[110] These inconclusive results likely will lead to additional research and perhaps to a new perspective on the issue.

In the meantime, it's clear that overconsumption of animal-derived saturated fats, in general, is not good for human health. Excess consumption certainly raises bad cholesterol levels and is associated with weight gain, obesity, diabetes and cardiovascular disease. In small quantities, taken with plenty of vegetables and fruit (and with exercise added to the mix), animal fats may not be so bad. Perhaps.

We also should say something about natural trans fats. Our ancestors probably consumed trans fats in milk and meat products, but these were natural trans fats, not the dangerous industrial trans fats. Research on natural trans fats (in the form of conjugated linoleic acids, or CLA) suggests that they may not be as dangerous as the industrially manufactured version—and may even be beneficial.[111]

So, like saturated fats, it may be that these natural trans fats are not harmful in small quantities. That said, more research is needed to be certain.

Until we learn more, my advice is that adults should limit consumption of saturated fatty acids and natural trans fats (especially from red meat products) to a small proportion of calorie intake. Providing you eat plenty of vegetables and exercise regularly, it may not be necessary to eliminate every trace of these fats from our diets. Moderation rather than elimination should be your aim, as there are more important food priorities to consider.

Vitamins

Vitamins are compounds that are essential for the health and growth of the human body, but they cannot be synthesized by the body itself.[112] Humans must obtain all vitamins from food sources, or if normal food sources are inadequate, from supplements.[113]

Appendix C contains a list of vitamins, with a description of their benefits and food sources.

Minerals

Minerals and trace minerals are naturally occurring elements that are needed to build cells and support body functioning for muscles, the heart, brain and digestive system. These simple substances play complex roles to keep you alive.

We usually ingest elemental minerals as part of a more complex chemical compound. Some minerals (macro-minerals) need to be ingested in relatively large quantities. The macro-minerals are: calcium, chloride, magnesium, phosphorus, potassium, sodium and sulfur.

Others (trace minerals) are required in tiny amounts, but although only small quantities are needed, they are still vital for health, and deficiencies can become dangerous. Appendix D contains the list of minerals and trace minerals we need.

Water: Hydration

Water is one substance we can't avoid. We can choose between different plant foods and different animal foods, but no matter what we eat, it all contains some water. More important than the water in our food is the water we drink—either as pure water or as a water-based drink.

Water is essential to the health of every body cell. Water keeps your joints and muscles moving smoothly and free of pain.

Brain cells function best when the cellular balance of water and chemicals is within the optimum range. Inadequate hydration leads to an inability to concentrate, confusion, memory lapses and even cell loss.

Hydration, of course, also benefits your skin health. We know it's important to keep skin hydrated by applying moisturizers. But you need to hydrate from the inside as well for the benefit of your skin (and entire body). Being hydrated from within helps to ensure that your collagen cells are properly moisturized, meaning your skin will be more elastic and look smoother. As a rule, try to drink 1 ounce of fluid for each 2 pounds of body weight. For example, a person who weighs 160 pounds should aim for 80 ounces (5 U.S. pints) of fluids per day.

In their quest for balanced and nutritious foods, people often overlook water. I include it in my list of "Foods That Are Good For You" later in this chapter.

FIBER

Fiber is essential for the health of your stomach and digestive system. Modern eating habits tend to be very low in fiber compared to traditional diets. Although modern nutritionists suggest we should eat around 25 grams of fiber per day, our ancestors (even the hunters) probably ate far more fiber. I recommend more than the guideline level to ensure the health of our digestive system.

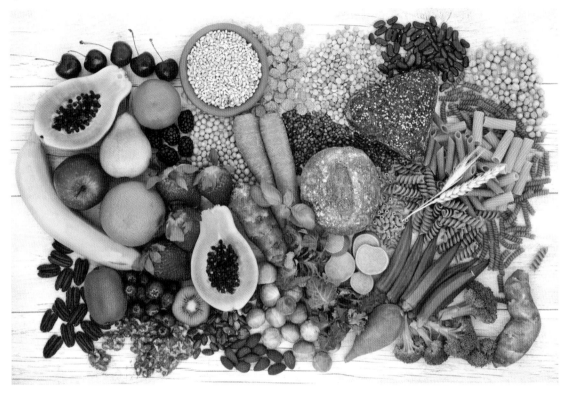

We need to consume both soluble and insoluble types of fiber.[114]

Soluble fiber attracts water and forms a gel as it passes through, which effectively lubricates the digestive system and lower intestine. Adequate soluble fiber is essential for stomach health, and some types are known to lower the risk of heart disease and type 2 diabetes. Soluble fiber is present in high quantities in oats, barley, nuts, seeds, beans, lentils, peas, leeks, onion, garlic, bananas, blueberries, apples and asparagus (and in slightly lower quantities in many other vegetables and fruits).

Insoluble fiber is important too. It adds bulk to our food and helps to fight diseases of the stomach and intestines. Most plants contain some insoluble fiber in their leaves and roots, and in the skins of their seeds or fruits. Good sources of insoluble fiber include whole grains, beans, peas, lentils, berries, apples, seeds and fibrous leafy plants.

All forms of fiber are forms of starch, and therefore fall into the category of carbohydrates. But unlike sugars and digestible starches, fiber does not contribute much energy to the body's system. Fibers are starches with almost zero calories. A plentiful intake of fiber helps the body manage its overall caloric food consumption—and therefore your weight.

The human digestive system cannot digest fiber efficiently, but some strains of stomach microbes can consume fiber and benefit. They are able to extract the energy locked in the fibers, and they use that energy to grow and multiply. The chemical by-products of that conversion process may be another reason why consuming fiber boosts health. The more fiber-loving microbes we cultivate, the healthier we become.[115]

OBTAINING NUTRITION

We obtain many of the nutrients we need for survival in everyday food, even in a relatively poor Western diet. We can survive that way, but the *Age Later* program has a higher purpose. It's not just about surviving; it's about thriving, so that we can live a longer, healthier life. To do this, our daily food intake should include a balanced quota of all the nutrients we need.

The *Age Later* food plan will provide more antioxidants, healthful nutrients and fiber than the average American consumes, while eliminating many of the damaging substances that so many people eat. You can achieve better results than a "normal" diet delivers by including generous amounts of foods known to be high in vitamins and minerals. All berries, nuts and seeds contain more of these nutrients per gram than regular vegetables. Some herbs and spices contain even more. At the same time, it's equally important to rid your daily routine of damaging foods, which can negate the benefits of a high-nutrient plan.

Even if you adhere to these guidelines, there are circumstances in which the *Age Later* food plan can use a boost. In that case, you may need to add carefully selected supplements.

HEALTHY CHOICES: CHANGING WHAT YOU EAT

The food recommendations in *Age Later* present plenty of menu options. To give you a preview of what lies ahead, here's a quick peek at my typical routine.

- Breakfast: I switch between a juice and eggs. My favorite juice is pressed from red and green vegetables, including red beet, kale, celery, apple, orange and ginger. I also like a shake with super greens, like Hush & Hush PlantYourDay with almond milk, which provides extra protein. My egg dish is made from just a small portion of egg whites, because I prefer to avoid the extra calories and cholesterol in the yolks.

- Lunch: Often, it's a salad without any fish or meat.

- During the day I sometimes eat fruits: blueberries, raspberries, strawberries, half a banana, apple, grapefruit, orange.

- Dinner: I always have a salad, usually with carrots and mozzarella, then a warm dish based on vegetables with some grains, and sometimes pasta. I never eat red meat or poultry, and very rarely do I eat fish.

You can see more of my favorite healthy living choice meal suggestions on my website (agelater-book.com).

FOODS THAT ARE GOOD FOR YOU

Leafy vegetables and fruits should top your list of nourishing foods. This is the foundation of your nutrition plan. Eat as many different kinds of fruits and vegetables as possible; they provide significant amounts of nutrients, antioxidants and fiber—which your body needs if it's going to run on all cylinders. Focus on these first. You can then add small amounts of other food groups—and still have a healthy food regimen.

All foods high in antioxidants will help to keep free radicals, inflammation and AGE production[116] under control. If you don't eat enough fruits and vegetables, you're missing out on the naturally occurring vitamins, enzymes and co-agents, which are essential for fighting free radicals and battling uncontrolled inflammation.

Plants provide some digestible carbohydrates, but they also contain useful amounts of carbohydrates in the form of soluble and insoluble fiber. The benefits of large volumes of both soluble and insoluble fiber are significant. Both are required to support the health of our digestive system, and the friendly microbes that help to run it.

Incorporate a variety of different healthy plant foods into your diet; from there, you may choose to add moderate quantities of other healthy foods.

The *Age Later* program encourages maximum diversity across food groups and within food groups: carbs, protein, fat, minerals, vitamins, fiber. I don't recommend one specific "diet." Instead, I recommend a set of healthy life choices that will help you to *Age Later*.

LEAFY VEGETABLES

All leafy vegetables are wholesome foods. My *Age Later* recommendation is to eat a variety of leafy vegetables, and at least two servings overall per day. At least one of those servings should be raw, in a salad. Leafy vegetables are rich in antioxidants, minerals, and soluble and insoluble fiber. Your options include spinach, chard, kale, collard greens, turnip greens, cabbage and dark varieties of lettuce. As a rule of thumb, intense dark colors often signal high levels of antioxidants and fiber, so add those to your shopping list. Also, since colors can reflect the nutrients inside, aim for a wide and adventurous palette of hues when it comes to your leafy vegetables.

FRUIT AND BERRIES

I recommend a healthy mixture of fruits every day. For example, have at least one banana, one apple, some berries or red/black grapes every day as a matter of course. Add different fruits for variety: citrus, papaya, pineapple, kiwi. There are no fruits you should avoid. All fruits provide antioxidants, minerals and fiber, plus some carbs and plant protein.

Berries, especially blueberries and blackberries, are on my list of high-nutrient foods; they provide lots of nutrition in a small package. Resveratrol, found in dark-skinned fruits, may inhibit the production of advanced glycation end products (AGEs).[117] Their vitamin C boosts the immune system, fights inflammation, and reduces the risk of heart disease and cancers.

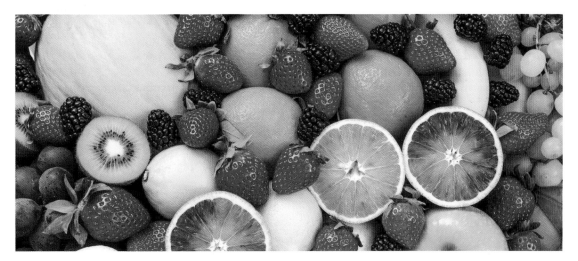

NUTS AND SEEDS

All nuts and seeds contain large amounts of nutrition for their small size and should be included in everyone's daily food intake. Nuts and seeds contain antioxidants and minerals in high quantities. Brazil nuts, walnuts and almond all have potent nutrients and are listed along with other valuable nuts and seeds in Appendix E: High Nutrient foods.

My *Age Later* recommendation is to start the day with some nuts and seeds for breakfast; perhaps include them in a serving of muesli, or along with berries and natural yogurt.

ONIONS AND OTHER ALLIUMS

I have nothing but good things to say about onions and their allium relatives: garlic, chives, leeks, scallions and shallots. Not only do they improve the flavor of almost any savory dish, but they are good for your health.

Onions contain vitamins C, K and B-6, along with a host of minerals and nutrients, including folate (B9), thiamine (B1), calcium, magnesium, potassium and manganese. They also provide plant fiber. Vitamin C is a strong antioxidant that helps to reduce inflammation in the body and improves many body functions, including collagen production. Onions also contain organosulfur compounds that assist the vitamin C to reduce the risk of cancers.[118]

The folates in these plant foods work to reduce levels of homocysteine in the body, which may help in improving mood and sleep patterns (thus reducing stress levels).[119]

Alliums also contain fiber in a form that the body converts to butyrates, which, in turn, provide food for beneficial bacteria.

All members of the allium family contain allicin, and garlic is particularly rich in this compound. Alliin, a derivative of the amino acid cysteine, occurs naturally in garlic; when the garlic is cut or crushed, the alliin is converted to allicin, which is responsible for that garlicky smell. Allicin reduces blood pressure and helps stave off airborne viruses such as the common cold and influenza. Allicin is available in pill form as a supplement (garlic capsules), but my preference is to eat lots of garlic. Allicin has been shown to combat the influenza virus and reduce incidences of the common cold in clinical tests.[120]

My recommendation: Include at least one or two members of this useful group in one or more meals every day.

WHOLE GRAINS

Grains are a useful source of carbohydrates, fiber and nutrients, but the fiber and nutrients are available only if the grains are actual whole grains—unhusked and not processed. The husks contain nutrients and fiber that are completely missing from processed grains. The fiber content means that the energy from the carbohydrates is absorbed more slowly than if you had eaten the equivalent amount in processed grains. This makes it easier to process the energy without causing a spike in blood-sugar level.

Whole grains contain less carbs for their weight than processed grains, and they also contain more fiber, protein and beneficial oils.

Fortunately there are lots of whole wheat and other whole grain products from which to choose, providing you carefully manage your intake. Real whole grain products give us more nutrients per serving along with the grain protein, plus the simpler processing results in more useful fiber. Consumption of adequate quantities of fiber is fundamental to good nutrition and bodily health.

Try working whole grains into your recipes. Do not eat white rice, which is high in empty calories and low in fiber. Instead, include one of these tastier and healthier choices: brown, red or wild rice; barley; farro (whole wheat); bulgur or dalia (cracked wheat); quinoa and other whole grains.

Wholemeal flour is better for you than white flour, so choose wholemeal bread and pasta over the white varieties. The grains still have been processed by milling, which reduces the nutrient value and makes the starches more accessible. If you can buy (or make) wholemeal bread that contains a proportion of unmilled actual whole grains, that is a healthier choice. Lots of commercial wholemeal bread contains unnecessary refined sugar and chemicals to extend shelf life, so read the label (if there is one).

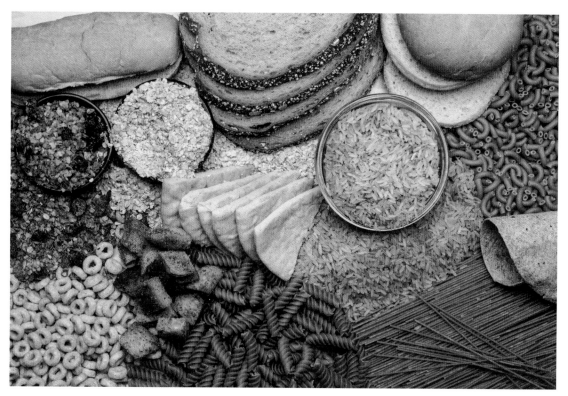

I encourage everyone to consume a range of nutritious and non-harmful foods, and that includes various whole grains. While whole grains are good, avoid highly processed grains (white flour products) and anything with additives.

My *Age Later* recommendation is to eliminate refined white flour products from your diet—and limit whole grain flour products (wheat and pasta) to around four servings per week. Whole grains that have not been milled into flour can be consumed more often. Brown rice, farro, steel-cut oats, quinoa, buckwheat and other whole grains provide lots of fiber and nutrients, and one of these at one meal a day makes sense as part of a balanced food plan.

Many people eat too many flour-based products. Humans evolved to consume grains in small quantities relative to other fruits and vegetables. After all, gathering and processing grains is more labor-intensive than gathering fruit and leafy vegetables. By eating only whole grains, you naturally will reduce your carb intake to something closer to the level that we have evolved to handle.

Unfortunately, too many people are avoiding the benefits of this useful food. In recent years we have seen an upsurge in people who have been convinced (by intensive marketing campaigns) that they are sensitive to gluten. Certainly there are people with celiac disease (an estimated 1 percent of the U.S. population) who suffer when they eat food that contains gluten—so, they must adhere to a gluten-free diet. But those who do not have celiac disease may not be as sensitive to gluten as they think. My guess is that the majority of people who eat only gluten-free foods are doing it unnecessarily.

Another condition that may be much ado about nothing in many cases is lectin intolerance. Grains are high in lectins, but in my opinion that is no reason to avoid them. Many natural foods contain lectins, and we shouldn't try to avoid them all.

I have provided more thoughts on the upsurge in gluten intolerance and lectin intolerance in Appendix F.

Anyone who suspects that lectin is causing them health problems should follow the *Age Later* food guidelines instead of excluding useful foods. Focus on fresh vegetables and fruit, eat only whole grains, cook high-lectin foods thoroughly, and eliminate refined sugar and white flour.

NIGHTSHADE PLANTS

Tomatoes, eggplants, peppers, potatoes and tomatillos are all beneficial foods, providing antioxidants, vitamins and minerals—perfect for inclusion in your nutrition plan.

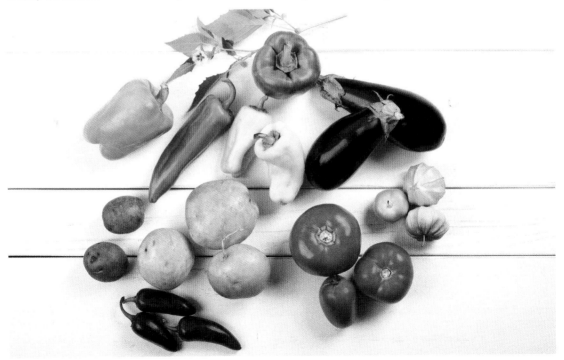

Although they all look and taste very different, these foods do have something in common: They are all members of the plant family Solanaceae, less formally referred to as nightshades. (This large and diverse family includes tobacco and belladonna, which contain toxins and certainly are not suitable for your food plan.)

Nightshades that we eat do contain some alkaloids, but not all alkaloids are harmful, especially in small quantities. These plants contain lectins too (but so does almost every food you can think of, including meat, fish and dairy). Some people with disorders of the immune or digestive systems avoid nightshade foods for that reason. For most healthy people, choosing fully ripe and fresh produce—and cooking these foods properly (especially potato and eggplant)—reduces the levels of lectins dramatically, enough to avoid digestive problems.[121]

Note that a high proportion of nutrients are either in or close to the skins of these foods, so it's often better to keep the skins on. I recommend eating one or more of the non-starchy foods in this group frequently, perhaps four to six servings per week. For more, see Appendix F.

BEANS, PEAS, LENTILS

Beans, peas, and lentils (often referred to as legumes or pulses) are high in fiber and a source of protein, minerals and vitamins. All three are a welcome part of a balanced diet, provided they're properly cooked; when freshly harvested and cooked, beans and peas are especially nutritious. All dried legumes must be thoroughly boiled or pressure-cooked until soft.

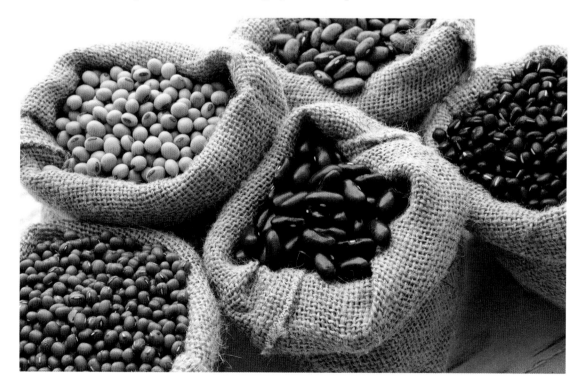

Although legumes are starchier than leafy vegetables, a proportion of that is in the form of indigestible starches. Not only do these starches release fewer calories, but they also improve the digestive system's overall health. I recommend eating beans, lentils and peas often, around four or five servings spread out over a week.

There are exceptions.

I'm not a fan of peanuts and soy, although I recognize that both have nutritional value. Both are high in plant proteins, and soy is one of the few to provide all essential amino acids. My concern is that peanuts and soybeans are intensively grown and often heavily treated with chemicals (fungicides, pesticides, herbicides).

In their commonly available form, salted roasted peanuts have too much saturated fat and usually too much sodium. Moreover, people typically eat more than the recommended serving size. Peanuts contain much more omega-6 than omega-3 fatty acids, which we should try to avoid if we want to keep our omega intake in balance.

Natural soybeans, cooked or fermented, are nutritious, but soy as it appears in many processed foods, has much lower nutritional value, thanks to heavy processing. Soy contains higher levels of phytoestrogens than any other natural food. Researchers have yet to reach a firm conclusion regarding the side effects of these plant hormones (in high levels), but we do know they mimic the behavior of estrogen in the body. That suggests a potential impact on human hormonal development; animal studies confirm this. Consequently, my opinion is that soy products should not be fed to infants and children—and adults should not eat soy in large quantities.[122]

Some people avoid all beans, peas and lentils because, uncooked, they contain high levels of lectins, proteins that are known to cause stomach irritation and digestive problems.[123] To remove most of the lectins from both dried and fresh beans, simply cook them properly—or choose fermented bean products. Fermentation products made from fermented beans, including soy, have been a nutritional staple in Asian diets for centuries. Fermentation reduces the lectin level and makes the beans more digestible while retaining most of the nutritional value. For additional insights, see Appendix F.

FISH AND SEAFOOD

The good news is that fish is nutritious, easy to prepare and easy on the digestive system. Fish and shellfish are high in protein, omega-3 fatty acids, vitamin D, B2 and lots of useful minerals including zinc, selenium, calcium, phosphorus, magnesium, iron and potassium. Shellfish like shrimp and lobster are rich in cholesterol, so I suggest eating crustaceans in small portions (and not every day).

Unless you've decided to become a complete vegetarian, there's mostly upside to eating fish. It's good for the skin, brain, hair, heart and your health in general; there's no easier way to acquire some of the key substances that you need to build a healthy body.[124] For many years, Japan has enjoyed the world's highest life expectancy (83.7 years in 2017)—and fish in the

Japanese diet is reason why its people live longer.[125]

There's some bad news too. Fish stocks in our oceans are being depleted at a record rate, leaving an increasing number of species on the endangered list.

In addition, thanks to human pollution of rivers and oceans with millions of tons of trash, [126]and mining, industrial and agricultural processes, fish today often contain trace amounts of mercury, pesticides, PCB (polychlorinated biphenyl) and other toxic chemicals. These substances can build up in the human body, just as they have built up over the years inside the fish we eat. Too much mercury can cause permanent, life-threatening damage to the kidneys and the nervous system.

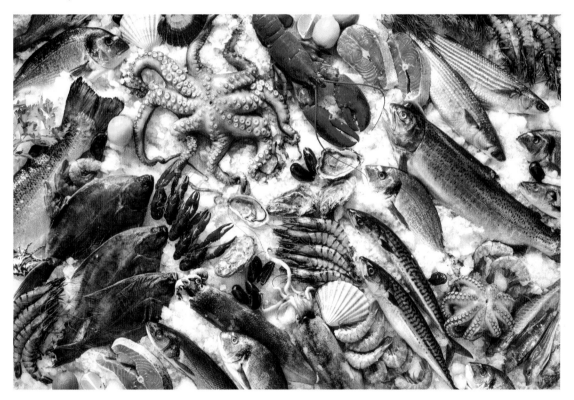

Controlling your consumption of fish allows your body to process the toxins and minimize buildup. I have a friend who was an avid consumer of fish, especially tuna. One day, he noticed that his hair was starting to fall out. Tests quickly revealed that he was in the early stages of mercury poisoning. He stopped eating tuna, his mercury blood levels started to go down, and his hair recovered.

The amounts of mercury and other pollutants in fish depend on the locality in which these fish live and breed. Some parts of the world are much more polluted than others. In general, fish that are higher up the food chain (ones that eat other fish) tend to have more toxin buildup. This includes sharks, swordfish, marlin, king mackerel, tilefish and tuna, which is a particular danger because it's so commonly consumed and because it's a consistent menu item for some people. I suggest avoiding these fish completely—if not for health reasons than because the populations of swordfish, and certain tuna and sharks are decreasing.

As for other fish, eat no more than 12 ounces overall per week, spread over two or three meals—unless you know for sure that the seafood you're consuming is low in mercury. Most nutritionists think that the benefits of eating small amounts of fish on a regular basis outweigh the risks from traces of pollutants.[127]

If you are concerned, research which fish are from sustainable fisheries and which are safest to eat.[128] [129]If we were all a little more patient and allowed declining fish stocks to recover, we would have a wider range of fish from which to choose.

If you don't eat fish, or only on occasion, consider taking omega-3 supplements. I eat fish maybe once a month. That's not because I don't like fish, but because I feel sorry for the fish. To ensure I get enough omega-3, I take supplements.

HERBS AND SPICES

Herbs and spices are intense: They have distinct aromas and tastes, and a little goes a long way. Better still, many of them pack a serious pound-for-pound punch when it comes to delivering nutrients and antioxidants, compared to other foods.

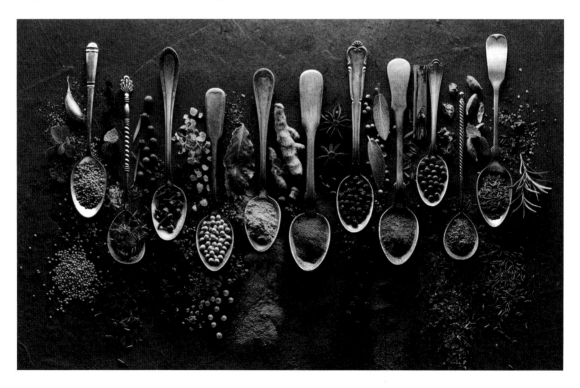

Herbs and spices have been used in every culture for thousands of years, and a wealth of knowledge exists regarding their use as remedies for ailments. For our purposes, we'll focus on their usefulness in maintaining health and as an antidote to aging. Even then, describing all the benefits in detail would require an encyclopedia.[130]

Increasing the use of herbs and spices at home can enhance a kitchen effort in need of help, gently push an already stellar dish to the next level—or simply add a little something fun to the mix. We use them because of their flavor intensity, but that intensity is there because herbs and spices contain a high density of nutrients. When you use these intense foods in cooking, they are automatically self-regulating. Use them freely, but keep sampling the dish as you cook. If you add too much, you will know.

My recommendation is to use all common herbs and spices freely in your cuisine. There are culinary conventions that link certain flavors to specific dishes, but you also can try herbs and spices in nontraditional combinations: turmeric in a shake or smoothie, basil on your bowl of berries and yogurt, cinnamon (real cinnamon) in your muesli. Have fun experimenting.

Also, research the benefits. I provide some information on the value of common herbs and spices in Appendix E (and also at agelaterbook.com).

DAIRY PRODUCTS

Dairy foods include:

- Milk

- Yogurt, kefir and other fermented milk products

- Butter

- Cheese

All milk-based products, whether from cows, goats or sheep, provide proteins, calcium, phosphorus, magnesium, potassium, zinc, and vitamins B2 and B12. Some milk products contain vitamin D as an additive. Milk contains carbohydrates, mostly in the form of the natural sugar lactose, as well as a large number of fatty acids (among them, omega-3 and omega-6 fatty acids). Milk does contain some natural trans fats, including conjugated linoleic acid (CLA)—but, unlike industrial trans fats, these ruminant trans fats are, on balance, beneficial.[131] Organic and antibiotic-free milk products balanced foods thanks to these useful nutrients.

One justified concern about milk products is that they are naturally high in saturated fats. Recent research suggests that saturated fats from milk are not as bad for you as animal fats from meat, but they're not as nourishing as fats and oils that occur in plants.[132] Also, it's not clear that low-fat versions of milk products are better for you than the full-fat versions when consumed moderately as part of a balanced food plan.[133] At this stage, compared to the dangers

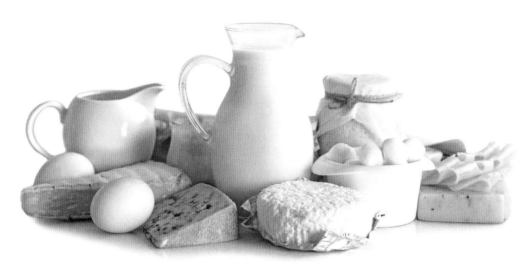

of carbs from refined sugar and white flour, saturated fats from milk don't seem so bad. That said, they shouldn't be consumed in large quantities.

Lactose intolerance and milk allergies are common throughout the world, which limits the value of this food for many people. Some milk products, low-fat milk and yogurt may contain added refined sugar. Check the labels and avoid versions that contain sugars in addition to the natural sugars found in all milk.

Yogurt, provided it's unsweetened and "live," contains natural probiotics that are helpful to your stomach flora and digestive system. The yogurt-making process results in a food that contains less lactose and more protein than milk.

Cheese has about the same amount of protein as milk but less lactose. Cheeses that have been aged tend to contain high levels of AGEs suggesting they should be consumed sparingly.

Butter contains even more saturated fat per spoonful than milk, and less protein and carbs. It provides all the nutrients that milk provides, and then some, but in a more concentrated form. Butter also has high levels of butyrate, which is good for stomach health. The fats in butter are definitely less harmful than the fats in margarine, but they fall short compared to plant oils and fats.[134]

Milk products are devoid of fiber, so ideally they should be consumed in the company of high-fiber plants; that's why yogurt and fruit, oatmeal and milk, bread and cheese, all tradition-al pairings, make digestive sense.

Milk alternatives (almond milk, rice milk, soy milk, coconut milk) are becoming more popular, but none has the same nutrient balance as milk from dairy animals. Nutrient contents vary from type to type, and from brand to brand, so check the labels. Their fats are derived from plant sources, so, from the fat perspective, milk alternatives do have added health value.

Moderate consumption of dairy products certainly can complement a complete and balanced food plan. Of all milk-based products, yogurt appears to offer the most benefits; a healthy suggestion is yogurt in combination with oatmeal, muesli, or nuts and berries. No matter which dairy products you enjoy, limit your intake to no more than one serving per day. Consumption of aged cheese and butter should be limited to occasional small amounts.

Those who prefer not to eat dairy, as with those who don't eat meat, will have to source the nutrients from plant foods—but many people around the world do that successfully.

Eggs

Eggs are traditionally included in the dairy group, along with milk and milk products, even though their characteristics are not exactly the same. Both contain a valuable range of minerals and vitamins but compared to milk, eggs provide more iron, selenium, phosphorus, and vitamins A, B12, D and folate (B9). Eggs and milk both provide complete proteins, but eggs offer more of them. On the other hand, eggs contain less calcium than milk.

All in all, eggs bring valuable nutrients to the table. However, they also bring lots of cholesterol and some saturated fats, mostly concentrated in the yolk. This has, in the past, caused nutritionists to ban or restrict egg consumption. More recent research suggests that consumption of saturated fats drives cholesterol levels in your body more than consumption of cholesterol itself.[135] On balance, I suggest that you restrict your egg consumption to no more than six whole eggs a week, mainly to keep your intake of animal saturated fats down. By eating just the egg whites, you avoid almost all the fat and cholesterol—and thus can safely eat more.[136]

To place the fat content of eggs in perspective, note that the saturated fat in one typical pork sausage (7 grams) is almost five times the amount in one hen's egg (around 1.5 grams).

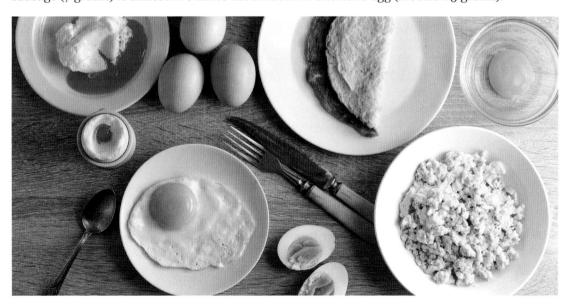

WATER

Let's not mince words when it comes to water. It's vital to your well-being. Maintaining adequate hydration levels from within helps in countless ways:

- Assists in the building of healthy collagen in the skin and in joints, improving skin health and joint functioning.

- Improves brain functioning; reduces confusion, improves concentration.

- Prevents the symptoms of dehydration: thirst, fatigue, lethargy and headaches.

That's just for starters. So, you definitely need to drink enough water. But how much is enough? Too much water intake can, in some circumstances, be dangerous.[137]

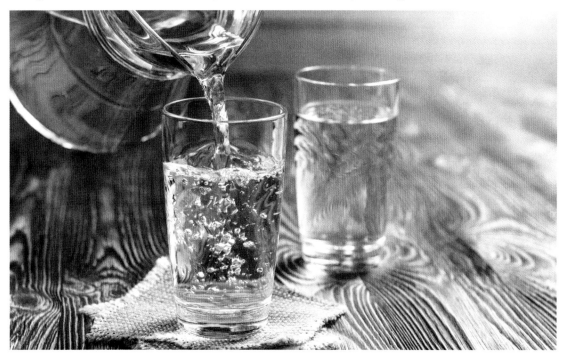

For years, the prevailing consensus has been to consume at least eight 8-ounce glasses of water a day. That amounts to 64 ounces or nearly 2 liters each day.[138] Recent research-based advice from the Institute of Medicine of the National Academies suggests an overall intake of 2.7 liters for women and 3.7 liters for men,[139] but that figure includes water extracted from food (especially fruit and vegetables), which typically amounts to around 20 percent of water intake. Adjusting the IoM recommendations accordingly puts their suggested daily fluid intake at around 2.2 liters for women and 3.0 liters for men—more than the traditional eight 8-ounce glasses but not far away.

For the purposes of the *Age Later* program, I suggest that adults should consume between 2 and 3 liters daily (depending on weight and level of activity), spread evenly through the day among at least six to eight drinks.

These figures are for guidance only. Adjustments can be made based on your individual needs. If you live and work in a hot and dry climate, you'll need more fluids than if you live and work in a cold, damp climate. Those who eat more leafy vegetables derive more fluids for their bodies than those who eat more dried fruits and nuts. Larger people need more water than smaller people.

The more you exercise, the more fluids you need to replace perspiration, however, not everyone sweats the same amount. If you engage in moderate or vigorous physical activity (which you really should), add an extra half-liter per session and replenish your fluids both during and after your exercise.

Your body processes fluids at a modest rate. Some people process faster than others. Try to balance your input with your output—and spread your intake across the day. A healthy average person can process no more than 1 liter every 60 minutes, so consuming more than that per hour, over say two or three hours, can be dangerous. At the very least, it will be uncomfortable.

Extended periods of hard activity (marathons, Ironman events, working in the midday sun) bring a special need to balance fluids and electrolytes.[140] Overconsumption of fluids in such situations can depress sodium levels, which stresses the heart.

Tea, coffee, sparkling water, milk or milk substitutes, soups, protein shakes, smoothies and so on count toward your daily quota, so it's not hard to reach your target every day. Most healthy people manage to consume enough liquids simply by drinking a glass of water whenever they get thirsty, but it's better for you to be proactive—and to have a routine that ensures you hit your target comfortably. If you become thirsty, you're already slightly dehydrated.

If, despite regularly consuming the recommended amount of liquids, you still experience severe thirst every day, consult your doctor. He or she probably will check you for hyperglycemia or other possible problems.

Warning: Don't count liquid from beer and other alcoholic drinks toward your total. Alcohol causes some dehydration as it passes through your body. Also, don't count sweetened sodas and other drinks that contain refined sugar and/or artificial sweeteners.

MODERATE YOUR INTAKE

STARCHY VEGETABLES

All vegetables are good. They all contain useful amounts of plant proteins, antioxidants and fiber. Starchy vegetables contain a higher-than-usual amount of carbohydrates, but most of them also provide the same useful nutrients. Some diets ban starchy vegetables because of their apparently high carbohydrate count.

Starchy fruits and vegetables come from various families of vegetables and include:

- Potatoes

- Yams and sweet potatoes

- Beets

- Beans, peas, corn

- Parsnips

- Pumpkin, squash

- Bananas and plantains

My opinion is that diets that refuse to accommodate these foods are probably being over-cautious. Much of the starch in starchy vegetables is in the form of "resistant starch" (or soluble fibers), which the human digestive system finds difficult to convert immediately to energy. The effective carb contribution is subsequently much lower than you might expect.

It's true that some of these foods also contain starch that is useful for energy—as well as, in some cases, sugars. Still, the energy-producing component of such foods is low compared to, say, white bread. Plus, the starches and sugars are in fairly complex forms, which resists the tendency to rapidly spike glucose levels.

For people of normal weight and health, a banana a day is a good idea. However, since most of us already get too much of our energy needs from carbs, and not enough from fats, my inclination is to be more moderate with starchy vegetables, limiting them to four or five servings total, spread out over a week.

Flour Products

Refined white flour is off-limits, but what about wholemeal flour? Flour that contains the wheat germ contains more fiber—along with nutrients that are not present in white flour. Bread and other products made from wholemeal flour are still relatively high in carbohydrates, but the fiber content helps to protect against rapid production of glucose in the blood. When wholemeal bread is eaten as part of a meal that includes vegetables and fats, it's even less likely to disrupt glucose levels.

I like to see people eating more plant-based oils, which provide a lot of energy. If you increase the vegetable fats you consume, you should reduce the energy you obtain from carbs. This is the main reason that I recommend moderation as far as eating bread, even wholemeal bread, which is relatively high in starchy carbs. I suggest no more than one serving per day.

Eating your daily bread is still OK—providing it's real whole grain bread.

To Meat (Or Not To Meat)?

Many humans are perfectly content with a diet that doesn't include meat. Others view it as an evolutionary staple, dating back to the caveman. They crave it when they've gone a few days without it. This craving, along with cravings for sweets and starchy foods is a product of training—and this training can, with a little effort, be reversed.

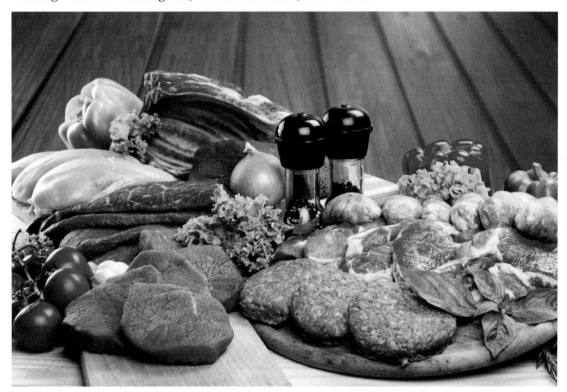

Eating meat, for me, is an ethical question. I choose not to for a variety of reasons, not the least of which is the suffering the animals endure. I'm also bothered by the impact of mass meat production on our environment, the dismal farming conditions involved, and the abundance of resources exhausted for livestock farming. There are lots of good reasons for not eating meat, and few for eating it.

There are no good reasons for eating meat every day, but many people do so without thinking twice about their selections. When you opt for a healthy salad for lunch, do you automatically ask for slices of chicken on top? Do you automatically associate breakfast with bacon and sausage? How about pepperoni on your pizza? Are you someone who believes that dinner is not dinner unless it contains a chunk of chicken, steak, pork or beef?

If you think about it, the unthinking eating of meat is just a habit, a habit that isn't good for you. And one that can be broken.

Our distant ancestors were hunter-gatherers and had to work hard for their meat, so the supply of meat was irregular. Humans survived in between on moderate meat intake (or none)—and lots of plants, like leafy vegetables, root vegetables, fruits, nuts and seeds. Maybe they added some grains, beans, fish, shellfish or insects, depending on what was available in their environment. Above all, our distant ancestors didn't eat as much as modern humans do.

The introduction of farming brought a change in the balance, with an increase in the consumption of grains and beans, because these were available in greater quantity once people learned how to farm them. The same applied to meat, which farming eventually made readily available for just about any meal. The introduction of domesticated animals on farms made meat an everyday product.

Today, many humans in developed countries regularly include meat and meat products as part of their diet. It's easily accessible in ways our ancestors never could have imagined—but it's not healthy, especially in large quantities.

We know that saturated fats raise bad cholesterol levels and are linked to diabetes and cardiovascular diseases. With that in mind, my recommendation is to cut out meat completely, or greatly reduce it. Animal fats, in general, are unnecessary and not good for us. If you must eat animal meat—beef, pork, lamb, poultry—try and change the narrative. Consider meat as a special treat, or even as a condiment, used in small quantities to add more interest to a dish.

I mentioned earlier that raw meat is high in AGEs, but cooked meat has even more. Generally speaking, we tend to prefer meat that is cooked at high temperatures (like a char-grilled rib-eye) or that's heavily processed (salami, pepperoni, bacon). Both varieties deliver large quantities of AGEs to our systems, which, as I pointed out earlier, is bad news for your skin or your body cells.

And then, there are fats. Not all fats are bad, and animal fats may not be as bad as we once thought. Nevertheless, they're not all good. Once again, if abstinence doesn't appeal, moderation is appropriate.

When you cut back on meat, or eliminate it, you'll need to compensate for the absence of substances that meat-eating delivers. Meat and fish provide human beings with a convenient package of materials needed to build our bodies: creatine, necessary for muscle development; gelatin, useful for collagen production; and proteins, vitamins and minerals.

We can derive a similar combination of proteins and amino acids—sans meat or fish[141]—by eating a healthy mix of nuts, seeds, beans and grains. That said, in the absence of meat, vegetarians should understand the importance of using multiple vegetable protein sources to ensure their diet includes the required amino acids.

Creatine, an amino acid, plays an important role in storing energy and delivering it to the muscles when needed. Fish can contain more creatine than steak, so fish is a solid alternative. However, the human body can build its own creatine from a diet that contains a rich variety of plant foods. So animal products, while convenient, are not required for creatine content.

If you're a professional athlete, or if you've suffered muscle atrophy for any reason, building muscle bulk and power from vegetables alone will be a challenge. See the notes on creatine in Appendix B, or in the list of amino acids at agelaterbook.com.

Gelatin is another component of meat and fish. It's also a transformed version of collagen; when it arrives in the body, gelatin is converted back to collagen. We need collagen in our skin, tendons, ligaments and bones, and gelatin has long been a primary source of collagen replenishment in our diets (for example, in the form of the meat-based broths and soups on which our ancestors relied). The amino acids needed to do the same job as gelatin occur in plants—but not in a single convenient source. That's yet another reason to include a broad mix of plant foods in your diet. Plant sources of various amino acids include seeds, grains, fruit, beans, avocados and green vegetables. I suggest you eat them all.

Meat and fish also are a ready source of nutrients, including some that aren't easily found in plant-based foods. Specifically, nand lysine are not common in plant-based foods; eat seaweed for iodine and walnuts for lysine.

Other nutrients found in meat are much easier to find in plants. For zinc, eat oatmeal, cashews, almonds, kidney beans and chickpeas; for iron, look to green leafy vegetables, beans, lentils, nuts and seeds.

Vitamin B12 is naturally available only from animal-based products (meat and dairy); it's not present in plant foods. We do have stomach bacteria that synthesize B12, and that provides a basic source of the vitamin to our systems. Our ancestors probably obtained their full quota of B12, and other B vitamins, from animal-based foods. Today, to reach the levels of B12 we need, we must eat meat or use supplements.

My recommendation: Don't eat meat or poultry. If you do, limit it to once every three months. For people who eat no meat, supplementation is even more important than for omnivores.

Omnivores who eat mostly fruit and vegetables with just small amounts of animal foods will come close to deriving sufficient amounts of all nutrients, but even they will benefit from taking some nutrient supplements. Vegetarians who consume dairy will be in a similar position, but may need more supplements. Vegans need to be well-informed about foods and nutrients—and manage their intake accordingly, with definite nutritional assistance from supplements.

As noted in the section on Supplements, I believe that everyone should take certain supplements daily. Vegans, vegetarians and omnivores all need supplements to truly thrive in this modern world.

Avoid These Foods!

There are some foods that have absolutely no redeeming nutritional value—but plenty of downside. Eating these foods becomes habit-forming; your digestive system desires them, anticipates the payoff and signals that to your brain. It's not uncommon, as you attempt to scale back on these substances, for your body to try to lure you into a bad-habit relapse.

There is no avoiding this period of withdrawal. In the meantime, increase your intake of healthy foods as you're cutting back on harmful foods. As your body (that is, your brain and your stomach microbiome) adjusts to the changes, you'll gradually begin to prefer the healthy alternatives. So, hang tough. If you persevere, you'll reach a point where the damaging foods actually lose their appeal.

This section contains information about foods that you should eliminate from your food plan. Every one of these substances is closely associated with accelerating the aging process and causing or contributing to life-threatening illnesses.

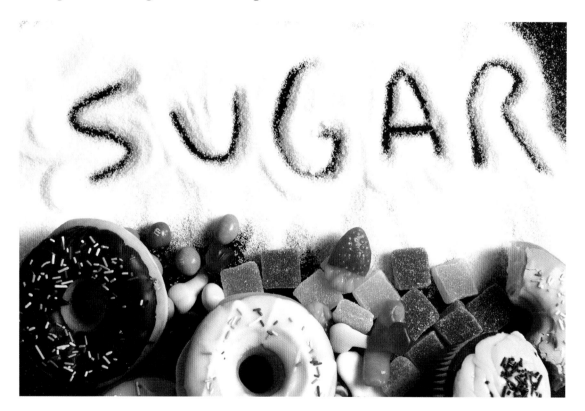

Eliminate Refined Sugar

Refined sugar makes people overweight and increases the risk of diabetes, cardiovascular disease and more. Humans need carbohydrates, including some sugar, but refined sugar is not the way to obtain them. It's an easy form of energy for the body. Too easy. It's processed quickly and causes blood-sugar spikes that our bodies don't handle well.

Spikes in blood sugar result in overproduction of AGEs, trigger inflammation and the mass-production of free radicals, and dump any short-term energy surpluses into fat.

Your body can handle modest amounts of sugar when it appears in a more complex form and is mixed with lots of fiber and other nutrients—like an apple. But refined sugar is a different animal. Maybe you can handle a small amount every day, but why risk it?

The safest path, and the healthiest path, is to remove refined sugar from your food plan. You don't need it. The natural sugars in fruits and vegetables should give you all the energy you need, and they provide it to you in a way that your body can handle.

You'll be surprised at how quickly you can adjust to food and drinks that aren't sweet. Before long, you'll find that you prefer the taste of non-sweet substances. There are countless food options that don't contain added sugar, so choose them instead.

Another suggestion: Start reading the labels of pre-packaged, manufactured foods. Heavily processed foods (ready meals, commercial sauces, spreads, breakfast cereals and canned vegetables) can contain absurd amounts of added sugar. Even some foods labeled "healthy"—flavored yogurt, fruit drinks, protein bars, bottled smoothies and low-fat processed foods—may contain significant amounts of added sugar. Avoid goods containing added ingredients like fructose, corn syrup, dextrose, sucrose or glucose.

As for candy, most of it is just sugar. That said, it is possible to buy chocolate that contains zero refined sugar, no artificial sweeteners and a high cocoa fat content. Since chocolate contains antioxidants and good fats, a morsel of that kind of chocolate every now and again won't hurt.

On the beverage front, eliminate all sugary drinks (like commercial sodas) and any drinks that taste sweet. Also, don't add sugar to tea or coffee. As mentioned in an earlier chapter, sweet cocktails deal your system a double blow—alcohol plus excess sugar.

If you need to snack between meals, avoid cookies, cakes and candies. Raw carrots or celery sticks work just fine.

It's not that refined or partly refined sugar is new to the scene; the production of sugar granules from sugarcane in India dates back more than 2,000 years. But our distant ancestors obtained nearly all their energy from the natural sugars in fruit and vegetables. The same can't be said today.

In early 18th-century Britain, a rich country at that time, refined sugar consumption was a mere 5 grams per person per day (around 4 pounds per year)—and that was an increase over the previous century.[142]

In the United States, use of refined sugar peaked at 100 grams per person per day in 1999.

Consumption dropped to 75 grams per day in 2008[143]—but that's still around 60 pounds per person per year, which is way too much. Refined sugar has become a basic industrial commodity, not a luxury.

Human beings in developed countries, for several generations now, have been trained since childhood to expect sweetness in their foods. Yet the human body can survive and flourish with no refined sugar at all. Every gram of refined sugar above zero is unnecessary—and today's average consumption levels are decidedly harmful.

AVOID WHITE FLOUR

Refined flour that's low in fiber is another relatively modern invention, and, like refined sugar, it's bad for us—and for similar reasons. Easily assimilated carbs make it too easy for the body to create AGEs and spread inflammation. When refined white flour was a luxury item, people consumed it in small quantities and on special occasions. Now, it dominates the baked goods market. Once again, this is an unnecessary product and, in excess, a harmful one.

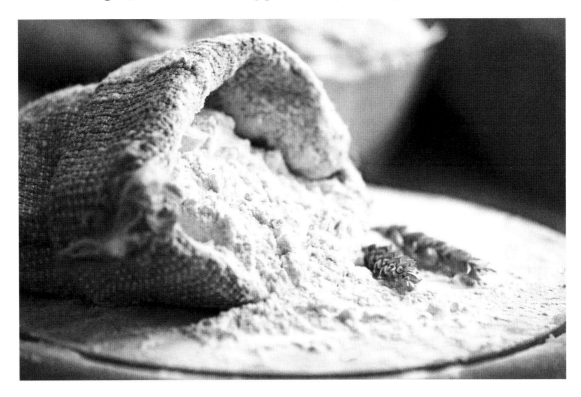

Our ancestors did not have access to flour in huge quantities; it was labor-intensive and expensive to produce. The technology to make white flour for the masses is relatively new.

All flour used to be wholemeal flour. Industrialization of agriculture meant that flour had to be transported over greater distances and stored for a longer time. Wholemeal flour that contains the wheat germ does not stay fresh for long. To extend the shelf life of flour, millers removed the wheat germ, the most nutritious part of the grain, as well as the husk (which contains fiber and nutrients). The result was white flour.

Modern white flour contains less protein and nutrients than wholemeal flour. White flour also is processed with a succession of chemicals that modify the color via bleaching, reduce the gluten content (for cakes and pastries), increase the gluten content (for bread) and extend the shelf life even further (through preservatives).

So, please, don't eat white bread, pastries, white flour bagels, cakes and similar goods. Most desserts should be off your list too.

Wholemeal flour, providing it is genuine wholemeal flour, is a different matter. The entire outer husk is included, with all its nutrients. That means more protein, more fiber, and a range of B vitamins (B1, B2, B3, B6). Wholemeal flour is mostly made from whole-wheat grains, but flour made from or including other whole grains also is nutritious (think barley, buckwheat and quinoa). Wholemeal flour that contains some entire grains or seeds is even better because it provides more healthy fats and minerals.

Many breads that appear at first to be whole-grain products may contain a mixture of flours— with whole grain only a fraction of the overall recipe. When you buy whole-grain bread, read the label. The word "whole" must appear consistently. If more than one type of flour is listed, each one should be described as whole-grain flour. Flours described as enriched, stone-ground, un-bleached and multigrain are often white flours. Those marketing words are intended to mislead you into thinking the bread is healthier than it really is.

Wholemeal flour certainly is far more nutritious than white-bleached flour, but it is still flour. The milling process makes the carbs more easily accessible, which raises the glycemic index, so some moderation is required.

In summary, remove these from your shopping list: white bread, white flour bagels and muffins (and similar products), cakes, cupcakes, pastries, supermarket pizzas, white-flour pasta and white flour.

Eat only 100-percent wholemeal flour products—and only then in moderate quantities.

DESSERTS: CHOOSE CAREFULLY

Do you have to think about it when the waiter asks, "Did you leave room for dessert?" You shouldn't. The answer, in most cases, should be no. I've already mentioned the dangers of refined sugars and refined flour products. Desserts can pose a double problem when both substances are present.

Many desserts on restaurant menus contain more calories than your entree. Typically, you're pretty full by the time the dessert question is posed. So why multiply the evening's calorie count by two when your stomach already is waving the white flag?

Being tempted into devouring a sweet dessert is a sure way of sabotaging your 80 percent eating discipline (see the section Changing The Way You Eat). Also, chances are high that you already have the energy needed for the rest of the day from your main course. Throw in extra sugar and flour, and it quickly will become fat in your body.

How about having dessert on a special occasion? Or as a reward? Don't include desserts in your reward system as part of the *Age Later* program. Your brain, your palate and your stomach all need to be trained to reject the sweet excess that makes refined sugar so attractive. If you need another reason to just say no, how about this: Daily desserts can lead to obesity, stroke and heart attack. In short, they can kill you.

If you really do have room for dessert, and desire something sweet, opt for simple fresh fruits and berries.

ARTIFICIAL SWEETENERS

Artificial sweeteners are fool's gold. They encourage your body's cravings for sweet foods and drinks, and some may even be harmful. Plus, there's no real evidence to suggest they help people lose weight.[144]

Modern marketing has convinced people that hyper-sweetness is acceptable. It's not. In addition to inflating your cravings, artificial sweeteners may affect the balance of your stomach microbiome.[145] Many of them don't taste very good either. When sprinkled on naturally sweet foods—like apples, bananas and berries—an artificial sweetener might undermine your enjoyment. It's possible that association will encourage you to bypass a once-favorite fruit in favor of a more damaging food. Artificial sweeteners are just not a good deal.[146]

You can find them in just about any product with the word "diet" on the label. They're in sodas, yogurts, desserts, cakes, some canned foods, and in lots of processed foods—including products specially designed for diabetics. Artificial sweeteners even show up in some wellness drinks, energy drinks and protein bars. No one, including diabetics, need artificial sweeteners— so be careful and read the labels.

It's much better to cultivate a taste for unsweetened products or naturally sweet fruits and vege-tables, like fresh blueberries or carrots. Still, that's easier said than done. Part of the reason it's a challenge to leave sweeteners behind is because they can change your sense of taste—a change you may not even realize has happened. But stay the course. Soon you'll be able to enjoy the real taste of food that's actually good for you.

FOOD COOKED AT HIGH TEMPERATURES

A number of foods contain compounds called glycotoxins, or advanced glycation end products (AGEs). Excessive intake of AGEs can contribute to inflammation and its related problems, including heart disease and diabetes. Many foods naturally contain AGEs at a low level. It isn't practical to avoid these substances completely, and in a balanced diet there's no need to do so as long as you keep AGEs at a level your body can comfortably handle.

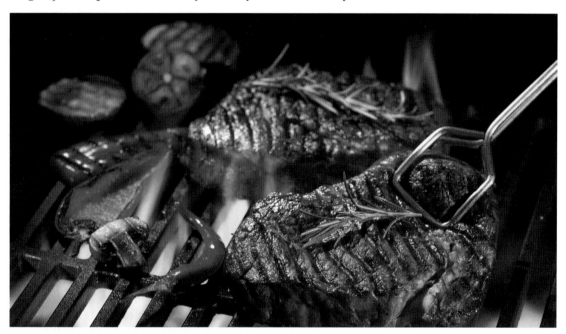

High-temperature cooking can dramatically increase the levels of AGEs in any food. Avoid foods that have been aggressively grilled, broiled, fried, roasted or seared. Anything that ends up with those black or dark-brown crunchy bits on it is bad news. Frying, by the way, brings additional dangers: industrial trans fats. Processed cooking oils and fats are likely to contain trans fats, and the high temperatures increase the level of trans fats—yet another reason to avoid all fried foods.

Cooking meat at a high temperature with no moisture will multiply the amount of AGEs by a factor of 10 to 100.[147] High-temperature cooking of meats also produces other chemicals, such as heterocyclic amines (HCAs) and polycyclic aromatic hydrocarbons (PAHs).[148] In high doses, these chemicals have been shown to have a carcinogenic effect in animals. Most preserved meats, such as bacon and sausage, contain nitrites[149]; the combination of nitrites, proteins and high heat results in the formation of nitrosamines, which also are known to be carcinogenic.

Cheese can be high in AGEs too, and it gets worse with grilling. All of this helps to explain why a cheeseburger with fries is not your best friend.

Fresh vegetables, grains, beans, lentils and milk are all naturally low in AGE products, but once again, their AGE content can increase if you punish them with frying or grilling.

Your best cooking choices are steaming and poaching. Sous vide is fine too. Gentle sautéing (no brown charring) is acceptable. Also, marinates that incorporate lemon or vinegar before cooking can reduce AGEs.

Whether you are cooking at home or dining out, choose food that has been prepared with added moisture and without intense heat. Don't automatically order fried or grilled dishes. Before humans invented temperature-controlled burners for cooking, we set fire to wood and let the resulting flames do the rest. We still eat too much food that relies on searing heat instead of gentle simmering. Try to change the balance. Broaden your palate with dishes that don't require cooking at high temperatures and see if you don't notice—and enjoy—the difference.

Avoid Processed Foods

Processed and packaged foods, especially meats, are much higher in AGEs than the original foods from which they are produced. That's because they are often processed at high temperatures and designed for long-term storage. High-temperature cooking and long-term storage both add AGEs to the AGEs already in the original foods. Highly processed food includes the usual suspects (like snacks, breakfast cereals and soft drinks) as well as any pre-made, packaged (frozen, canned, microwavable) goods from the supermarket.

Processed vegetable oil is higher in AGEs than the plant seeds from which it's made, thanks to the processing. That's why you should always use cold-pressed oils, not the aggressively processed products.

High-temperature processing is not the only thing wrong with many processed foods. Look out for, and avoid, excessive sodium, dubious chemical preservatives, refined sugar, refined starches, artificial sweeteners and containers that use BPA.[150]

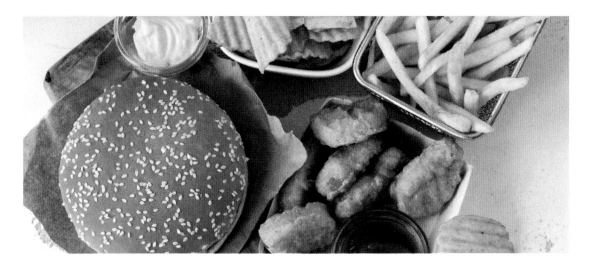

Then, there are trans fats. Margarine and vegetable shortening, and anything containing partially hydrogenated vegetable oil, contain industrial trans fats. Many vegetable oils contain some trans fats, unless they have been obtained by a cold-press process. As always, read the labels. Until recently, cakes, cookies and anything fried contained significant amounts of trans fats—and many still contain small quantities.

While the U.S. is on course to eventually ban trans fats in all commercial foods, there is still plenty of it around. No matter what happens at the legislative level, it's possible to restrict your intake. To avoid most of the industrial trans fats in packaged food—just avoid packaged food. If you find it necessary to buy packaged food, avoid anything that has "partially hydrogenated vegetable oil" on the label, even if the label also indicates zero trans fats.[151] Also, as mentioned before, avoid all fried foods.

Junk Food

No need to mince words when it comes to the snacks so many people find irresistible: Almost every product that one would categorize as junk food is bad for you. That's because junk food contains most, if not all, of the dangerous substances we've already discussed—from refined sugar and white flour to artificial sweeteners, AGEs and industrial trans fats. Naturally, they're also highly processed.

Most of the items that fall into this category go without saying—but are a few examples for the record:

• Fried fast food

• Sodas

• Chips, pretzels and similar snacks

• Pre-packaged, pre-cooked meals

• Burgers, hot dogs and just about all food and drink sold in a sports stadium

Healthy Choices: Changing The Way You Eat

A Permanent Transformation of Your Eating Habits

It's time to change not only what you eat—but the way you eat. Eating the right food is not about dieting. It's about changing, permanently, your relationship with food. If you want to be healthy for the rest of your life, you need to adopt healthy eating habits now and sustain those new habits forever. Achieving this, like so many other aspects of living a healthy and longer life, means forming new habits—good habits—and saying goodbye to bad habits.

To be clear, I don't classify this approach to food as a diet. Many people associate the word "diet" with a short-term effort, one accompanied by inconvenience and even suffering. Changing your eating habits is not a short-term fix. Also, there's no need to suffer: Trust me, you're going to enjoy your new eating regimen.

Along the way, you will train both your mental subconscious and your digestive system to crave and look forward to healthy foods—and to become less stimulated by the thought of eating food that is bad for you.

Calorie counting, keeping records and setting targets are not really necessary, but for some people they help with motivation, with accelerating the process of acquiring new habits, and with building the self-discipline to stick to your new habits. Once you've counted and measured for just a week or so, you will start to acquire a good sense of the quantities that are appropriate. What's more, if you exclusively stick to the recommended foods, quantities and methods, you are unlikely to overeat. This way of eating healthy food is designed to be largely self-regulating.

FORMING NEW EATING HABITS

Just as your brain has a mind of its own (the subconscious), your digestive system has something similar (neurons in your stomach, plus your personal microbiome). Your conscious mind is challenged to educate your subconscious, your gut and your microbial flora, all at the same time.

The colony of microbes in your stomach is a living entity that has evolved to look after itself, first and foremost. As a secondary thought, it will look after you—because if the colony keeps you happy, then the colony will be happy. The problem is, sometimes what the colony wants and what you need may not be aligned. For example, if your gut is overpopulated by microbes that love sugar, the colony will release chemicals that urge you to eat more sugar.

If you defy those microbes and eat less sugar, they will be unhappy for a few days, which may leave you unhappy. But stay true to your new habit for just a week or so, and the balance of microbes in your stomach will change. Microbes that prefer a less sugary environment will start to flourish; your craving for sugar will diminish as your microbe population evolves.

Similarly, if you increase your intake of fibrous plants, you may experience some discomfort for a few days. But those fiber-loving bacteria are lurking there somewhere, and as you feed them more fiber, more of them will be produced. As the fiber-loving population increases, you will grow to appreciate fiber all the more.

You need to train your microbiome to serve your interest. If your gut is dominated by sugar-loving microbes, then you will eat sugar and risk suffering cardiovascular and neurological diseases. But you're smarter than the microbes in your stomach. They will do your bidding if you stick to the program. If you repopulate your gut with fiber-loving microbes, your stomach health will improve and your susceptibility to diseases will decrease.

This part of the *Age Later* program doesn't even require seven weeks. Adhere to your new eating habits for just two or three weeks, and your brain, digestive system and microbiome will be fully reprogrammed.

It's the springboard for a new relationship with food. You'll change the way you shop at the supermarket, the way you order off a menu, the way you snack in between meals. You will know what foods and preparation methods to select, and which ones to reject. What's more, you will enjoy your choices.

NO ROOM FOR TREATS?

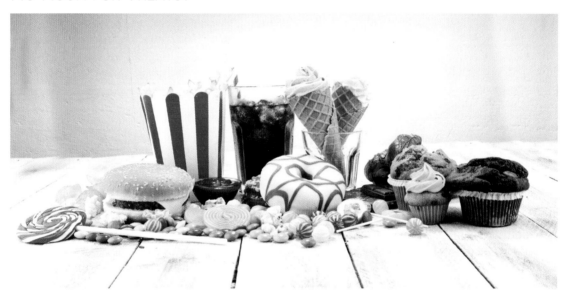

Perhaps you're wilting at the thought of giving up one of your favorite tasty foods. No more broiled steaks? No more Stilton cheese? No salami? No bacon sandwiches? Not even roasted potatoes? For much of the developed world, these items are regarded as normal, everyday foods. But in the quantities too many people consume, these foods also are harmful. Still, some of you might wonder whether it's necessary to cut them out entirely. What about an occasional treat?

Here's my take on treats: We need to redefine the line between foods that we eat as part of our basic diet and those that we eat mostly for pleasure. Fifty years ago, chicken was a special-occasion food. Today, fried chicken is an inexpensive and common meal. At one time, going out for a steak was a big deal for people. Now, there are traditional steakhouses, fine-dining establishments, casual restaurants, chain restaurants and sports bars that serve steaks.

Industrialization has served us well in many ways. On the plus side, it has made food more affordable so that fewer people go hungry (at least in the U.S.). But the ability of people to discriminate has been blurred: We can get high-energy foods with little effort; restaurants offer huge portions of food, and people either devour it all or take some home in a doggy bag. Foods that we'd be better off not eating at all (or in small quantities) have become everyday staples. There's something very wrong here.

Treats used to be treats for a reason. We didn't have easy access to them. And, in some cases, they were expensive. But just because they're cheaper and accessible today doesn't mean we can't change the way we view them. Cakes, pies and ice cream may not be expensive in terms of dollars, but they can be expensive in terms of our health. They can shorten our lives if we turn them into staples of our daily diet.

So, bottom line: Can you have treats or not? First things first. Let's start by changing your habits. Create a food plan that includes a full menu of delicious fruits, vegetables, grains, beans and lentils. You want your body and digestive system in such good shape that it can handle an occasional treat. Perhaps then you will enjoy that slice of cake even more because it's no longer a regular part of your diet.

But don't be surprised if, like many people who turn to healthy living choices, those special treats don't seem so special anymore. You may find that your body has changed—and with it your desire for daily treats.

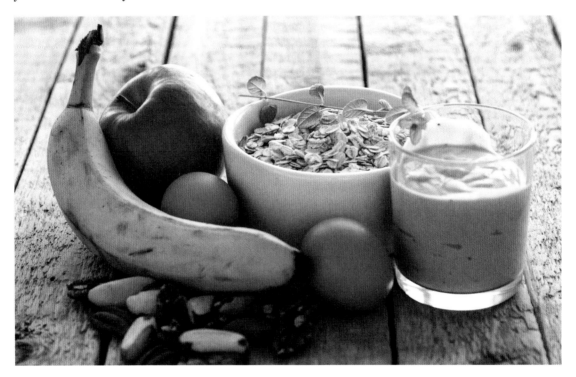

Don't Skip Breakfast

Your mother, or maybe your grandmother, probably told you, over and over, that breakfast is the most important meal, and you should never skip it. They were right. People who eat a healthy breakfast are more alert during the day, more productive and generally better able to manage their weight.

Breakfast wakes up your digestive system and increases your metabolic rate. A higher metabolic rate ensures that you have the energy to be active; in so doing, you convert carbs to energy (instead of to fat) and when you run out of carbs, you start to burn fat. Without breakfast, your metabolism stays low and you're less active, so you naturally need less energy.

If you don't have breakfast, you'll be so famished by lunchtime that you'll probably eat more than you should. Not only does that leave you with a sluggish after-lunch feeling, you'll probably gain weight. A breakfast that contains a small amount of carbs and is high in protein buffers that sense of hunger, so you can eat a moderate lunch and keep going during the afternoon.

What is a healthy breakfast? It needs to include protein, carbs and fiber, which can come from some combination of whole grains, fresh fruit and vegetables, beans, lentils, eggs, egg whites or dairy. Those products all include some carbs, to provide energy for the day, as well as fiber.

Here are a few examples of healthy breakfast choices as part of the *Age Later* program. Of course, I always recommend organic food, whenever possible, but nonorganic is okay, too.

- Protein shake made from vegetables and fruit, like Hush & Hush's PlantYourDay (hushandhush.com)

- Red and green vegetable juice (fresh-pressed) containing red beet, kale, celery, apple, orange and ginger

- Whole-grain muesli with fresh and dried fruit, nuts, seeds and plain unsweetened live yogurt

- Cooked steel-cut oatmeal with fresh fruit, nuts, seeds and plain unsweetened live yogurt

- Scrambled egg whites, tomato, whole-grain bread

- Avocado (half) on whole-grain bread, with olive oil, sesame seeds, spices, plus some fresh fruit

For more breakfast ideas, visit agelaterbook.com.

ABOVE ALL, EAT LESS

Changing the way you eat is first and foremost about eating less food, which studies throughout the world have shown to be healthier than eating too much. Overeating is linked to higher risk for cancer, cardiovascular disease, diabetes and (of course) obesity. Even if you are comfortable with your weight, your health can benefit from a more disciplined approach to eating so that you never overindulge.

You might reasonably ask, how much is too much? Your body will tell you, if you pay attention.

Unfortunately, many of us don't pay attention.

We all recognize that feeling of satiety when we've had enough (or too much). The problem is that we reach the point of being full before that feeling of satiety tells us to stop. This is because your stomach is a bit slow to signal when you're really full enough.

By training ourselves to eat less—and by becoming more in tune with how our body works—we won't need flashing red lights to tell us to put down the fork.

THE 80 PERCENT RULE

It's said that the ideal point to stop eating is when you're around 80 percent full. In Japan, they call this approach Hara Hachi Bu,[152] and they practice it widely. I call it the 80 percent rule, although there's really no magic in that figure. To put it another way, just stop eating before you're full. Millions of people in Japan and around the world eat this way, so there's no reason why you can't do it too.

Learning to judge when you are almost full does take some practice. When you've consumed enough to curb your hunger, but not enough to feel completely full, stop. And then wait 20 minutes. If you feel hungry again, then you stopped too early. If your stomach still feels beyond full after a 20-minute wait, you probably kept eating too long. If you feel satisfied, neither hungry nor stuffed, then you got it about right. You'll soon get the idea, and the 80 percent rule will become yet another good habit.

Applying the 80 percent rule means that the amount of food on the plate in front of you is irrelevant. It's about eating an amount that's right for you at that time, not the amount that someone else has decided you should have. Be prepared to ask for to-go boxes at restaurants. Doesn't it feel good to be in control?

RAW FOOD OR COOKED FOOD?

My healthy living choice recommendations include eating both cooked and uncooked food, every day.

Salads and fresh fruit provide their full quota of vitamins and other heat-sensitive nutrients in the uncooked state. Raw fruits and vegetables contain a range of antioxidants and enzymes, and other good things, along with digestible and indigestible fiber that is good for your beneficial stomach bacteria.

You can enjoy tomatoes in salads and in cooked dishes too; don't worry about which is better, because they both have benefits. An uncooked tomato contains more vitamin C than the same tomato cooked. But a cooked tomato provides more accessible lycopene.[153] Try slicing some fresh tomatoes into your cooked pasta sauce just before serving.

Cooking improves the digestibility or many foods, including meat, and reduces the energy and time needed for the body to extract nutrients and amino acids. But that only helps if the nutrients are not sensitive to heat. Your stomach has to work overtime to process certain raw foods (for example, grains, red meat, beans, potatoes and eggplant). Some undercooked foods can cause digestive problems because of the presence of lectins (see Appendix F). The energy used to digest a chunk of raw meat amounts to around a third of the energy available from the meat itself. Anthropologists speculate that one of the reasons humans have bigger brains than other primates is because humans learned to cook. Cooking kills potentially damaging bacteria and viruses in products that are susceptible to infection.

On the other hand, overcooking fruit and leafy vegetables can reduce the level of nutrients significantly.

Set a goal of consuming a mix of cooked food, and raw fruit and vegetables, every day. Fruit for breakfast and dessert is a good start. Salads are good, but try not to limit yourself to simple green salads. Aim for a mix of different colored greens (generally, the darker the better), and remember that adding raw vegetables, fruit, nuts and seeds make appetizers and main-course salads much more interesting.

More Tips for Controlling Food Intake

Eat slowly: Leisurely eating brings benefits—more time for intelligent conversation between mouthfuls, more opportunity to savor the food you're eating. Also, by eating at a moderate pace, you give your digestive system a chance to send an "almost full" message to your brain before it's too late, which helps you apply the 80 percent rule.

Eliminate between-meal snacks: Snacking between meals is just a bad habit for many. If you can't break the habit straight away, then aim to control it. I find nibbling celery, carrots or nuts fills the psychological need for something to munch on between meals. Between-meal snacks should obey all the rules that define your main meals—like no refined sugars, no baked goods, etc.

Build self-control at the buffet: All-you-can eat restaurants can be terrible for you, or they can be your friend, depending on your attitude. Buffet eating has a bad reputation, and justifiably so. But you also can choose exactly what to eat—and how much—at a buffet. Yes, I know, look at the guy with a mountain of fried shrimp, fried chicken tenders and french fries on his plate. But that's not you: You're going to follow the *Age Later* guidelines, make the healthiest choices, and take one small helping at a time. You're going to eat slowly, and stop when you're comfortable and before you feel full.

Go upmarket: When you dine out, consider going to some expensive restaurants. (Perhaps you already eat only at fine-dining establishments; if so, this tactic won't work for you.) The idea is this: Go to a fancy restaurant, but stick to your normal dining-out budget, and order accordingly. You'll eat less food, and it probably will be more interesting and of a higher quality. You won't end up spending additional dollars—and you'll have some new foodie adventures to share with your friends.

SUPPLEMENTS

WHY WE NEED SOME SUPPLEMENTS

Everyone needs to take some food supplements. Even if you follow the *Age Later* food plan, I still recommend supplementation. There are several reasons. First, based on my experience, I estimate that around 90 percent of people in the U.S. are deficient in one or more essential nutrients. This is often because their food intake is poor, with too much junk food and not enough fresh fruit and vegetables—but there are other factors.

A lot of commercially available vegetables are not as nutritious as they used to be; their content of natural minerals and vitamins is lower than it was in the past due to soil depletion (caused by over-intensive farming practices) or by long-term storage.[154] Also, many people just lead busy lives that interfere with their eating habits, force them to skip meals, or eat less nutritious meals. Some people don't have access to a wide range of healthy foods and have to make do with what they can purchase locally. Other people, for whatever reasons, eat restaurant meals every day, or snack on the go, so they have no real way of knowing for certain that those meals are delivering adequate nutrition. And some people are not as good at absorbing vitamins and minerals as others.

The *Age Later* program does not aim merely for average health: We need to raise the bar and achieve an optimum level of health. For most people today, regular food intake is not sufficient to achieve that.

For all those reasons, taking daily supplements makes sense for everyone. I believe that we can all do better by giving our bodies additional amounts of important nutrients. The most efficient way to do that is by consuming carefully selected supplements. If you have your blood checked regularly, you will be in a much better position to identify where you're falling short in the nutrient department, and where you're doing fine.

MY PERSONAL LIST OF DAILY SUPPLEMENTS

This is my list of recommended daily supplements, with suggested amounts for adults. Those quantities will give your system a boost without reaching levels that might be wasteful, counter-productive, or dangerous.

Supplement	Typical Adult Dose	Notes
Calcium	1000-1200 mg/day	Take vitamin D3 at the same time
Ginseng	100-400 mg/day	Asian ginseng is more potent than American versions
Magnesium	400 mg/day	It's important not to take too high of a dose, otherwise you could experience an upset stomach and diarrhea

Omega-3	Three 1000 mg capsules, spaced through the day	Although omega-3 is plentiful in fish oil, flax oil and linseed oil, our scope for eating more fish is limited, these days, so take a supplement
Resveratrol	200-500 mg/day	Resveratol may interact with blood thinners and aspirin so do not mix them
Vitamin B5 (Niacin)	15 mg/day	B5 is necessary for the synthesis of coenzyme A. Vitamin B5 deficiencies are rare.
Vitamin B6 (Folic acid)	2 mg/day	Vitamin B6 is often used in tandem with other B vitamins
Vitamin B9	200 mcg/day	Especially important for women who are pregnant or likely to become pregnant
Vitamin B12	100 - 500 mcg/day in two or three separate doses	Vegans receive no vitamin B12 directly from their food, and the natural B12 provided by gut bacteria may be insufficient, so B12 supplementation is especially important for vegans
Vitamin C	One 1000 mg capsule per day	Take your vitamin C at the same time you take vitamin E, as the combination seems to be more effective than either alone
Vitamin D3	1000 IE per day	You should have your vitamin D blood level measured every year and adjust supplementation if needed: Aim for a blood level of 30mg/ml. Take vitamin D at the same time as calcium, to help calcium absorption
Vitamin E	15 mg of natural alpha-tocopherol per day	Take vitamin E along with vitamin C
Zinc	15 mg/day	Excess zinc interferes with magnesium absorption, so don't exceed the recommended dose

Everyone's needs are slightly different. You can find all of the vitamins, nutrients and minerals listed above, and then some, in Hush & Hush TimeCapsule—it's my favorite all-inclusive nutraceutical. Discuss supplementation with your health-care provider or with a nutritionist, and create your own daily formula (taking into account the quality of your regular diet and the results of blood tests).

Multi-Nutrient Supplements

Combinations of nutrients in a single package make life simpler. Here are some combinations that you might consider. Multivitamins are convenient and save time, but many don't contain sufficient nutrients to meet the *Age Later* recommended doses. So check the nutrient levels on the label and compare them with the recommendations above, and add additional supplements if necessary.

- My heart protection cocktail includes fish oil (for omega-3) with vitamin D3, B6 and B12.

- Vitamin B complex: A single tablet makes it easy to get all your B vitamins. I recommend a daily vitamin B complex supplement containing all of the B vitamins listed earlier: B1, B2, B3, B5, B6, B7, B9 and B12. Members of the vitamin B family are needed in adequate amounts for human health. Taking B6, B9 and B12 together provides an extra protection against stomach cancer.

- Calcium, magnesium, zinc and vitamin D3.

MICRONUTRIENT BLOOD TEST

Blood testing is one way to be more confident of your real needs for nutrient supplements. Regular blood tests, the kind that your family doctor might order for you, are designed to track parameters that may indicate the early presence of diseases, such as cancer and heart disease. Specialists order specific blood tests to decide the best treatments for diseases and to monitor progress. These are valuable tests, but for nutritional purposes we need the information provided by a different type of blood test.

Our aim is to avoid diseases and to reduce the impact of growing chronologically older, so I recommend a blood test that isn't typically suggested by your family doctor—but that one day soon probably will be. This new test measures levels of micronutrients in the blood and provides insights into where your intake of specific nutrients might be too low. We're not all the same: Some of us absorb nutrients more efficiently than others. We all have freedom to choose the foods we eat, and some of us make poor choices.

A micronutrient panel will allow you to identify specific nutrients that may be at unacceptably low levels in your body. With this information, you can make some informed decisions about what you eat, and what you might need to supplement. A few years ago, such blood tests may not have been reliable, but analytic methods improve all the time—and today these tests are meaningful and helpful.

A good micronutrient blood test panel will include measurements of:

- Vitamins: A (retinol), B1 (thiamin), B2 (riboflavin), B3 (niacinamide), B6 (pyridoxine), B12, C, D3, E, K2, biotin (from B7), folic acid (from B9), pantothenate (from B5)

- Minerals: calcium, chromium, copper, magnesium, manganese, zinc

- Amino acids and derivatives: asparagine, carnitine, cysteine, glutamine, glutathione, serine

- Fats, fatty acids and derivatives: alpha-lipoic acid, coenzyme Q10 (CoQ10), oleic acid

- Others: choline, CoQ10 (both sometimes classified as vitamins), inositol

- Carb metabolism: glucose, glucose-insulin interaction, fructose sensitivity

FOOD PLAN OVERVIEW

FOODS YOU SHOULD EAT EVERY DAY

Category	Examples	Frequency
Green leafy vegetables	Spinach, kale, chard, lettuce	Uncooked (in a salad) once a day, plus at least four times a week cooked

Berries	Blueberries, blackberries, red and black grapes, blackcurrants, strawberries	At least one serving per day
Nuts and seeds	Walnuts, almonds, brazil nuts, flax seeds, chia, sunflower seeds, pumpkin seeds	At least one helping of mixed seeds and nuts a day (add to morning muesli, and always include walnuts)
Onion family	Onions, garlic, shallots, chives	At least once a day
Water and unsweetened water-based drinks	Water, green tea, tea, coffee, herbal tea	Your daily target for fluids should be 1 fluid ounce per 2 pounds of body weight. For example, a person who weighs 160 pounds should aim for 80 ounces (5 U.S. pints) of fluids per day.
Olive oil	Olive oil for salads and cooking	Every day (I prefer Italian oil from Tuscany)
Fermented milk products, live	Yogurt, kefir (live, unsweetened)	Every day

Foods to Eat Often

Category	Examples	Frequency
Cabbage family	Cabbage, broccoli, cauliflower	At least four servings per week, including at least one uncooked
Whole grains	Farro, bulgur, brown rice, red rice, oats, barley	At least four servings per week
Legumes	Beans, peas, lentils	At least four servings per week
Nightshade family	Tomatoes, peppers, eggplant	At least four servings per week
Starchy vegetables	Potato, sweet potato, squash	Up to four servings per week
Whole wheat flour products	Whole wheat bread, pasta	Up to four servings per week

Foods To Eat Only in Moderation

Category	Examples	Frequency
Fish (not fried, not endangered)	Salmon, sardines, trout	One or two servings per week (more if the fish is known to be mercury-free)

Alcohol	Wine, beer, aperitifs, liquor	No more than two drinks per day if red wine with a meal is one of them. Otherwise, no more than one drink per day. No liquor; nothing stronger than wine.
Dairy	Eggs, milk, butter, non-aged cheese	No more than four servings per week

FOODS YOU SHOULD NEVER EAT, OR HARDLY EVER

Category	Examples	Frequency
Poultry	Chicken, turkey, duck, quail	Seldom; no more than once in three months
Red meat	Beef, lamb, pork	Seldom; no more than once in three months
Shellfish	Shrimp, mussels, clams, oysters, langoustine	Never. Too many heavy metals, including mercury.
Processed meat products	Sausages, bacon, salami, ham	Never
Processed oils, margarine	Canola, peanut, safflower oils	Never
Fast food	Burgers, fries, hot dogs	Never
Refined sugar products	Sodas, candy, sweetened desserts, danish pastries	Never
Refined white flour products	White bread, cakes, buns, danish pastries	Never

Chapter 8

MIND AND BRAIN

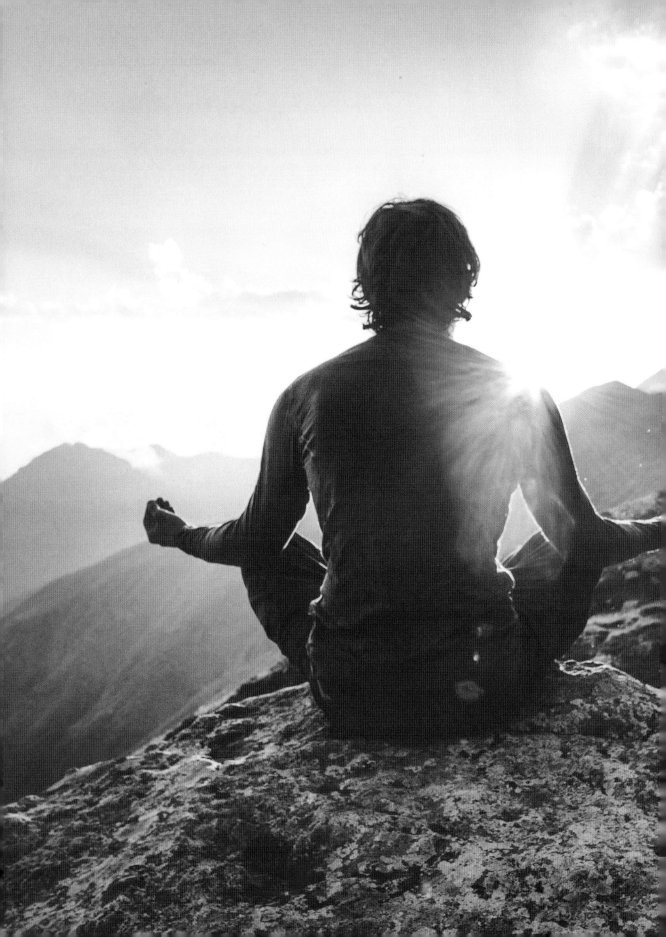

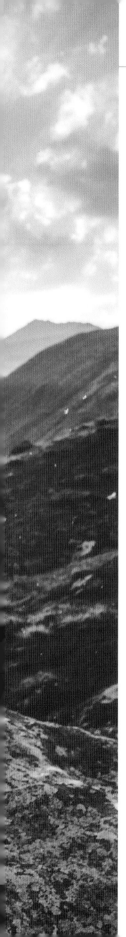

MIND AND BRAIN

The healthy living choices necessary to *Age Later* are intended to rejuvenate more than just your skin and body. It's equally important to develop routines that boost the effectiveness and overall well-being of your mind and brain.

But don't think for a second that your psychological state has nothing to do with your physical health. Your mind can affect your body. And visa versa. Indeed, the two are deeply intertwined.

Every healthy living choice I have suggested in earlier chapters can make a positive contribution to mental and neurological health. Physical exercise and good nutrition benefit brain cells just as much as they benefit other cells in the body. Certain foods, for example, can improve your mood; physical activity can alleviate stress. Exercise that engages the brain as well as the muscles provides a double benefit.

In addition to appropriate food and exercise, there's more you can do to build and maintain the health of your mind and nervous system. Those healthy choices are the focus of this chapter.

In a world that seems to grow more stressful by the day, it becomes even more important to understand and employ techniques that can manage and reduce our tension levels, tackle the negative impacts of stress, build our mental resources, and help cope with events in the world around us. This combination of fortifying our mental awareness, stability and control contributes to a state of mind I describe as Inner Peace.

INNER PEACE

Inner Peace is a positive state of mental well-being, in which a human being maintains a level of awareness that brings balanced tranquility and self-possession, even if the environment around is changing and potentially disruptive.

Inner Peace is a fundamental part of the *Age Later* program. Achieving it requires the elimination of negative factors in your life by relieving anxiety and avoiding dysfunctional behavior, while at the same time working to strengthen mental control and stability.

Inner Peace and mental health are not one and the same thing, but Inner Peace does require mental health. The World Health Organization offers this definition of mental health: "It is defined as a state of well-being in which every individual realizes his or her own potential, can cope with the normal stresses of life, can work productively and fruitfully, and is able to make a contribution to her or his community."[155]

This is a good starting point. Mental health, especially when defined broadly like this, is one of the requirements for achieving Inner Peace.

Happiness is also part of what we mean by Inner Peace. For many of us, happiness is often determined by events external to ourselves. If an individual finds joy because of an event or achievement—and then loses that feeling until the next happy occurrence—does that really contribute to Inner Peace? Probably not. Instead of looking only to external factors to bring happiness, Inner Peace is associated with the ability to find some level of contentedness, satisfaction or acceptance no matter what challenges life brings.

So, it seems that Inner Peace involves more than mental health, and even more than a state of happiness.

Inner Peace is tied to the ability to maintain one's emotional and cognitive balance no matter what else is going on. This ability is linked closely to a concept called homeostasis, which is the property of biological and other systems to regulate their conditions in spite of changes in the environment.

Homeostasis is a useful concept in many branches of science.[156] The human body has certain homeostatic capabilities, for example, as it strives to maintain consistent levels of inner temperature, sodium content, oxygen and so on. Economists regard homeostasis as a key characteristic of economic and financial systems: A homeostatic economic system is internally stable, despite the presence of disruptions in the outside world. In the *Age Later* program, we strive for homeostasis in the workings of the human body by recognizing, for example, that the right food and exercise can make the body more resilient against the assaults of the environment.

Inner Peace, as a homeostatic state of mind, does not imply a lack of interest or concern regarding events in the world. What it means is viewing those events more objectively and with a sense of proportion.

The implication is that while we should be aware of what is going on in the world around us, we should avoid thoughtless responses to those external events. Instead, we should aim for appropriate and mindful responses through self-control. Inner Peace is what enables humans to be imperturbable, steady, dependable, tough-minded, self-controlled and self-sufficient.

By contrast, humans who lack Inner Peace tend to be panicky, unsteady, unreliable, thinskinned, undisciplined and needy. Most people find themselves somewhere in-between, and it should be our objective to move closer to the self-sufficient end of the spectrum.

By raising your overall level of mental fitness, and working toward Inner Peace, you'll find that incidents and events that used to create anxiety and irritation are easier to handle. Imagine what a difference this can make in your daily life.

THE PATH TO INNER PEACE

It's time to take stock of your state of mind. You may feel that you're coping well with the stresses of life, that you have inner tranquility, that you're mentally on top of your game, and that you're leading a thoughtful and intellectually stimulating life. If that's the case, congratulations on achieving something quite rare today.

On the other hand, if, like so many people, you yearn for a life that is less stressful and more fulfilling, then please pay attention to the health of your mind and nervous system, and follow the advice in this chapter.

There is no single path to Inner Peace. It may be better to think of Inner Peace not as a destination, but simply as an attitude of mind that reflects your choice of paths. Different cultures around the world have developed useful approaches to acquiring a sense of mental equilibrium, so, individuals can choose the methods that work best for them. The goals are always the same: to strengthen your mental resources, to develop habits of thinking and behavior that maintain mental balance, and to learn to control your responses to events and circumstances that push your emotional buttons.

Each of the topics in this chapter will help you to achieve those goals.

- Mindfulness training and practice can give you the tools to maintain awareness of your thoughts and emotions, leading to more mental control and balance.

- Learning to manage stress will help you deal with situations and relationships that typically cause anxiety.

- Sufficient restful sleep provides an opportunity for your brain to repair and reconstruct neural networks; this helps to boost mental well-being and overall health.

- The health of your nervous system can affect your state of mind and the way you respond to stress, so you need to develop habits to protect and improve your nervous system with mental exercise, physical exercise, socialization and nutrition.

Along the way, you may feel that you need support or even just occasional encouragement. Sharing your thoughts with sympathetic friends and family certainly can make a difference. Working alongside others in mindfulness sessions or yoga classes also can provide support.

If your anxiety continues to get in the way, and you're making slow progress (or no progress) in taming it, you may need to seek counseling from a trained therapist or psychologist. There's no shame in doing that, especially if it clears a roadblock toward attaining a higher level of Inner Peace.

None of this is easy, but most people will be able to use my suggestions to embark on paths of exploration that will lead them closer to Inner Peace. This simple introductory approach can produce new habits that will build mental and emotional strength. It's my hope that you're able to take these disciplines further than I can explain in one chapter of *Age Later*.

Let the journey begin.

MINDFULNESS

There are many meditative disciplines that can help individuals build mental control and balance. I have chosen to emphasize mindfulness meditation because it's easily accessible, it's compatible with many religious beliefs, and its effectiveness has been validated by extensive research.

As you'll read in the next section, mindfulness is now established as a beneficial activity for a myriad of reasons. However, mindfulness alone isn't the answer to all problems. If that's your expectation, expect to be disappointed.

The *Age Later* program approaches mindfulness exercises as a useful and proven way to achieve a balanced positive mental attitude, one that will help you focus on changing all of your habits for the better.

BENEFITS OF MINDFULNESS

The roots of mindfulness can be identified in many world religions, and the practice of mindfulness meditation draws from other forms of meditation, such as guided meditation and transcendental meditation. Today, mindfulness is taught in both religious and secular contexts. The secularization of mindfulness, and its adoption as a mainstream form of therapy, has resulted in more scientific interest to objectively assess its value. As a result, there is now wide research that confirms that mindfulness meditation and mindfulness-based therapies bring many benefits.[157]

- Enhancements in self-insight

- Reduction in stress and anxiety

- Reduction in symptoms of depression

- Reduction in rumination (worrying over problems without getting closer to a resolution)

- More control over emotions and emotional responses

- Improvements in working memory

- Improvements in focusing

- Improved self-observation (which leads to improved control of responses to stressful or negative situations)

- Improved relationship satisfaction

- Improvements in immune system functioning

- Improvements to cardiovascular health due to reduced stress.[158]

Just as I encourage people new to physical exercise to do something each day to get the ball rolling, I encourage people to take that first step with mindfulness. Almost everyone who starts to exercise regularly begins to see the benefits and actually enjoy the workouts. It's the same with meditative mindfulness.

That said, if the mindfulness exercise starts to feel like a chore or an obligation, then your own mind isn't in the right frame to appreciate and receive its benefits.[159] Whatever you do, don't give up. Focus on something else for a short time, and then come back. Consider why you have a negative attitude to becoming healthier in body and mind. Then try again.

Trust me, the gain outweighs the pain. Mindfulness meditation will improve the way you handle day-to-day life—and add value to everything in the *Age Later* program.

LEARNING TO BE MINDFUL

While most people do not need formal therapy programs to learn mindfulness, it's worth mentioning again that its value is widely recognized by medical and psychological professionals. Mindfulness training is even used in psychological therapies for people experiencing significant mental or physical difficulties.

Mindfulness Based Stress Reduction (MBSR)[160] (mindfulness:MBSR) is used as an adjunct to other physical and mental therapies, and is proven to be effective.[161] It's an intensive program, focused on patients who suffer from chronic stress or chronic pain, that incorporates group sessions to deliver training in mindfulness techniques. The first MBSR program was initiated at the University of Massachusetts in 1979,[162] and today MBSR group therapy is available in many locations.

Mindfulness Based Cognitive Therapy (MBCT) uses mindfulness principles to give people with a history of depression the skills to help avoid relapse.[163]

Being mindful is not some kind of trick. Anyone can be mindful, and some people are naturally more so than others. Some of the important aspects of mindfulness include:

- Awareness of your mind, what you are thinking, how your thoughts come and go.

- Awareness of sensations, what you hear, see and feel, and how you receive and interact with those sensations. In other words, awareness of how your body and mind interact with the world.

- Taking notice of your emotions, understanding where your emotions come from, how they affect your thoughts and behavior, how your emotions impact other people as a result of your behaviors.

- Taking notice of your attitudes to people and situations, your preferences, your urges and cravings, your dislikes and fears—and replacing your unthinking responses to those things with mindful responses.

- Acquiring the discipline to insert some space between your thought processes, emotions and urges, and your actions in the physical world.

Anyone can learn mindfulness techniques from a trained local teacher, or you can study the principles online and make a lot of progress independently. Mind-body practices such as yoga, tai-chi and qigong, and many forms of meditation, can help to build mindfulness.

However, we will focus here on the techniques of mindfulness meditation. Note that these are not exclusive choices: You can learn any or all of these disciplines and benefit.

For most of us, the best path into mindfulness meditation probably is with a teacher. Start with an Internet search. Talk to some friends; maybe someone knows an instructor. There likely are people in your community who advertise their services. The most important thing is to feel comfortable. Meet with your potential teacher. Find out how long he or she has been practicing meditation; the longer the better. It takes several years of meditation practice before someone is ready to train as an instructor. If your teacher just learned to meditate a couple of months ago, look elsewhere.

Another option is to join a yoga class. Yoga is beneficial in its own right, and when you make some friends in the group, you are likely to find people who are informed about mindfulness and meditation.

If you can't find a teacher, or if you would prefer to start on your own, there are many sources of information. Some simple exercises to get started are outlined in this chapter as part of the "Mindfulness Exercises" section. Visit your bookshop to find an array of how-to material for beginners and advanced practitioners.[164] You'll also find helpful sources online[165]—in fact, you can take meditation courses online.[166] This may help as an introduction to the discipline, but some people will miss the personal attention that can be important to building this habit.

Whether you acquire mindfulness skills through training or go it alone, consider using a mindfulness smartphone app.[167] Apps may be no more than simple timers for your meditation sessions, or they can provide a broad selection of guided meditation sessions. At agelaterbook.com, you can find information about some of these apps.

Mindfulness also is connected to activities that lead us into a zone of complete focus on the moment—and awareness of self in that moment: creating or appreciating music, art or literature; solving a math or science problem; visualizing and executing a golf shot. The learned ability to focus in these areas builds mindfulness skills. In turn, mindfulness skills improve your ability to focus and be "in the zone." Mindfulness training and engaging in activities that demand concentration turn out to be mutually reinforcing.

At this point, I suggest that you give mindfulness meditation a try. It's been around for more than 2,000 years in one form or another, yet Western medicine has only recently become serious about understanding what it is and how it works. That's no reason to be skeptical. Mindfulness is an important component of the *Age Later* program; as you learn how to apply it to your daily life, the investment will begin paying handsome dividends.

MINDFULNESS EXERCISES

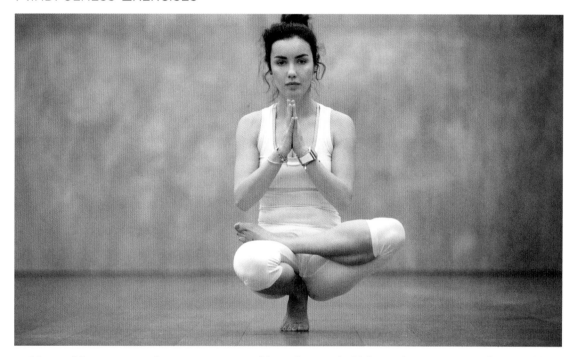

My goal is not to teach everyone everything about mindfulness in *Age Later*; that would be a book unto itself. Hopefully, especially for beginners, I can provide some simple mindfulness exercises and tips so that you begin to understand the power of this technique. At this level, the aim is simply to improve mental control, focus and balance—and not deal with significant psychological conditions that might need expert support using formal MBSR or MBCT programs.

We start with a mindful breathing practice, in which you can develop your mindfulness abilities in a quiet and protected space. This is about building your mental muscles through mindfulness techniques that will allow you to bring calmness and control to situations that you may not have created.

MINDFUL BREATHING PRACTICE

Would you enter a marathon race without any training or practice? Would you accept a challenge to play a high-stakes game of Texas Hold'Em with no knowledge of that variation of poker? Maybe, but you'd probably leave the game a bit lighter in the wallet. We learn about and practice things like this in order to develop skills that allow us to better perform.

This is why we start learning about mindfulness with a simple breathing exercise. You should do this every day, perhaps before you warm up for that day's physical exercise.

Focus on breathing until you're ready to move on to a different daily mindfulness exercise. Exercising when you don't really feel like it is part of the training; it's just as important to push through when strengthening your mind as it is when strengthening the body.

This exercise was adapted from material on the Berkeley University Greater Good In Action website.[168] The Berkeley website also contains an audio track that you can use to work through this practice exercise.

Set a timer to indicate the finish of your session. Choose a gentle alert tone.

Find a relaxed position, whatever feels comfortable. Sit on a chair or on the floor, anywhere you can sit straight but relaxed. Rest your hands on your knees. You can close your eyes or focus on something in the room, whichever you prefer.

Take a minute to relax and notice your body. Notice where the tip of your tongue is and change the position to something comfortable. If your jaw feels clenched, let it relax and separate your teeth. How are your legs and arms positioned? Move them to somewhere comfortable so that they feel balanced.

Observe the shape, position and weight of your body. Consciously relax any body parts that feel tense: shoulders, wrists, fingers. Breathe.

Tune in to your breath. Feel the natural flow of breath—in, then out. In, then out. Don't force your breathing; just observe it. Keep it natural. Where is the focus of your breathing sensation? It might be in your nostrils, in your chest, perhaps in your stomach. Focus on that, and continue to breathe naturally. Pay attention to the feeling and sensations of breathing, one breath at a time. Observe how when one breath ends, the next breath begins.

You may notice that your mind will start to wander, and you are no longer paying attention to your breathing but something completely different. That's normal. Make a mental note that your mind has wandered, and gently direct your attention back to your breathing.

Continue for five to 15 minutes. Continue to pay attention to your breathing. When other thoughts intrude, gently return to focus on your breathing.

When it's time to stop, direct your mind back to your body. Observe your whole body again, and relax some more. Congratulate yourself for your achievement. Promise yourself you'll do it again tomorrow.

Managing Stress and Anxiety

We tend to want to forget about stressful situations we have encountered in the past, yet those situations are raw material, rich with learning opportunities. By calmly reviewing a past stressful situation, you can prepare yourself better for future stressful events. The exercise below is one example of a specific mindfulness exercise intended to focus on helping you manage your response to stressful situations. There are many more along similar lines.

If you practice mindfulness regularly, whether those exercises are aimed at specific stress reduction or not, you may find that your growing mental control and calmness will significantly reduce the intensity of your responses to challenging situations. Certain situations of danger and conflict always will cause a certain amount of stress. Mindfulness will not eliminate that stress entirely, but it will help you control the way that stress impacts your behavior, your mind and your body. Special supplements, like Hush & Hush MindYourMind, can also help alleviate stress and instill a state of calm.

Here's one way in which you can help prepare your mind to handle stress-inducing events.

Form a mental image of a recent event that caused you to feel stressed and anxious.

Replay that event in your mind, and try to recall your feelings at the time. Try to reproduce those feelings of anxiety, shame, fear, doubt or hopelessness. If your body reacts physically, then you're on the right path.

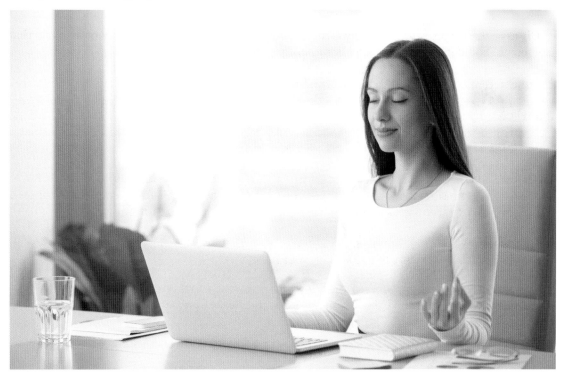

Notice your emotions. Admit how you felt. This is mindfulness in action. Admit your pain and recognize those emotions. Tell yourself what it was like. Be mindful of what it was like.

Recognize that your emotions at this point are entirely normal. Other people have felt like this, and many are feeling these emotions right now. You are a human being, and this is how human beings react.

Be mindful of all the circumstances surrounding the event. If your stress was caused by the behavior of others, recognize that, and forgive them for causing you pain and anxiety. The stress they caused almost certainly was a by-product of their own fears and anxieties. We're all human. On the other hand, if you were the cause of the stressful event, forgive yourself with an open heart, and learn from your recollection of the behavior.

Forgiving yourself and forgiving others helps to put those emotions in perspective. It also allows you to assess what really happened and to consider what you could have done differently to eliminate that stress. You must take responsibility, even if someone else caused the problem. Tell yourself that if a similar situation arises, you will understand better how to handle it. If you have to think rather than react emotionally, you will be up to the challenge. If you need to be solid and mature in the face of someone else's childish behavior then that is what you will do.

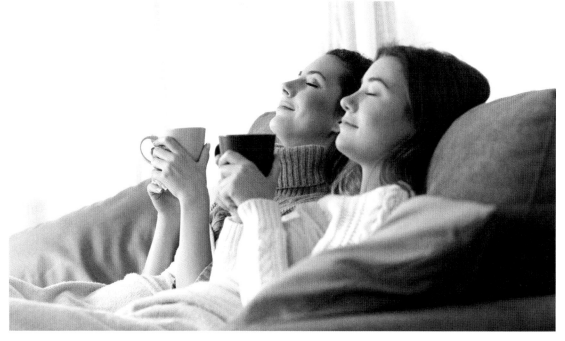

TAKING CONTROL OF YOUR EMOTIONS

Emotions can be complicated and unpredictable, and "being emotional" is sometimes associated with immaturity or lack of control. Still, our emotions have evolved for a reason; they're an important factor in human interactions. Your aim should be to understand and manage your emotions, not to eliminate or bury them.

For example, anger and frustration, which often can be negative and destructive, also can be used in a controlled way to change things in your life for the better. Sadness, which is not the same thing as depression, can help people understand what is important to them and can help develop a sense of proportion.[169] Empathy for others has its roots in a mix of different emotions, and to suppress those emotions diminishes your capability of understanding the motivations and behaviors of others. You need empathy in order to get along with other human beings. From a practical viewpoint, you might notice that the most effective sales people, business managers and politicians all bring a degree of empathy to their dealings with others.

Setting aside time for mindfulness exercise every day will open windows and provide insights into your emotional self, as well as into your calculating brain. It's all part of the same system. Being aware of your emotions, working out what triggered them and why, is a necessary first step. From there, your awareness will grow into an understanding of how your emotional reactions influence others, for better or worse, and how the emotionally-driven behavior of others affects you.

Mindfulness means you take notice.

A mature understanding of your emotions will enable you, in times of stress and anxiety, to make some space between the valid emotions you experience, and the urge to respond without consideration. Mindfulness does not reduce your emotional senses, but it does help you control those spontaneous reactions that, sometimes, can make matters worse.

Changing Your Attitude to Others

Your first response to the notion of "changing your attitude" may be that you're quite happy with your attitude and your perspective on the world. Even so, it's worth taking a fresh look at your perspectives now and again, and mindfulness will help and encourage you to do this. What if your attitudes color your behavior in such a way that you are not making the most of yourself? What if those attitudes are doing harm to you and to others?

Your attitude to other people, and to the world in general, is a complex combination of perceptions, intuitions and prejudices. If you find that your perspectives are dominated by feelings of negativity, irritation and frustration, do yourself a favor and give yourself an attitude upgrade. Day-to-day life has its share of challenges. The planet is populated with people of all stripes, including some who just rub you the wrong way. And, sometimes, everything that can go wrong, does. But living in negativity suggests that nothing can be done, and that not much is good and worthwhile.

A mindful approach to your attitudes requires you to assign some mental space to assessing your attitudes in different situations—and weighing whether your attitudes are likely to help improve the situation or make it worse.

Start this process by examining your relationships with people who are close to you. Have you become dismissive toward them? Hypercritical? Hypersensitive? Are you supportive or are you an obstacle?

It's within your power to change the attitudes and linked behaviors that adversely impact those close to you. That is, if you want to. If you don't, it's important to understand why. If you have a relationship that has become toxic, you should decide to repair things—or else move away from the relationship.

This all starts with being mindful about what really is going on. Take notice of your attitudes, and of the behavior that those attitudes cause, before taking steps toward a more sustainable relationship and peace of mind for yourself and those around you.

Before Bed

Insomnia can have many causes, as we'll discuss later in the section on Sleep. One common difficulty is that the brain insists on thinking and re-thinking the happenings of the day, or what might happen tomorrow.

You can calm those thought processes with Hush & Hush MindYourMind or by doing some simple mindfulness exercises before you go to bed, or even when you're in bed.

You could try the breathing exercise described earlier, for about 10 minutes. If you do this in a comfortable seated position, you are more likely to remain awake, allowing your mind and your body to derive full benefit from the duration of the exercise. Then, when you go to bed, you'll be relaxed and tranquil. As always, focus on your breathing, become aware of your body and how your body makes contact with the chair and the floor. Be ready to notice when your mind starts to wander, and gently bring your thoughts back into focus.

You can use this exercise to relax even more when you're in bed. Focus in the same way, but don't set a time limit. When the body is ready, and you're truly relaxed, then you will fall asleep.

Many smartphone mindfulness apps contain specific exercises for just before bed, and you may wish to try them. But the basic breathing exercise works for many people to still the mind and encourage sleep.

Managing Stress and Anxiety Levels

Stress and anxiety hinder your mental well-being. Mental stress causes biological changes in the body. If you have an argument with a friend or work colleague, it's not the argument that increases your blood pressure and heart rate. It's your response to that argument. You may not be able to alter the nature of your co-worker. However, you can adjust your own response to that person's stress-inducing behavior with mindfulness, along with an understanding of the physiological mechanisms of stress.

Everyone can benefit from learning about stress reduction and stress management.

Not all stress is bad. There are occasions when a surge of adrenaline can be helpful, but, in keeping with the overarching goals of *Age Later*, let's aim to better control our reaction in those situations.

STRESS CAN SHORTEN YOUR LIFE

Do you ever find yourself unable to manage stress? Do you have feelings of being under siege in more than one area of your life?

The bad news is that stress can reduce your effectiveness and sap your energy. The worse news is that, if it goes on too long, it can kill you. Research has found a definite link between mental well-being and the incidence of coronary heart disease.[170]

Constant stress packs a double whammy in that it leads to habits that further undermine your health. People sometimes respond to daily tension by using substances that seem to relieve the pressure: tobacco, alcohol, soft drugs or hard drugs. All of these affect the body as well as the mind, and long-term dependencies can cause severe damage. As it applies to dealing with stress, substance abuse reduces the ability to strategically avoid problems, and it diminishes your coping skills when unexpected events occur.

Chronic stress affects your body in many ways, including increased blood pressure and muscle tensions that result in persistent pain. Stress impairs heart functions and blood circulation. Your brain needs oxygen and so reduced blood circulation is bad for the brain too.

When we are stressed, our brain and nervous system react as if we are facing danger. Thanks to evolution, our body's internal circuitry prepares us to either take on an adversary or to run away—aka, "fight or flight." Your body releases hormones into the bloodstream that increase your heart rate and raise your blood pressure. You become more alert and ready to call on energy supplies for your muscles. When facing a physical confrontation, this natural body response improves your ability to either escape, or to win a battle—to that end, the body's fight-or-flight response has been critical to survival through the centuries. It's also useful if you're playing a tough tennis match, skiing challenging slopes, giving an important speech, or performing in front of 20,000 fans at Madison Square Garden.

There are times when the fight-or-flight response does more harm than good. Damage can occur when this automatic response occurs repeatedly without a satisfactory resolution, or when it morphs into extended anxiety. The body's response leads to permanent stress of our mental capacities and of our physical selves. Persistent stress has been linked to heart attacks and strokes.[171] Although evidence that stress might cause cancer is not conclusive, there is evidence that, once cancer is present, stress can increase the rate at which it spreads through the body.[172]

Severe stress also can signal part of your brain (the prefrontal cortex) to temporarily shut down, handing over control to other parts more concerned with emotion than reason. While this is a protective mechanism inherited from our distant ancestors, and sometimes does serve to protect, it also can lead to regrettable actions. If prolonged or repeated, brain functioning can be affected. In particular, it can impair concentration and control of impulses.[173]

As most of us realize from personal experience, stress also increases our susceptibility to everyday ailments, such as colds, coughs and stomach disorders. We live in an environment rich in pathogens. Some of us sail through, seldom falling ill. Others catch every new bug. There is evidence that psychological stress can affect your skin's protective barrier, thus reducing your resistance to illness.[174]

Troublesome skin conditions also are linked to mental strain. Most cases of hives are linked to stress, which can cause quiescent conditions such as eczema and psoriasis to flare up.[175] When your skin's barrier function is affected, your skin's integrity is compromised at all levels.

On top of all that, stressed skin just looks older.

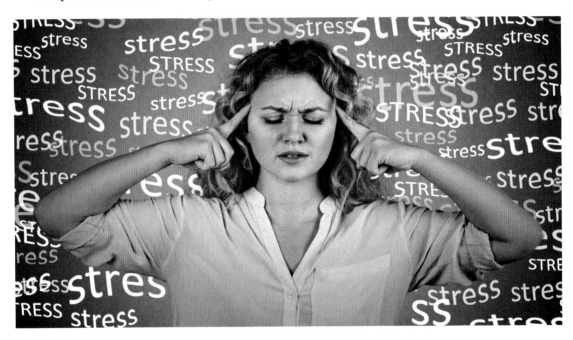

GOOD STRESS AND BAD STRESS

Not all stress is unhealthy. If humans lived lives devoid of tension or nervousness, they probably would not learn as much or earn as much. They wouldn't embark on potential relationships, and they wouldn't play competitive sports or games. In short, we might lead very boring lives. On the surface, there's not much to separate pleasurable excitement from severe anxiety: The pulse rate goes up, perspiration increases, and perhaps there's some breathlessness. The difference is that recurring anxiety damages health, whereas pleasurable excitement generally does not.

In reducing stress we need to focus on eliminating the negatives—and perhaps adding more pleasure and excitement. That's why we need to know the difference between good stress and bad stress.

Not all anxiety-inducing situations have the same impact on our minds and bodies. Some kinds of stress give us a short-term boost and make us alert. When the stress goes away, we have a sense of achievement and well-being. That kind of stress is generally good for us.

Sometimes, stress makes us nervous and unhappy, and even when the original cause of the stress is gone, we remain uneasy, even depressed. That kind of stress is not good. Bad stress makes you less effective, less energetic and unwilling to face new challenges.

It's easy to tell the difference between a good stressful experience and a bad one. One indication is that good stress often makes people smile, even laugh, especially when it's over. Bad stress always feels like a burden. Apart from the presence or absence of smiles, there are at least three significant differences between the circumstances that result in good stress or in bad stress:

Who is in control? Who makes the decisions? In a bad-stress situation, a person will feel that he or she has no control over what happens next. In a good-stress situation, the person will feel empowered. Even if they're not totally in control, they understand that there are options available.

Is there a sense of achievement? Bad-stress situations often are characterized by a feeling of frustration or futility; the dominant thought is, "What's the point of all this?" Good stress is always associated with a sense of achievement: an exam passed, a work task accomplished, a mountain climbed, a wedding proposal that results in her (or him) saying "yes."

When will it end? In a bad-stress situation, a person will see no clear end in sight, and that adds to the frustration. In a good-stress situation, there is a desirable or useful result in view, your levels of the hormone adrenaline increase just enough, and there is a surge of happiness along with a distinct sense of a job well done.

Good stress occurs when your nervous system triggers the fight-or-flight response, you take action, and then it's over—for better or worse. Your body returns to normal.

Bad stress occurs when your nervous system triggers the fight-or-flight response, you take action—and the problem lingers on and on. Your body keeps boosting your adrenaline levels in response. If this happens frequently and persistently, you'll feel relentlessly stressed.

For example, let's say an impending hurricane is inching closer to your community. In the hours before it hits, there is danger in the air, anxiety levels are high and adrenaline surges. But when the storm is over, those who emerge relatively unscathed feel good about themselves.

For those dealing with storm fallout that lasts for weeks or even months, it's a different story. They may have no electricity, polluted water, and difficulties obtaining food and supplies. How do those people feel? They remain at high anxiety levels as their bodies deliver adrenaline every day to handle new problems and setbacks. People lose their tempers and argue. It's nothing but bad stress.

THE STRESSFUL WORLD WE LIVE IN

We live in a world that causes its own share of modern-day stresses. In another era, hunter-gatherers worried about their next meal.

Today, we fret over too many emails in our inbox, we grow frustrated sitting in traffic, we lose it when we spend 10 minutes sifting through voice prompts to reach a human cable company representative. Add to this, the concerns we all have about making a living, raising children and tending to our relationships.

Back to those emails for a second. For many people, a significant cause of stress is our inability to unplug and disconnect. Others expect us always to be available, so we're compelled to be tethered to our smartphones, tablets and computers. In my opinion, this is the number one cause of excessive stress for a lot of people living in the U.S.

There is (and always has been) a lot of violence in the world. Today, even if that violence does not directly affect us, modern media channels give these events unprecedented visibility. And that adds yet another, less noticeable layer to our baseline anxieties. Even without considering crime, the stress associated with living in densely populated cities is significant.[176]

The World Happiness Report 2017[177] provides insights into causes of stress and unhappiness worldwide. Some of these causes are under the control of governments and corporations (or more accurately those who run these institutions). Around the world, humans' sense of well-being is heavily affected by concerns about such things as social cohesion, trustworthiness, financial security and health care.

We all ask variations of the same big-picture and day-to-day questions: Will I be employed next week? Can I pay the rent? What happens if I get ill? What crazy task will my boss ask me to do tomorrow? If we have answers that reduce uncertainty, those stresses fade. When we don't, those stresses build.

Although things happen to us and around us that are not directly under our control, we can decide how to respond. If we make a conscious effort to respond in a way that doesn't add to the stress—better still, if we find our Inner Peace and make decisions that ease tension—it can lead to healthier mental wellness for ourselves and even diminish the stress levels of those around us.

HOW STRESSED ARE YOU?

Do you know what causes stress in your life? You probably know the obvious triggers, but you may not be aware of how subtle things can affect your stress levels, or if your base level of stress is high or low.

There is no single indicator of stress, and no easy-to-use anxiety meter that you can wear like a watch. Two metrics that can give an indication are blood pressure (BP) and heart rate variability (HRV).

High blood pressure, or hypertension, has long been associated with stress, although high BP also can be caused by poor condition of the cardiovascular system. Nevertheless, a rise in blood pressure can be the body's response to a stressful situation; if the stressful events are repeated or continuous, the body stays in a state of fight-or-flight readiness, and blood pressure remains high. There is more information about blood pressure at agelaterbook.com.

Low resting heart rate variability is associated with stress. A normal sympathetic nervous system is always working at a low level, ready to leap into action when needed (like if you're in a fight-or-flight situation). Repeated stressful events can cause the sympathetic response to always be on, at a higher level than is healthy, and continuously feeding the body with the hormones and chemicals associated with stressful situations (even when nothing stressful is happening). That means that the heart rate is always being kept at a steady rate (low variability) because the sympathetic response is flooding it with signals. So, when a low heart rate variability is measured in a resting person, it may indicate high levels of mental stress, but (as with BP) many other factors can cause low HRV, such as cardiovascular disease, diabetes, cancer and more.[178] Still, monitoring HRV over time may well help to indicate whether baseline stress levels are worsening or getting better.

Note that HRV is naturally lower during strenuous exercise or during periods of actual mental stress. That's why the resting HRV level is the measurement we use for overall health and well-being.

There is more information about HRV at agelaterbook.com.

While HRV promises some insight into stress levels by direct measurement of the body, a more traditional way of measuring stress, and probably the most common used by psychologists, are measurements based on a self-assessment scale called the Perceived Stress Scale (PSS).[179] The PSS documentation is freely available[180] and self-assessment is straightforward, but it does involve some calculation.

It's even easier to visit one of the many websites that offer online tools for self-assessment based on PSS.[181] On some of these websites you can expect to be offered stress-related training and other services, but don't let that add to your stress. (Please note that these online questionnaires are not intended to replace professional diagnosis or consultation; they possibly can provide some insights and an indication of the presence of problems but not much more. If you are seriously concerned, obtain professional advice.)

MANAGE YOUR RESPONSE TO STRESSFUL EVENTS

Everyone reacts to stressful situations. But you've no doubt noticed that some people react with greater intensity than others: more pronounced, more dramatic, more emotional.

An emotional reaction has the potential to heighten an already stressful situation, kind of like throwing gasoline on a fire. Learning to control your emotions and react with calm and reason is one of the keys to a lifestyle guided by the principles in *Age Later*. With some persistence you can learn to do this. The awareness provided by mindfulness will help you observe your reactions and measure your response. Regular practice will build awareness and self-control, so you are less likely to be driven to over-react.

To some, the notion of controlling emotions is almost nonsensical. After all, we are taught that logic and emotion are two different things, that some people are ruled by emotion, others by reason. Some people think that emotions are more natural, and that we should follow our emotions, while reason is just cold calculation. Others think exactly the opposite: Cold logic should determine our response to events, and emotion should be held at arm's length.

The reality is that emotion and logic always are intertwined when it comes to deciding what actions to take in any circumstances. If we ignore our ability to work out the most effective response, our uncontrolled emotional reaction can make a bad situation worse and even more stressful. On the other hand, if we try to ignore the natural emotion that we feel, our reason can lead to making decisions that fail to account for important human factors.

Everyone has emotions, and every one has the capability of understanding how to work out the most effective reasoned response. There's no excuse for relying on just one at the expense of the other.

Reduce Stressful Distractions in Your Life

There are a lot of things that create stress that are avoidable. The most avoidable sources of stress are due to anger, frustration and anxiety caused by events we can't control. Sometimes, the fact that we can't control the events is what causes the anger, frustration and anxiety.

None of this is to say that we can't change the narrative when it comes to things that tend to push our buttons in the modern world.

Do you have to be available online at all times? Actually, that's a choice. But if it's one you make, don't be surprised if your stress levels escalate along the way. Obviously, the nature of your work and social environment may dictate how much time you spend connected to your phone and computer. At work, you can be firm about expectations regarding when you're available and who has access to you. Make it clear that you have important things to do—like tending to work without being interrupted. In your social life, take a clear, objective look at how much time you spend online and how much good it's doing you. Avoid paying attention to the trivial matters that dominate the web and social media—in other words, stop wasting time on nonsense. You'll be amazed at how many minutes and, maybe, hours that you free up—while reducing your personal stress levels.

Social media has a unique way of driving emotions. It's a place for some people to share photos of their children—and for other people to rage against anyone who doesn't share their views. How much time are you willing to invest on the endless flow of verbiage, videos and images? Give yourself some slack and live with less anxiety.

Be mindful that some of the assertions and opinions that push your buttons aren't even valid, let alone relevant to your day-to-day life. It's possible to choose not to have an opinion on something you know nothing or very little about. Public figures appear to feel obliged to do so and they must find ways of living with that stress. But don't feel the need to take a position in the absence of information. To the contrary, you should feel that there is a moral requirement to learn the facts before taking sides.

This isn't to suggest that you should never engage or get involved in discussions that matter to you personally or to your community. But your mindfulness training requires you to do so with awareness. Choosing a side without knowledge is not responsible.

I realize that our politicians don't help much. They have learned to create fear and anxiety in order to persuade people to their point of view. It's their job to do that, or at least it's the way they have been conditioned to see their jobs. As ordinary citizens (which the vast majority of us are), we can choose not to behave in the same polarizing way as our politicians.

Earlier I mentioned the stress-related topic of rumination, a term psychologists use to describe worrying about problems without getting closer to a resolution. Many social-network-driven issues are of that nature. If you lie awake at night trying to solve these problems, you will have less energy during the day to truly understand what's going on around you, a prerequisite for taking a stand and taking reasoned action.

These are just a few examples of how your own emotions can drive you in a stress-inducing direction, one that can negatively color your response to similar situations in the future.

Mindfulness can help you avoid that kind of downward spiral.

RELATIONSHIPS: SUPPORTIVE AND TOXIC

Relationships with other people often are a source of pleasure and satisfaction, but relationships also can be toxic. And toxic relationships cause stress.

A toxic relationship is characterized by, from one side, unreasonable demands, unreasonable expectations, inconsistency and even bullying. On the other side, there may be a feeling of frustration and hopelessness. Toxic relationships are almost always caused by an unequal power relationship, or a constant struggle for domination.

Despite living in the shadow of bullying bosses or domineering partners, or needy and energy-sucking friends, people often choose to stay around. They feel a sense of obligation that the dominant participant does not have.

We all owe it to ourselves to recognize when a relationship is toxic—whether the toxin comes from a boss, a work colleague, a supposed friend or a partner. Then we must decide whether it is possible to mend the relationship. If that's not possible, it might be time to abandon it.

Every situation is different, so generic advice may not be helpful. Mending a toxic relationship requires a complete change of attitude from you and the other person. You need to clear the air and commit to being honest with each other. You need to define the terms of engagement: What kinds of behaviors are acceptable, what kinds of behaviors are not acceptable. That much we can say with confidence.

To repair a relationship, everything depends on both parties being ready to mend things. Sometimes that's just not the case, and you can't find a path to agreement. Then it becomes a question of escalation (HR, counseling, legal action, arbitration) or exit. If a toxic relationship is dominating your life, you won't be able to fully benefit from the *Age Later* program. Either way, you need to take action, even if it means seeking advice from a trusted third party. The most stressful option is to do nothing. Sometimes, being indecisive is worse than making a poor decision. Whether your indecisiveness is because you wish to avoid confrontation, or simply because you can't see a perfect way out, don't allow the toxic relationship to linger.

Once you have repaired it or moved on, it's important to review what happened and be objective about it. Learn something from the episode so that you avoid the same problem down the road. This, too, may require some third-party assistance, perhaps with a professional. From there, it's time to move forward and embark—with optimism—on the next chapter in your life.

THE VALUE OF SLEEP

Everyone sleeps. Sleep is both natural and essential, and it contributes significantly to your mental well-being and your physical health. Yet more than a third of adults have sleep problems.[182]

Adults typically spend (or should spend) one-third of their lives sleeping. Those hours of slumber are not wasted; sleep-time is when essential maintenance of your body takes place. If you don't enjoy seven to nine hours of sleep in each 24-hour period, you won't perform at your best when you're awake. Sleeplessness leads to increased exhaustion and a reduced ability to cope with the events of the day. Furthermore, lack of sleep, whether it's caused by stress, overwork, a frenetic social life or other factors can directly lead to medical conditions that include obesity, heart disease and diabetes.[183]

There really is no substitute for sleep, so taking steps that ensure a peaceful nighttime rest is another healthy living choice you need to make.

WHY DO WE SLEEP?

Think of sleep as a session of intensive offline maintenance for the body. These are some of the internal tasks that take place while you're fast asleep:

Your brain is creating new cells to replace dead cells, and building new neural connections. This is one of the ways that information you've acquired is stored. Sleep plays an essential part in learning, skill acquisition, and the building and embedding of cognitive skills such as problem

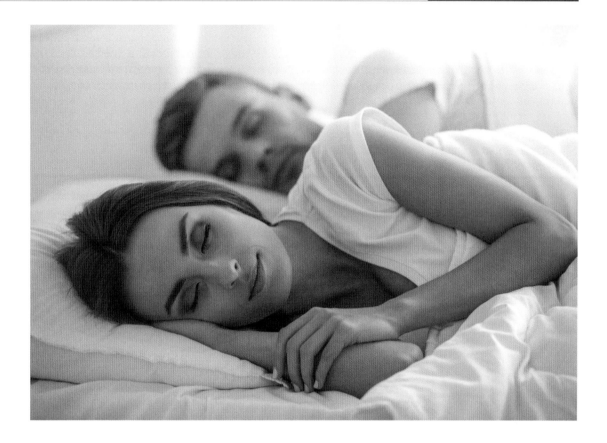

solving and pattern recognition.

The flow of cerebral fluid in your brain increases during sleep[184] in order to clear out dead tissue and toxins. Your body, meanwhile, is busy repairing damage to your circulatory system, building new blood vessels and fighting inflammation in your cardiovascular system, your brain and other organs.[185]

Your immune system never stops functioning, but during sleep it gets a chance to catch up. There is evidence that sleep plays a role in building your immunological memory and countering low-grade inflammation.[186]

During deep sleep, the body releases growth hormones that foster the building and repair of muscles and other tissues. The same mechanism ensures normal development in children and young adults.

Sleep influences the way your body reacts to insulin, the hormone that controls your blood glucose level, and thus helps to determine your risk for diabetes and stroke.

How Much Sleep Is Enough?

Most adults need between seven and nine hours of sleep each day. Some people claim to be able to get by on just three or four hours sleep. If their claims are correct, they probably are heading for some kind of mental disturbance. It's more likely that their three or four hours in bed are supplemented by naps and snoozes during the day, and slumbering in front of a TV for a few hours in the evening.

You can tell if you're not getting enough quality sleep if you frequently:

- Fall asleep, doze or have to fight against sleep when you're stuck in traffic, watching TV, reading a book or sitting at a desk trying to get some work done.

- Have persistent difficulty getting to sleep when you go to bed.

- Wake in the middle of the night and are unable to go back to sleep.

- Have difficulty getting out of bed, and routinely feel tired and grumpy during the day.

- Overreact emotionally to small difficulties.

If you are concerned about the amount and quality of sleep you are getting, you might be interested in learning a bit more by completing the questionnaire provided by the World Sleep Survey,[187] which covers a number of different perspectives. (Please note: This online questionnaire is not intended to replace professional diagnosis or consultation; it may provide some insights and an indication of possible problems, but not much more. If you are seriously concerned, obtain professional advice.)

Sleep Deficiency

Lack of sleep or disturbed sleep patterns can lead to:

- An increased risk of heart disease,[188] kidney disease, obesity, high blood pressure, diabetes and stroke

- A higher chance of neurological illnesses, as a result of insufficient clearance of dead tissues and toxins

- Low-grade inflammation throughout the body

- Immunodeficiency[189]

- Less resistance to common infections, such as colds, coughs and flu, and to allergens

- If that isn't enough, lack of sleep also manifests itself during daytime in ways that decrease our performance and increase risk:

- Lack of sleep reduces alertness and increases nervous system response times, which results in higher risk of driving accidents, household accidents, injuries caused by machinery and sports injuries. The risk of injury is increased not just for the fatigued person but for others in the vicinity.

- Tiredness affects your mood. People who are tired are more likely to be depressed, less likely to be enthusiastic, and may lack the ability to focus and concentrate.

- Tiredness leads to mood swings and emotional responses, which can negatively impact the way we interact with people.

- Tiredness affects judgment; so tired people are more likely to take unnecessary risks.

There is a definite pattern of dysfunction related to tiredness, and it's not surprising that people who do not get enough sleep suffer from additional stress as a result. We also know that a person experiencing stress and anxiety finds it more difficult to sleep. That can lead to a sleep-stress-sleep cycle,[190] in which lack of sleep causes more stress, which results in restless (or no) sleep, and so on.

Breaking an ongoing cycle like this requires, first and foremost, stress reduction.[191] You can't wave a magic wand and eliminate stressful events, but the various recommendations for stress reduction that appear later in this chapter will go some way toward reducing stress. We need to replace the downward sleep-stress-sleep cycle with an upward self-reinforcing trajectory that results in more sleep and less stress.

How to Sleep Longer and Better

Around one-third of adults in the U.S. don't get enough sleep,[192] so if you feel you have a sleep problem, you're not alone. In addition to working on mindfulness and stress reduction, it might improve things by just changing the way you approach sleeping. Here are some examples.

Exercise More

My number one tip for sleeping longer and better is to get more exercise. If you don't exert yourself, you will not sleep well. No matter what else is going on that might be disrupting your sleep, the first step is to increase your physical activity. Body movements demand more oxygen, and that oxygen reaches all parts of your body, including your brain. Your body uses more energy, and that causes genuine sleepiness. Exercise also reduces stress and anxiety, which in turn encourages beneficial sleep. I suggest avoiding vigorous exercise within an hour of bedtime to allow your heart rate to settle—and to allow your body to ease into its bedtime routine.

A CALMING BEDTIME ROUTINE

If you work and exercise right up until bedtime, your mind and body will be fully engaged, and thus it may take longer to fall asleep. Similarly, if you become absorbed in stressful activities just before bed, you'll still be thinking about them while your eyes are closed. Watching TV or browsing online just before bed (or even in bed) can fool your brain into believing it's not time to sleep: The blue tinted light in these devices is not helpful, so if you have problems sleeping, that could be one of the reasons.

Start winding down at least an hour before you go to bed. Stop working, shut down the computer, switch off the TV. Connect your smartphone to its charger (outside the bedroom) and leave it there. If you are feeling stressed, a warm bath and a warm drink (herbal tea) can be relaxing. Also, anxiety levels can be reduced with a short meditation session before sleeping, or even a calming nutraceutical like Hush & Hush MindYourMind.

SLEEPING ENVIRONMENT

Consider your sleeping environment. It should be quiet, welcoming, comfortable and dark, with curtains or shades that block outside light. Many bedrooms are busy with unnecessarily bright LED indicator lights on various devices: You can put some sticky tape on them to block or dim the light. If you have an LED clock, turn it away from you, or replace it with an old-fashioned clock.

Some people sleep better when pulling the sheets back from a properly made bed, so making your bed in the morning should be a daily habit.

How old is your mattress? Mattresses don't last forever. If yours is more than 10 years old, it's probably time to get a new one. But it's not just about age. A well-designed and well-made mattress will last longer than a less expensive one. If it's been well maintained (regularly turned and vacuumed according to instructions) it also will last longer. If it's been damaged by spills or been used like a trampoline, it will wear out. Lumps and sags and squeaks mean that you need to buy a new one.

TIME DISRUPTIONS

Disruptions to your daily patterns of behavior can affect your sleep for several days. Examples of time disruptions include changes to your working hours at either end of the day; traveling across multiple time zones; twice-a-year changes to local time (daylight savings); partying until way past your normal bedtime. All of these can cause sleep disruptions for more than one night. Interruptions to normal schedules can have an impact on your sleep quality, even though you may not be conscious of it.

Many people handle time changes with ease, but others who already have erratic sleep patterns can find that a small change has a disproportionate impact. Many of these disruptions are unavoidable if you're leading a busy life, but you still can do something to reduce the impact. A good approach, if possible, is to plan ahead. Get plenty of sleep before the change happens, and gently adjust your sleeping hours in small chunks as you approach the date of the change.

CIGARETTES AND ALCOHOL

If you smoke cigarettes, you are more likely to have unsatisfactory sleep patterns. The remedy is to quit smoking, although it's understood that words alone won't change this habit. As for drinking alcohol immediately before bed, it generally reduces the quality of your sleep. Sometimes alcohol can bring on drowsiness, but it doesn't encourage good sleep. If you keep within the "moderate" levels of alcohol consumption described earlier, and avoid alcohol within a couple of hours of going to bed, you may improve things. But the best course of action, if you have sleep problems, is not to drink alcohol in the evening (or at all) until your sleep patterns improve.

CAFFEINE

When someone needs to fight drowsiness, they tend to drink a caffeinated drink. Coffee, tea, and caffeinated sodas all work to keep people awake, so it's hardly surprising that caffeinated drinks, before bedtime, are disruptive to sleep. Try and drink caffeinated drinks in small quantities, and only in the morning and early afternoon. It helps to allow at least eight hours between your last cup of coffee and going to bed; that gives the caffeine time to work through your system.

AN OVERACTIVE BRAIN

Too much thinking can be a problem. Even without high levels of stress some people lie awake thinking through problems, or just trying to do work. You should try to avoid working in bed. One approach is to use meditation or relaxation techniques to remove focus from these thoughts and encourage sleep. Another approach is to get out of bed and work when this happens—and then come back to bed when you actually feel sleepy.

Productive thinking in bed is not so good, but too much useless thinking is an even worse problem. Trying to solve things that you can't do anything about is a waste of your sleep hours. For example, if you're anxious about a forthcoming event (a speech, an interview, an appearance on a talk show), don't ruminate endlessly over your anxiety. If you can do something (like write notes about the next day's activities), then do it immediately to defuse the anxiety. If you can't do something, then do some mindfulness meditation, or find a brain challenge that allows you to displace your anxiety-forming thoughts.

NAPS, SIESTAS, AWAKENINGS

Having more than one session of sleep during the span of a day is nothing to worry about. It's quite natural for some people, and there's no rule that your eight hours of sleep must be in one continuous stretch.[193] If you nap during the day for, say, half an hour, that might even be good for you.[194] Siestas are part of the culture in many countries, allowing people go to bed later and still get up early without suffering a sleep deficit. Some people routinely wake up in the night, do something for a couple of hours and then go back to bed and sleep. If you feel that works for you, then don't become anxious about it.

MAINTAINING A HEALTHY NERVOUS SYSTEM

Your brain is at the core of your identity. Your nervous system is an extension of your brain; it works in concert with the brain to sense the outside world and allow you to function as a human being. Your brain and nervous system are effectively you. No matter what else you do to maintain health and stay more youthful, it doesn't amount to very much if you don't have a brain to appreciate your new healthy life.

The relationship between brain functions and what we think of as "the mind" has been a topic of philosophical and psychological research for generations, probably since humans started to be aware that they were humans. For the purposes of this book, I won't get into that. All we need to focus on, for the purposes of *Age Later*, is the idea that the health and performance of our body, skin, mind and brain are all intertwined. Looking after one component helps the others.

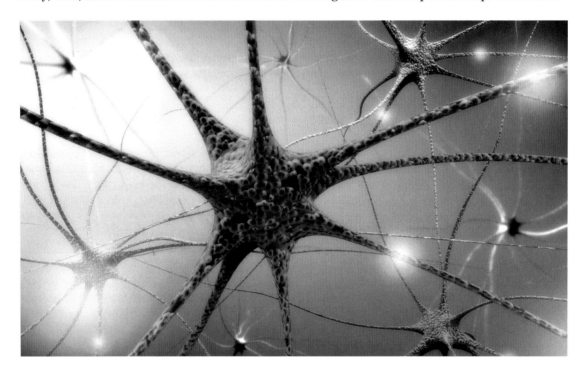

A PLAN TO MOVE YOUR BRAIN UP A NOTCH

Your brain is uniquely yours, so make the effort to draw up an action plan for brain health that's unique to you. Everything you decide to include in your mental fitness regimen should be a personal pleasure for you.

Earlier in this chapter, I provided suggestions for mindfulness, stress reduction and sleep. All of these contribute to the physical health of your brain at the same time as they build psychological strength and stability.

In earlier chapters of the book, I outlined healthy living choices for food and physical exercise. Following these choices will contribute to the health of your nervous system, just as they will improve skin and body health.

But there's even more you can do—and should do—to boost your brain's performance and extend its life. You can find ways to exercise your mental muscles that also result in measurable improvements to your brain cells.

Just living in a complex world exercises the mind. But sometimes things can get so complex that people's brains start to shut down instead of functioning at maximum capacity. In this section, I offer suggestions that will help you cope with that complexity, help prevent shut-downs, and also boost the long-term health of the brain.

THE WORKINGS OF THE HUMAN NERVOUS SYSTEM

We now know enough about the workings of the brain and the central nervous system to be confident that the onset of illnesses such as Alzheimer's and Parkinson's can be prevented or delayed if action is taken early enough.

So, let's do a deeper dive into those workings.

We tend to think of our brain as the control center of the body because that's where most of the conscious thought takes place, including how you're processing the information in this book. The brain is connected to the entire nervous system, which is spread throughout the body, and control of the body is distributed throughout that entire system. This vast network consists of your brain, the nerves in your spinal column, peripheral nerves everywhere else in your body, and your sensory system, which detects what's going on in the outside world and inside your body.

The body contains, and depends on, a complicated communications system, much like the Internet—except smarter and more reliable. Specialized body cells called neurons play an important part in building the communications infrastructure, connecting to the brain, to muscles, the sensory organs, and to the other organs of the body. Neurons are connected to each other through extensions called axons that send signals, and dendrites that receive them. The point at which a dendrite from one neuron connects to an axon from another is called a synapse. In addition, various endocrine glands (pineal, thyroid, adrenal and so on) signal their wishes by injecting chemicals into the bloodstream. In this way, our blood conveys chemical messages throughout the body, another part of the communications complex.

Using this network, the body can sense its own status and behavior, a process called interoception.

The external world provides its input through the sensing processes that allow us to experience the world: perception. Our perceptive senses enable us to see, hear, feel, taste and smell. Neurons capture this information and the collected data allows us to understand and navigate the world around us.

The nervous system constantly sends signals to motor neurons that trigger muscles to contract or relax. Other neurons (interneurons) act as relays to pass information throughout the nervous system to yet other neurons, sometimes to hundreds all at the same time.

Patterns of neuron connectivity within the brain and throughout the entire nervous system influence how we respond to stimuli and what we remember. As we acquire knowledge, the patterns of neural connectivity are constantly being modified and updated. Neuron patterns reflect who we are and what we know.

Neurons are plentiful in our bodies. A typical healthy human nervous system contains around 100 billion neurons of many different types.[195]

Neurons are not the only vital components in our nervous system. We also need to consider glial cells (or glia). Estimates vary, but it seems likely that there are at least as many glial cells as neurons in most human brains.[196] Not only are glial cells plentiful, experiments have shown that many brain functions depend not just on neurons, but on glia.[197]

Glia play a role in performing such housekeeping functions as managing the delivery of nutrients to other nervous system cells, cleaning up dead cells, building and maintaining the protective sheathing around axons, managing the creation of synaptic connections between neurons, and closing down neural pathways that seem to be redundant or unnecessary. Once again, if you don't use it, you do lose it.

Glia ensure the blood and oxygen supply to the brain is maintained.[198] Glia communicate with each other—and with neurons. They also eavesdrop on signals between neurons. The purpose of all this interaction is not entirely understood, but it seems clear that glia play some role in human brain functioning (and therefore cognition). Perhaps they contribute to logic, creativity and decision-making.[199]

Glia and neurons are widespread through the body, in the central nervous system and in the peripheral nervous system. So, as we think about brain health, we really need to think about the health of the entire nervous system, which reaches almost everywhere in our bodies.

What Can Go Wrong?

There are many ways in which the nervous system can become degraded: cells die; glial cells prune pathways but may make mistakes; axon sheathing may deteriorate faster than it can be renewed. Your nervous system is yet another collection of cells, so the entire nervous system can suffer from oxidation and inflammation, just like all the other cells in the body.

Feelings of stress and anxiety cause your nervous system to respond aggressively by producing adrenaline. If prolonged, severe stress can affect brain functioning, which can result in impaired concentration and reduced control of impulses.[200] Managing stress is an essential part of maintaining a healthy brain.

Damage to (or deterioration of) the nervous system can cause a wide range of problems, including slow reflexes, forgetfulness and confusion. These problems may be temporary, or sometimes they may be early symptoms of dementia, a broad label for a range of neurological diseases. Dementia is characterized by some or all of the following symptoms: severe memory loss, impaired reasoning, language difficulties, inability to focus and even personality changes. Dementia may be caused by cardiovascular disease, thyroid problems, trauma, vitamin deficiencies, or one of a number of diseases involving abnormal protein cells in the brain—specifically, Lewy Bodies disease (LBD), Parkinson's disease and Alzheimer's disease.

Actions You Can Take

Although symptoms of neurological diseases can sometimes be alleviated, once many of these diseases have taken hold, there is no cure. Still, some lifestyle changes can improve cognition and help delay (or even avoid) these diseases.

For example, a two-year trial in Finland (2014)[201] (FINGER project) revealed that changes to diet and exercise resulted in measurable improvement in cognition. It is also suggested that ongoing mental activity and social activity can play a part in maintaining the nervous system and avoiding deterioration. Many other studies confirm these findings. As a result, the Alzheimer's Association concurs with the notion that combatting cognitive decline requires a multifaceted and holistic approach.[202]

Research into nervous system health has identified a few key factors that together may delay, stop or even reverse, a decline in nervous system functioning. These include: active thinking and cognitive exercise, social interactions, stress reduction, physical exercise and nourishment.

Active Thinking and Cognitive Exercise

Active thinking is my way of describing the proactive aspects of our patterns of thought. This involves trying to solve problems, engaging in activities that work the brain hard, learning new skills and interacting in a positive way with human beings. (Interacting with animals can be helpful too.)

Why You Need Active Thinking

All active-thinking activities engage and exercise parts of the brain that are important for cognition; as you exercise these capacities, your powers of cognition improve. If you don't exercise these capabilities, they will grow weaker. The brain needs this type of mental exercise as much as the body needs its physical exercise. The value of mental workouts is increased when approached in a mindful way, with focus and awareness.

Stretching our brains slows the organ's aging. To improve brain performance, or even to maintain its current level of performance, we need to put the brain through some rigorous paces—and regularly.[203] As with your physical muscles, there are two complementary ways of doing this.

First, be mindful of how your normal everyday activities can be used to contribute to your daily cognitive activity, and take steps to introduce more thinking and more cognitive challenges into your everyday life.

Second, as with your physical muscles, take purposeful action in the form of regular mental workouts.

You need to do both to retain and build neurological health.

Mental Workouts

Mental workouts (or cognitive exercise) involve purposeful effort to tackle mental and intellectual challenges. Don't go easy on yourself. Just as with physical exercise, the intention is to challenge yourself and stretch your limits. Choose activities that challenge you in all these areas: memory, speed of thought, creativity, flexibility, focus and attention.

Regular mental workouts can take on a variety of forms. Your mental equivalent of the physical exercise machine might be solving a logic puzzle, a word puzzle or a crossword. Your workout might involve reading a detective novel, playing a computer-based brain game, or trying to solve a mathematical theorem or a problem in economics. There are many websites that offer tiers of increasingly difficult exercises and problems, some of which require pure logic skills and others that rely on quick reactions. Both can boost your cognitive capabilities.

You may decide to design or create things: clothing, electronics, woodwork, painting, sculpture, landscapes. The combination of mental effort and manual effort is particularly helpful.

Perhaps you read a lot or listen to music? Have you thought about stretching your brain by writing, or by playing music, or even composing music? When did you last attempt to paint a picture? We now understand that getting physical exercise is good for us even though our goal isn't to become a professional athlete. The same goes for the brain. These exercises are invaluable, even if you have no intention of playing the piano at Carnegie Hall.

Games played with others also provide useful exercise: Scrabble, bridge, chess and many others. If you play against another person (rather than against a computer program), you'll earn a check in the socialization box too, providing you don't take it too seriously. When a game ceases to be fun, or stops being a challenge, be bold enough to move on to something new to keep up the cognitive work-rate.

Most of all, try different things to stretch different mental muscles. If your mental exercise is too easy, then it's not exercise; only you can judge whether you're stretching or coasting. Exercise your brain regularly, and your mental muscles will grow in strength, your ability to focus and concentrate will improve—and you'll enjoy how good it all makes you feel.

Active Thinking in Everyday Life

Earlier, I suggested that you should find reasons to walk sometimes instead of driving the car.

Your mental fitness also demands, at times, that you choose the tougher path to make sure your brain is sufficiently exercised.

Your natural curiosity plays a huge role in this. Being inquisitive means not ignoring things you don't understand, always trying to find out more and constantly seeking answers. When your brain isn't being challenged, look for something more demanding. Tap into that desire for continuing knowledge. This process should never stop.

This mirrors what humans do in the early years of life. Babies, children and adolescents all have an innate urge to learn. Even as adults, we continue to experience new cognitive challenges—raising a family, balancing our budgets, learning new work skills, improving our athletic prowess, starting hobbies, taking an active role in a charity organization. When we're learning, and especially when we're working hard to learn, our brains remain flexible, and we're more likely to stay in good condition.

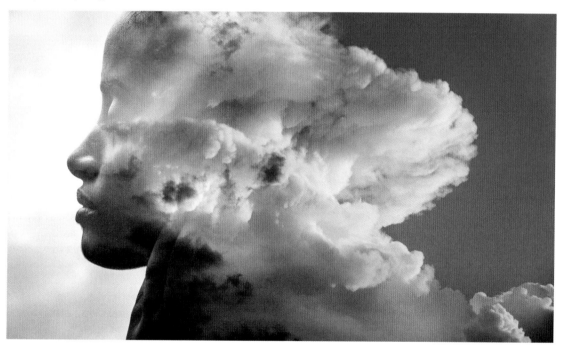

Then what happens? When people become older (maybe 30-something), they often develop the, perhaps, faulty notion that they have acquired wisdom. It's a dangerous time in our lives, especially if we ease off the throttle when it comes to learning.

A person might be bored at work yet fail to look for some way to make the work more exciting or mentally stimulating. If that's you, try and actively fight against boredom—because boredom is wasting your brain.

Do you do the same things every evening? Surf the same Internet sites? Watch the same TV shows? Read the same news sources? Listen to familiar music?

Perhaps some of us come to believe that getting older (by year count) necessarily and inevitably brings a reduction in cognitive ability and mental dullness. If you believe that, it will become true—and, in due course, you can wave goodbye to mental agility.

On the other hand, you can choose not to ease off: Keep up the mental effort. You can recognize that "old in years" does not mean "old in mental capability." With that attitude, you are well-positioned to keep learning, proving to yourself and others that our brains are big enough for the job at any age.

Here's an exercise that will, I hope, make you think. You probably know two or three people who, despite their years, seem to be just as mentally sharp as they always were. People, say, in their 80s or 90s? Engage one of these mentally agile individuals in conversation. Ask them what they like to do to fill their days. Take mental notes. At some point, ask them how they managed to stay mentally sharp. Learn from that.

My experience is that a universal characteristic of mentally agile older people is that they never stopped being curious, asking questions, learning things, doing things and interacting with other people. Perhaps your research results may differ; if so, you'll have learned something new. Plus, you will have stretched a mental muscle in the process.

At the same time, you'll have exercised yet another mental muscle, the one that enables you to get along with people, which is a nervous system skill too. Active thinking involves thoughtful discussions and debate with others.

It's called social interaction.

Social Interaction: Thinking Together

There is a connection between cognitive health and socialization. Exercising your mind proactively with others will stretch your mental processes more than exercising your mind in isolation.

For example, watching a play or movie, or reading a book, gives your brain something of a workout (which is a good thing). But it may be more of a gentle stroll around the park than a serious mental strength builder. If you read the same book, or watch the same movie, with the intention of discussing it with friends soon after, that will help you to be more mindful as you read or watch the film. You'll pay more attention to the content, the style and the hidden messages. Expressing and defending your opinions, and listening to the opinions of others, is all healthy for the brain. It helps the brain perform its basic functions: receiving information, processing and analyzing the inputs, identifying patterns, forming an opinion, and testing that opinion ... over and over.

The same kind of mental activity goes on when you play games, especially ones played with other people. Games played face-to-face with other humans add an extra layer of cognitive stretching, all of which is good. You not only have to work out the next move, but you have to engage with the other person's way of thinking to choose the best moves ... over and over.

"Over and over" is important for physical exercise, and it's important for mental exercise too. In interacting with others, you will be opening yourself up to a wider range of mental activities. Thinking in the company of others forces you to construct and reconstruct discussion points; it makes you focus on the way you think as well as on what you think. If you approach it with the right attitude, it should make you question the basis of your own opinions. These mental and social efforts will improve your brain functions.[204]

EXPANDING YOUR SOCIAL INTERACTIONS

For some people socializing is easy; for others it feels like hard work.

Even if you're someone who has plenty of friends and lots of opportunities to socialize, consider a review of your social habits. If you find yourself doing the same things with the same people, introduce some changes. Suggest new things to do together. Your relationships need attention and different stimulations to keep them fresh.

You can (and should) have social interactions of many different types. Socializing can be having a conversation with a complete stranger for a few minutes at a coffee shop, or meeting someone on a hiking trail, or joining a club of some kind. Or maybe it involves going on vacation with five close friends (and working hard to make sure everyone enjoys it).

You shouldn't expect every social contact to turn into a friendship. You should attempt to be mindful when you meet new people, look for value in the interaction without even thinking about potential friendship.

I suggest that you don't do things just to find friends. For example, don't just join a club or a class to find friends. Join up so you can pursue a deep interest or passion, and have fun sharing your knowledge with others. If doing that introduces you to some new friends, regard that as a bonus.

Every conversation starts with someone saying something. Make sure that the someone who starts a conversation is you—at least some of the time.

Also, don't forget to reveal your passions sometimes. If there are topics in which you are seriously interested and knowledgeable, mention them. But don't go on about those things if there's no positive reaction.

You don't have to socialize with people you don't like. Still, behave in a civilized way when you do have to talk with them. Not only is that the mature way to behave, but it also helps you manage your own stress levels.

Ask for advice. Sometimes you might feel that to keep your friends close, you need to be the one who always offer help. It turns out that asking someone else for advice (when genuinely needed) is a way of becoming closer to that person.

Finally, in the quest to get to know someone, don't act a part. Be yourself when interacting with others by being open about your preferences and opinions (without forcing them on others). Pandering results in unproductive or even toxic relationships.

Oh yes. And whatever you do, don't break the rules we're establishing in *Age Later*. Stick to your new habits, your good habits: healthy food, no smoking, zero or moderate alcohol.

Physical Exercise for the Brain

Physical activity improves cognition, to the extent that there is now some evidence that exercise can significantly lower the risk of neurological diseases, including dementia.[205]

Exercise will strengthen your heart and improve your blood circulation, and the brain is one of your biggest customers for oxygen in the blood. Increased blood flow also helps to clear out dead cells and unwanted substances.

Beyond the suggestions for exercise I provided earlier, it's worth noting that some physical exercises make heavy use of the nervous system components responsible for balance, coordination and spatial awareness. If you use those components regularly, those sensing organs will become more capable.

Other physical activities that engage functions of the brain when it comes to acquiring a complex skill, or solving a succession of tactical or strategic challenges, also boost cognition. Aim to take part in sports and activities that provide cognitive strengthening by exercising multiple areas of the brain at the same time you exercise multiple parts of your musculature and joints. Examples of enjoyable activities that provide this kind of multiple benefit include: yoga, tai-chi, badminton, squash, tennis and golf.

Food for the Brain

Brain health is linked to body health. This notion has been around for centuries,[206] and it is still true. Not surprisingly, the same foods and eating habits that are good for your body also are good for your brain.

The evidence is becoming stronger in favor of an eating regimen that benefits cardiovascular health, which in turn helps to maintain brain health.[207] This seems logical: A healthy heart and circulation delivers more blood and oxygen to the brain when it needs it. Also, a heart-friendly diet is rich in antioxidants and will prevent excess inflammation. This benefits every cell in the body, including the cells of the entire nervous system.[208]

The Finnish trial I mentioned earlier prescribed a Mediterranean diet. A Mediterranean diet features whole grains, fruits and vegetables, little or no red meat, fish and olive oil. This diet is rich in antioxidants, omega-3 and fiber. I also recommend eliminating refined sugar and refined flour products, and adding more fiber in the form of beans, peas and lentils (in addition to whole grains).

Some amino acids are now being more clearly associated with cognitive function. Food products rich in serine, for example, have been shown to protect the nervous system.[209]

Omega-3 fatty acids are very important to brain health. EPA can reduce symptoms of depression; DHA makes up about 8 percent of brain weight and is vital for brain development and functioning.[210]

Your brain also needs to be hydrated. Without enough water in your system, you will experience headaches, and you may find it difficult to concentrate. Serious dehydration can affect short- and long-term memory loss.

Our new and growing understanding of the role of stomach microbiome may eventually provide additional insights into how the condition of our own personal collection of microbes influences brain and nervous system health. We already know that the microbes in our stomach constantly interact with our bodies, and with other microbes, and release a wide mix of chemicals into our systems.[211]

Some research[212] confirms that several microbiome mechanisms can influence the functioning of the central nervous system, thus providing affirmation of findings that food intake (and, consequently, the health of the microbiome) has the capability of altering mood, pain sensitivity, and levels of stress and anxiety. It also can affect the path of normal brain development.

There are indications that differences in microbiome content may contain clues to the origins of neurological diseases, but that research is in its early stages.[213] Taken together, these early research findings suggest that a diverse and healthy microbiome containing a majority of bacteria that we know to be generally beneficial, may also affect brain and nervous system health.

All of this research provides evidence that the food recommendations in *Age Later* are valid—not just for general health, but for neurological health too. For confirmation, take a quick look at the MIND diet,[214] which has been formulated as a combination of the Mediterranean diet and DASH[215] specifically to delay brain and neurological degeneration. You'll notice that these recent recommendations for neurological health are broadly in line with the *Age Later* healthy living choices for food.

Protect Your Nervous System

Your Vulnerable Nervous System

Your nervous system is vulnerable to physical damage. Your brain, your sensory organs and your internal neural networks often are exposed to potential harm. Our bodies evolved to be fairly resilient against a wide range of traumatic injuries, but modern life has provided more means of physically injuring our nervous systems, as well as more ways of protecting them.

The nervous system can become permanently damaged by physical trauma caused by accidents or injury. This is of particular importance for the brain and spine: together they form the Central Nervous System (CNS).

The Peripheral Nervous System (PNS) is the term often used for everything in the nervous system apart from the brain and spine. Every part of the PNS is vulnerable, including the eyes, ears and the other sensory organs[216] that we use to perceive the world outside (as well as the sensors we use to track what's going on inside our body). Each sensing system consists of versions of your own unique human cells, connected to and working as a part of your whole nervous system.

The unhealthy substances you ingest can damage your nervous system (CNS and PNS); this is physical damage too, it just happens over a longer period of time.

Your nervous system may be less capable of repairing itself compared to other body parts. Break a leg, and in four to six weeks, you might be playing tennis again. At the very least, your chances of healing and returning to the courts are excellent. Damage your brain, just one time, and we can't be 100 percent sure of a happy outcome.

So please look after it.

Protect Your Neurological Assets

If you ride a bike or motorbike, if you climb mountains, or ski or snowboard—or do anything else where your head is vulnerable—wear a helmet. A good helmet can make the difference between a trivial event ending in some bruising and permanent vegetation.

One injury can be enough, but persistent small injuries will do damage too. In a survey (by autopsy) of 111 deceased National Football League players, 110 were found to have chronic traumatic encephalopathy, a neuro-degenerative disease linked to repeated head injuries.[217]

Is there a message there?

Your spinal column contains a big chunk of your internal communications, and when it's damaged, it's difficult to repair it completely. Most spinal injuries involve car and motorcycle accidents. (If you're a motorbike enthusiast, I probably can't persuade you to change that habit, but I can suggest that you ride carefully.) When you're in a car, wear a seatbelt. The seatbelt doesn't guarantee that you will not damage your spine or your head, but it will reduce the risk of damage and reduce the extent of likely injury. An airbag plus seatbelt combination is even more effective.[218]

Your senses also form part of your nervous system. When you discover that your sense of hearing or sight is impaired, it means that your sensory system cells have been damaged or are unhealthy. Protect your senses with sunglasses, goggles, dust masks and other sensible measures. You also should have the operation of all these senses professionally checked on a regular basis.

Avoid Substances That Damage Your Nervous System

Any bad habit that diminishes circulation reduces oxygen to your cells, which causes physical damage. Cigarettes, cigars, pipes, hookahs, joints, vapor sticks or anything similar will damage your brain, thus aging your nervous system more quickly. Assume that anything bad for your heart also will be bad for your brain.

Lead dissolved in water is a natural result of using lead pipes and soldered joints in water supply systems. Lead in water has been proven to damage the brain and nervous system.[219] Potentially, in some locations, there may be other substances in drinking water that can damage your neurons, such as mercury and other toxins.[220] Wherever you are, be safer by installing a water filter for your drinking supply.

All mind-altering drugs, by definition, alter the brain. That often means changing the physical state of your brain and nervous system. Some of those changes might be transient, but experts can't be sure. What experts do know is that habitual use of drugs will eventually damage your brain or nervous system. This is true whether the drugs are legal or illegal: They will all harm your nervous system eventually.

Drugs are not the only way to change your nervous system for the worse. Other addictions can create brain chemicals that also alter the nervous system. Visit my website (agelaterbook.com) for more about addictions.

Physical Exercise For Inner Peace

All physical activities are useful in tackling stress, but some exert an added calming influence, which takes even more steam out of the pressure cooker. If it feels less stressful it often is less stressful. That calming influence also helps to create a frame of mind with more resilience, so that events with high-stress potential actually turn out less stressful.

The calming effect of such exercises is achieved through requiring mental concentration in concert with physical movement. In all these activities, the benefit is maximized when you succeed in focusing exclusively on what you're doing and thinking during the activity. This level of concentration takes practice, which is why it's a good idea to work with a teacher, at least at first.

Exercises and activities that help to achieve calmness and reduce stress include:

- Yoga

- Tai chi and qi gong

- Mindfulness movement

- Walking in peaceful, beautiful surroundings

- Deep breathing

- Rhythmic exercises

- Massage

- Laughter

Earlier, we discussed mindfulness as a discipline for achieving focus in meditation, and for simply clearing the mind. Part of the skill in mindfulness is to achieve awareness of the present, and not to be distracted by random thoughts.

That same skill also is helpful in getting the most from these calming exercise activities. For example, when taking a stress-reducing walk in the park, focus on your surroundings and what is happening in the world of nature. Look at the people you pass with interest. Think about your own body and your breathing. Don't diminish the therapeutic benefit by devoting the time to thinking about work or planning dinner.

If you're being massaged to loosen up your body and your mind, then be mindful of what is happening to your body, and what is going on in your mind. Resist any thoughts of what you need to do at work tomorrow.

The same applies to all of these activities. Immerse yourself and focus for maximum benefit. Apply mindfulness methods to all of these activities.

The ability to focus on the now is a skill worth mastering; we never want our emotions to push us into situations where we're the cause of added, unnecessary stress. The physical and mental exercises suggested in *Age Later* can quiet our minds and help us find better ways to manage real-world interactions.

Chapter 9

In Conclusion

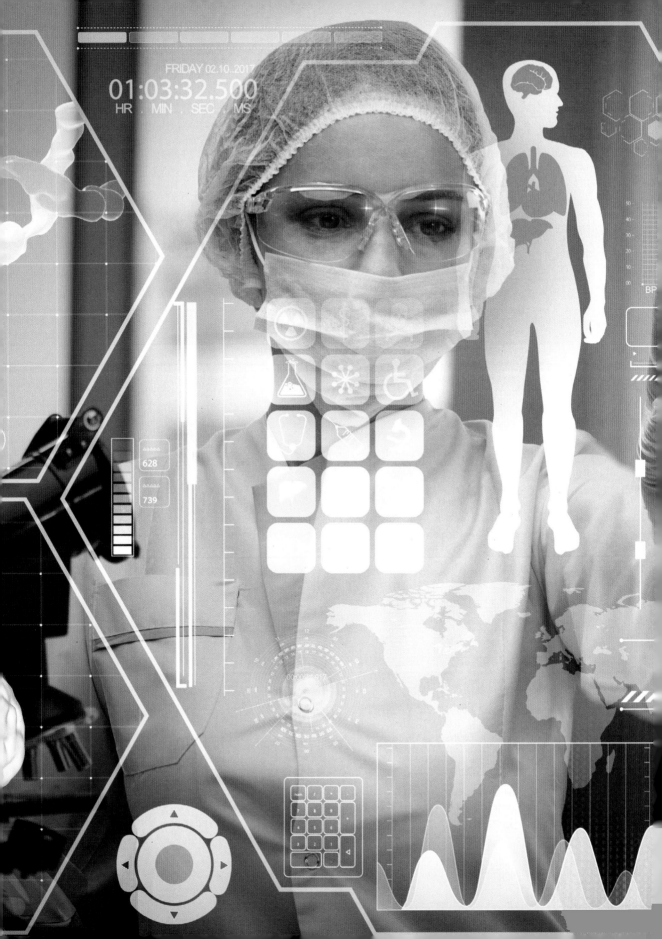

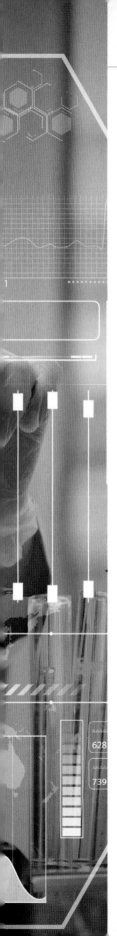

A Simple Message

If you want to look younger and live a longer life, then the *Age Later* program is your golden ticket. You're about to exchange bad habits for empowering, life-altering habits. Eat nutritious foods, and avoid beverages and substances that undermine your health. Exercise regularly. Take care of your skin, because it won't look after itself. Pay attention to the health of your brain, and seek a balanced and productive mental approach to the world.

How many of you have heard these suggestions before? Many of the ideas in *Age Later* have been promoted for years, so it stands to reason. But here's the question: Are you finally ready to listen? Are you willing to open your mind to the possibility of a new life—a better, healthier life?

Times have changed. Years ago, people said that smoking tobacco wasn't so bad, that eating lots of meat was essential for growth and health, that sunning yourself on the sand for hours offered health benefits, and that refined sugar was a great invention.

Today, we know which assertions are right, and which are mistaken. We know that exercise is vital to the body's needs and that tobacco kills. How? Through extensive experimentation and statistical analysis carried out over the years. Those long and detailed researches underpin all of my recommendations.

We now know so much more about how the body works, how it can flourish and what will accelerate and curb the aging process.

The evidence out there should give you confidence to take action, now.

What the Future May Hold

The process of scientific discovery hasn't come to an end. What comes next? No one can be certain, but here are just a few possibilities for you to mull over.

Gene Therapy

The last 50 years has resulted in significant advances toward our understanding of human genetics. With the mapping of the human genome, we have been able to identify genetic sequences associated with thousands of genetic-driven diseases. Now, with the development of tools and methods to investigate genes, edit DNA and replace genes in body cells, we are poised to move gene therapy from an experimental technique to a mainstream method.[221] Many diseases and conditions are not genetic in origin, so gene therapy will not work for those. But around 4,000 diseases are known to have some genetic component, including early-onset Alzheimer's, Huntington's and Parkinson's.

Gene therapy involves replacing small sections of DNA that are known to cause potential illness with segments that are not harmful. This is done with chemical editing tools such as TALEN and CRISPR.[222] The DNA is then embedded in body cells, which are transported to the appropriate part of the body. The cells grow and divide, spreading the repaired DNA naturally through all the cells in that area. It's even possible that replacement of all body cells will become common: By implanting the cells in bone marrow, cells with defective DNA gradually will be replaced with fresh cells that contain the edited DNA.

As gene therapy becomes mainstream, it will become safer, cheaper and more accessible. Then we can expect to hear discussions about other genetic interventions, to address non-life-threatening illnesses and conditions.

BIOELECTRONICS

Some people who have suffered chronic back pain for years are now walking around almost pain-free thanks to the insertion of a tiny electronic device in their lower back close to the spinal cord.[223] Spinal Cord Stimulation is now an established tool for alleviating certain types of back pain, but it is just an example of an early step in the area of bioelectronics. Blocking pain signals using electrical pulses can specifically target small regions of the body in ways that are not possible with drugs. Better still, the imbedded device is free of the dangers connected to some pain-killing medications, including addiction.

As researchers map the myriad pathways of the human nervous system, they not only will find out what nerves are involved in various human functions but also those that carry messages triggered by certain drugs, where those messages go, and how they affect different parts of the body.[224] Perhaps we can develop implanted devices that will block some of the signals created by drugs so that the drugs only affect the exact parts of the body that need that specific drug. The next generation of bioelectronics devices may even do more than just block signals: They may be able to simulate the signals of drugs and cause the same results with no chemicals.

This is all speculative, of course, but let's take this speculation one step further. Suppose someone is having problems managing food intake. They can't control their cravings for, say, sugar, pastries, alcohol or fried chicken, potentially causing severe and life-damaging problems. The vagus nerve carries messages from the digestive system to the brain. What if those messages can be monitored and modified with a bioelectronics device? Could we use bioelectronics devices to suppress cravings for fried chicken—and replace them with a craving for a spinach salad, with walnuts and olive oil?

Harnessing Microbes

The study of the complexities of our microbe started relatively recently with the initiation of the Human Microbiome Project, so we've only started to explore ways in which we can work with those microbes to improve health. Seeding our systems with new microbes is now common: That's what probiotic pills aim to do.

Yet, as our understanding of the roles of individual species develops, we may be able to produce more targeted specific microbial treatments—not just to cure illnesses but to generally improve health.

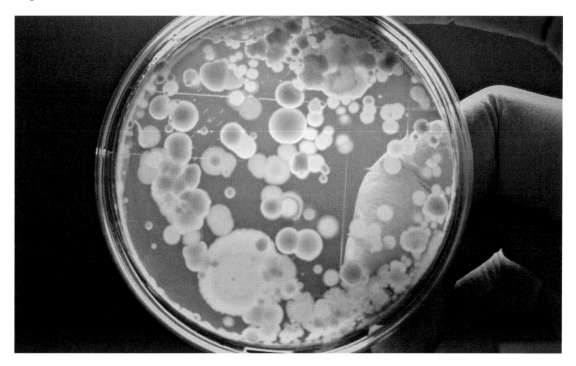

As we improve our understanding of each member of our microbiome (and their roles), we can expect to see some interesting developments. It's even possible, that we will find it useful to genetically engineer some of our microbe population to be less harmful, or more beneficial, or even to perform functions that we haven't dreamed up yet.

Still Learning About Cancer

We have made great strides in treating cancer, but we have yet to piece together the entire puzzle regarding its metastasis—that is, when the first cancer cells spread from the original tissue to other tissues. Detecting a cancer before that happens dramatically improves the chances of successful treatment.

Traditional thinking was that metastasis happens directly as a result of a specific cell mutation, and so identifying those mutations might lead to ways of preventing metastasis. Using genetic sequencing tools to search for those mutations revealed that a wide range of different cells could metastasize. Further research suggests that it's not a special mutation that causes metastasis, but that other factors such as the tumor's size and location come into play.[225]

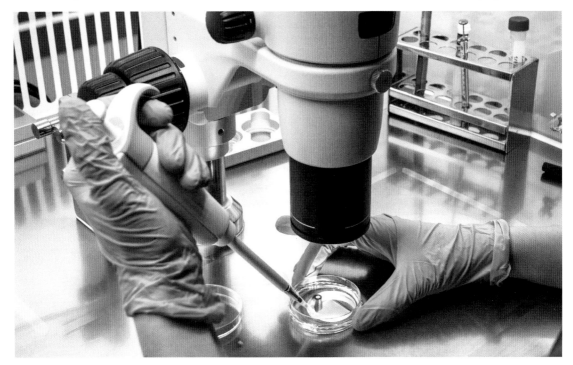

Moreover, we now know that the direct ancestors of cancer cells that eventually spread to other body locations may be present in a tumor months, years or even decades before metastasis. Sometimes, they can be identified at a point where a tumor would not be diagnosable.

This new model of metastasis was discovered by scientists from several different specialist disciplines working together: human biology, evolutionary science, gene sequencing, computer analysis and modeling (and probably others that I don't know about). No one can tell yet what new discoveries and interventions may develop from this work, which is continuing.

Real-time Monitoring

We already have access to wearable technologies that monitor basic metrics such as distance walked, heart rate and heart-rate variability. Continuous monitoring of other key biometrics is now common for people with heart disease or lung problems. The future will bring the ability to measure, record and analyze a range of human health metrics in real time, effectively providing us with a detailed blood chemistry panel combined with measurements of circulation, respiration and other life processes.

These future wearable devices will provide early warning of health problems, of course. However, they'll also allow you to monitor what happens to your body in response to your daily decisions. The metrics of your body functions change when you exercise more (or less). As you eat sugar-rich foods, you can observe your blood glucose rising. This will be a tool not so much to control your life minute by minute, but more of a feedback mechanism that will encourage more healthy living choices. Advances in artificial intelligence technologies can make these devices inexpensive and potentially (under your supervision) a smart extension to your own human feedback mechanisms.

The future will bring many more of these cross-disciplinary investigations and discoveries. As scientific methods evolve, so will our research into the mechanisms of aging and illness widen and accelerate. We have come a long way, yet there is still great potential for further discoveries.

LET'S DO THE MATH

According to the Organisation for Economic Co-operation and Development (OECD), life expectancy for the United States was 78.8 years in 2015 and 78.6 years in 2016—nearly two full years below the OECD average. So why are we going backward when most industrialized nations are seeing a yearly increase in life expectancy? In addition to an overall lack of mental well-being, experts point to the addiction crisis in this country as among the major reasons; between 2000 and 2014, there was a 137 percent increase in opioid-related deaths in the U.S.

However, as we have explored in *Age Later*, there are several other factors to consider. Though Germany's average life expectancy tops the United States by nearly two years (80.6), it lags behind other European countries. A European Union commission calculated that 28 percent of the burden of disease in Germany in 2015 could be attributed to behavioral risk factors—diet, smoking, alcohol and lack of physical activity.[226]

Based on research and hard scientific evidence, I've come up with my own calculations regarding longevity. Depending on the healthy living choices you make, I estimate that your individual life expectancy can fluctuate as much as 30 years.

Stop and think about that.

How long you ultimately live depends on decisions you make when it comes to exercise, mental health, skin care and nutrition. Each healthy or unhealthy living choice you make has the potential to add to your life expectancy—or subtract from it.

Depending on the deliberate choices you make in your day-to-day life—regardless of genetics, environment and other outside factors that you cannot control—you can decide to live one, two, five, 10, 20, maybe 30 years longer.

The blueprint is in your hand. Change your destiny.

The End of the Book,
The Beginning of Your Journey

You've reached the end of the main themes outlined in *Age Later* (there are still several appendices, packed with additional information, to complement those themes). But this is just the beginning of your journey. Please keep going. As you become healthier and more fit, return to the book periodically and make some additional healthy living choices, perhaps those that you felt were too daunting the first time round.

Even if at first you commit yourself to just a few important decisions, you will feel the benefits. Then you will feel enthusiastic to come back and do more.

One day soon, your friends will start telling you that you look great—and they'll ask you what you've been doing.

You'll say that you've been making some serious healthy living choices. Maybe you'll suggest the *Age Later* program to your friends—especially if they welcome the idea of looking better, and leading a longer, healthier and more active life ... after just seven weeks.

Here's to living younger, longer.

For additional information, frequent updates
and to share your experience, please visit agelaterbook.com.

APPENDICES

APPENDIX A: ALCOHOL CONSUMPTION

This is what the evidence is telling us about the links between excessive alcohol consumption and illness:

- Abuse of alcohol eventually will cause liver damage and may result in permanent damage when the liver cells are scarred beyond repair (cirrhosis).[227]

- Alcohol consumption increases the likelihood of throat and mouth cancer, even at low levels of alcohol consumption.[228]

- Alcohol consumption during pregnancy can lead to birth defects in children, and may be the leading cause of birth defects in the U.S.[229]

- Heavy drinking affects functioning of the brain and may cause permanent brain damage.[230]

- Consistent heavy drinking can result in significant weight gain,[231] and even moderate levels of alcohol in a high-calorie form (sweet cocktails, beer) eventually can cause weight gain.[232]

- Heavy drinking raises your blood pressure and creates an increased risk of cardiovascular disease.[233]

- Excessive alcohol consumption is linked to depression. In some cases, the depression may be caused by alcohol consumption; in others, the depression may have led to alcohol abuse, which could then lead to a reinforcement of the depression.[234]

- Heavy alcohol consumption increases the risk of Type 2 diabetes.[235]

The factors listed above directly address issues of illness, physical health and aging. They do not take into account the social, financial and mental problems that can accompany alcohol abuse or those afflicted with Alcohol Use Disorder, which amounts to around 7 percent of the adult population in the U.S. It also doesn't address the number of drunk driving deaths and injuries each year—and other deaths and injuries directly or indirectly related to alcohol consumption. Needless to say, it's impossible to defend excessive drinking.

On the other hand, light to moderate drinking (within the normal medical guidelines) does not seem to be associated with major health issues. In some contexts, it even may decrease the risk of serious illness. Note that these reductions do not compare moderate drinking with heavy drinking: The comparisons are between moderate drinking and abstinence.

- Moderate drinking may have some benefits for brain health, including reducing the risk of dementia.[236]

- Light to moderate drinkers (women) are likely to gain less weight over a long period than abstainers.[237]

- Light to moderate consumption of alcohol provides cardiovascular protection predominately through improvements in insulin sensitivity and HDL, resulting in less risk of cardiovascular disease.[238]

- Moderate alcohol consumption may reduce the risk of type 2 diabetes.[239]

- Red wine contains lots of antioxidants and may bring health benefits when consumed in moderation.[240]

- Beer and (to a lesser extent) red wine are good sources of available dietary silicon, which is good for bone health.[241]

APPENDIX B: PROTEINS, AMINO ACIDS AND DERIVATIVES

Alanine is one of the structural building blocks for a range of proteins. It is concentrated in meat and dairy products. Alanine does not have to be included in our food; the human body can use other amino acids to make it.

Arginine is an amino acid that is used to build proteins. All high-protein natural foods contain some arginine, and those foods usually contain some components the body can use to make its own arginine. Foods containing arginine include meat, dairy, poultry, pumpkin seeds, soy, chickpeas, lentils, parsnips and beets. Arginine relaxes and widens blood vessels and may prevent cardiovascular disease and ailments associated with blood circulation. Excess arginine may have some unacceptable side effects.[242]

Asparagine is an amino acid that is very common in both plants and animal proteins. Human bodies make asparagine from other nutrients. Plant sources of asparagine are asparagus, potatoes, nuts, legumes and soy. Excess asparagine is implicated in accelerating the spread of breast cancer, but there is no evidence that it causes tumors to form.[243]

Aspartic acid (aspartane) is an amino acid that can be synthesized in the human body. Natural foods that contain aspartic acid include fish, vegetables, dairy, whole grains, eggs, meats, beans, nuts and seeds. (Aspartame is an artificial sweetener that uses aspartic acid in the manufacturing process.)

Carnitine is found in almost all plants and animals. It is synthesized in the human body from the amino acid lysine and, in turn, is used in many metabolic processes.

Creatine is an amino acid that is made naturally by the human body in the kidney and liver, for which it requires inputs of the amino acids arginine, glycine and methionine (all available from a wide range of plant foods). Creatine is essential for muscle mass and muscle strength.[244] Creatine is stored mostly in muscles (including heart muscles) where it is readily available to contribute to the production of energy for the muscles. All mammals and fish make and use creatine, and so when we eat meat and fish we add to our creatine supply. There may be a role for creatine as a supplement for people who experience loss of muscle power as they age, but it should not be used over the long term; if you're taking other drugs, check with your doctor about how they interact with a creatine supplement.[245] Creatine is a very popular supplement among athletes and body builders, but overuse may cause problems.[246]

Cysteine is an amino acid that is used for cell-building, specifically as a source of the useful antioxidant glutathione. Cysteine is naturally present in meat and poultry, eggs, some dairy products (yogurt, whey, raw milk) and a variety of fruits and vegetables. In addition, your body can make some cysteine itself, providing it has a supply of foods containing methionine (eggs, sesame seeds, cheese, Brazil nuts, meat, fish, grains). Cysteine, usually in the form of N-acetyl cysteine, has a number of valuable medical uses,[247] but it has side affects and its use as a medicine usually requires medical supervision. Cysteine deficiency can have a genetic cause or dietary. Consuming cysteine supplements unnecessarily can cause a range of problems. My recommendation is not to supplement with cysteine unless you know you are cysteine-deficient—in which case, do so in consultation with your health advisor.

Glutamine, an amino acid that can be synthesized in the human body, plays a role in a number of important body functions. It strengthens the immune system, it's a source of energy for cells, it helps to build proteins—and more. A wide range of natural foods include glutamine: meat, fish, dairy, eggs, beans and a range of vegetables, fruits and grains.

Glutamic acid is an amino acid that can be synthesized in the body. It is present in almost all proteins. Natural sources of glutamic acid therefore include all types of meat, eggs and dairy products. It also exists in plant protein, and wheat gluten is high in glutamic acid. Mushrooms and walnuts also are good sources. Glutamates formed from the acid are concentrated in many traditional processed foods, such as hard aged cheeses, soy sauce, fish sauce and kombu.

Glutathione is a valuable antioxidant. It is derived in the body from the amino acids cysteine and glycine.

Glycine is an important amino acid, found in almost every part of the body: skin, connective tissue, nerves and muscle. Glycine is important for skin health, muscle development and nervous system functioning.[248] The body can make its own glycine from foods containing serine and threonine; it also can make use of glycine that occurs in food. Good food sources for glycine include fish, meat, dairy, beans, green leafy vegetables, cauliflower, cabbage, pumpkin, banana, kiwi fruit and more. There's a long list, so most healthy people can meet their glycine requirements from a balanced food intake. There may be a role for glycine in treating some ailments.[249]

Histidine (an essential amino acid) aids in the manufacturing of hemoglobin and blood cells, blood pressure regulation, and forming the myelin sheath that protects nerve cells—plus, it acts as an anti-inflammatory agent to protect tissues throughout the body. It can help resist infections, especially in combination with zinc. Histidine deficiency is linked to arthritis and a slowing down of the body's regeneration and repair mechanisms. Histidine is synthesized in plants and in microbes, but all animal products receive it from the plants they eat. Good sources are soy beans, chicken, beef, wheat germ, salmon, root vegetables and various leafy vegetables.

Isoleucine is an essential amino acid and is instrumental in converting food into protein.

It's involved in energy production and conversion, and regulation of blood sugar. It naturally occurs in all meat and fish, dairy products, seaweed and soy.

Leucine, an essential amino acid, helps to build and maintain muscle mass and other body tissues. It's available in meat, milk products and soy products.

Lysine is an essential amino acid that is involved in collagen building, calcium absorption and blood cell creation. The most abundant food sources of lysine are animal products: meat, poultry, eggs and fish. Cheese, nuts and soy also contain lysine. Sardines, Parmesan cheese and walnuts are especially high in lysine. Researchers are finding promising results regarding the role of lysine in the control of AGEs in diabetics and maintaining neurological function.[250] Lysine is popular as a cure for cold sores (herpes simplex). While this treatment has not been adequately researched in clinical trials, it seems that there may be a plausible mechanism for this to work.[251] For omnivores following *Age Later* guidelines, there is probably no need to supplement lysine. But vegans may find it a challenge to consume enough lysine without consuming a lot of calories. That problem can be addressed with adequate exercise.

Methionine is an essential amino acid involved in the production of protein; building blood vessels; growing healthy hair, skin and nails; and tissue repair. It also contributes to DNA and RNA production. Food sources include eggs, seeds and nuts (especially Brazil nuts), fish, meat and grains. It is required for the absorption of selenium and zinc.[252] The body also can use methionine to produce cysteine.

Phenylalanine is an essential amino acid found naturally in milk, cheese, eggs, nuts, meat and soy. Phenylalanine increases noradrenaline (norepinephrine), which supports cognition, memory and nervous system health. Phenylalanine can be used by the body to make tyrosine, which may have a protective effect against anxiety and depression.

Phosphatidylserine is a phospholipid present in cells throughout the human body. It is present in cell membranes and is essential to brain health and cognitive functioning. It also plays a role in blood clotting. It is present in many plant and meat foods, but it also can be derived within the body from serine and fatty acids.

Proline is an amino acid used in protein-building. It is common in meat products and plants, but the body also can make it from glutamate.

Serine is an amino acid that plays a part in building protein in the body and the brain. There is some evidence that serine might help to protect the nervous system.[253] Serine is one of the amino acids that the body can use to make glycine, which is of importance throughout the body. (The body also can reverse the process and make serine from glycine and threonine.) The body uses serine to make phosphatidylserine, an ingredient in the nerves' myelin sheaths. While serine is important, too much serine can be toxic to the nervous system.[254] Serine, like most amino acids, is plentiful in meat and fish products, including cheese and eggs, but some plant products are rich in serine too: seaweed and marine algae, dark green leafy vegetables, tofu and soy products, many seeds (carob, chia, mustard, sesame, pumpkin, squash), chickpeas, peanuts and whole grains. A healthy food plan should deliver sufficient serine.

Threonine is an essential amino acid and is one of the amino acids that the body can use to make glycine, which is of wide importance throughout the body. Threonine also may play a role in nervous system functioning and is prescribed as a medicine for some nervous system disorders. Most high-protein foods are natural food sources of threonine: nuts and seeds, seaweed, fish, shellfish, meat, eggs, soy, leafy green vegetables and dairy products. Avoid threonine deficiency by consuming a wide range of protein sources.[255]

Tryptophan: Your body uses tryptophan (along with vitamins B3 and B6) to synthesize serotonin, which regulates appetite, mood, sleep and pain. Tryptophan can be administered to encourage relaxation or sedation. Conversely, deficiency can result in anxiety, depression or even symptoms of dementia. Tryptophan occurs naturally in dairy products, soybeans, meat, fish and grains.[256] Tryptophan is an essential amino acid.

Tyrosine is capable of crossing from the bloodstream into the brain, where it is used to make adrenaline, which directly affects alertness and well-being. Folic acid (vitamin B9), copper and vitamin C also are involved in the process of making adrenaline. While tyrosine along with vitamin C can make you happy and awake, in the absence of vitamin C, tyrosine may result in lethargy. For full benefit from tyrosine in your food, don't forget the vitamin C. Tyrosine is a precursor for thyroid hormones and melanin. Tyrosine can be obtained from protein-rich foods: cheese, soy products, meat, fish, seeds, nuts, eggs, milk products and grains. It also can be synthesized within the body from Phenylalanine.[257]

Valine, an essential amino acid, is involved in building muscles and in repair and restoration of tissue. It helps to maintain a healthy nervous system and therefore supports mental alertness and coordination. It also encourages relaxation and calmness. Like most other amino acids it can be found in soy products, milk products, meat, fish and vegetables.[258]

APPENDIX C1: VITAMINS

Vitamin A helps prevent UV damage, stimulates skin cell renewal and encourages fibroblast production, which helps make your skin firm and resilient. Your daily intake of dark green, red and orange vegetables provides beta-carotene, which your body readily can convert to vitamin A. Eggs and dairy products also contain vitamin A. With a healthy food intake, food supplementation of vitamin A typically isn't necessary. You should have a blood test to measure your vitamin A levels before deciding to supplement.

Vitamin B1 (Thiamine) is found in many foods: grains, beans, nuts, seeds, yeast and meat. There are several medical uses for thiamine, including digestive problems, boosting the immune system and neurological health. Most people get enough thiamine in a varied food plan. When thiamine deficiency is diagnosed, supplements are available either as part of a B complex or in a multivitamin.[259]

Vitamin B2 (Riboflavin) is an antioxidant and plays an important role in energy conversion and red blood cell production. Riboflavin is naturally present in many foods: organ meats, poultry, dairy, vegetables (especially leafy greens), fresh fruit, almonds and mushrooms. It's also added as a supplement to some processed foods such as breakfast cereals and breads. Riboflavin needs can be met easily from a varied diet, but if supplementation is necessary, it seems that every multivitamin and protein shake contains riboflavin.[260]

Vitamin B3 (Niacin) is found in green vegetables, grains, beans, nuts, seeds, milk, eggs, yeast, meat and fish. It's added as a supplement to some processed foods such as breakfast cereals and breads. There are several medical uses for niacin, including diabetes, skin-condition problems, circulation problems, neurological disorders and much more. Most people get enough niacin in a varied food plan. When a niacin deficiency is diagnosed or suspected, supplements are available either as part of a B complex or in a multivitamin.[261]

Vitamin B5 (Pantothenic acid) plays a vital role in metabolism and cell formation. B5 is needed to support all life processes; it's available in many plant and animal foods, including beans, eggs, milk, meat, mushrooms, and in varying amounts in almost all vegetables. That said, I still recommend that everyone take a B complex supplement that includes B5.

Vitamin B6 (Pyridoxine) is involved in brain and nervous system development and health. Food sources include fish (sardines and salmon, especially), meat, poultry, organ meats, nuts, seeds, lentils, starchy vegetables (including potatoes), chickpeas, bananas and fruits (except for citrus products).[262] A varied diet including these foods should provide enough vitamin B6 for a healthy person. Supplementation may be prescribed for kidney diseases and some other conditions.[263]

Vitamin B7 (Biotin) is an important vitamin because the body does not hold it in reserve. B7 supports enzyme activity, so it's involved in conversion of food to energy, extraction of nutrients from food, and providing nutrients required for healthy hair and skin. B7 also plays a role in ensuring healthy nervous system functioning, and it may help with mental processes. B7 in sufficient amounts is needed to make use of the muscle-building amino acids leucine and isoleucine. You'll find B7 in a variety of foods, so there shouldn't be a need for supplementation except in special circumstances (pregnancy, genetics) or illness. Biotin is available in small quantities in just about every plant food. Larger amounts can be found in organ meats, egg yolks, oily fish, almonds, sweet potatoes, oatmeal, bananas, apples and cheese. Because of its presence in many foods, problems due to insufficient biotin intake are rare.[264][265]

Vitamin B9 (Folate, Folic acid) plays an important role in building DNA and healthy cells. It's vital to nervous system health and helps reduce the chance of Alzheimer's. Supplements usually contain folic acid, which the body can convert to folate. We know folic acid deficiency is linked to birth defects, so it's almost standard for pregnant women to supplement natural sources of folate with folic acid supplements. For everyone else, food sources of folate should be sufficient. Try green leafy vegetables, broccoli, peas, grains, tomatoes, bananas, apricots, cereals and meats. Moderate folic acid supplementation is beneficial for everyone, especially pregnant women, but excessive amounts will not provide extra protection—and too much might be harmful.[266]

Vitamin B12 is a group of nutrient compounds that all contain the element cobalt (so the B12 group is sometimes referred to as cobalamins). Vitamin B12 supports some essential body processes: DNA synthesis, renewing red blood cells, and neurological functioning. Foods containing vitamin B12 are all animal-derived products: fish, meat, poultry, eggs, yogurt, cheese and other dairy products. Bacteria that synthesize B12 can be found in the stomach. Some processed foods such as breakfast cereals and bread may be fortified with vitamin B12. Vitamin B12 deficiency may cause fatigue, anemia, loss of appetite and weight loss. Severe cases may cause neurological problems and, eventually, nerve damage.[267] Omnivores and lacto-vegetarians should be able to easily ingest sufficient B12, because the quantities required are very small. It's recommended that vegans eat B12-fortified products or B12 supplements made from bacterial action.[268]

Vitamin C is widely available in all fruits and vegetables. It's a powerful antioxidant and essential for cell health throughout the body. In the normal course of events, a healthy human should be able to obtain plenty of vitamin C from a varied food intake that includes lots of plant foods. But when vitamin C is low, the body becomes more vulnerable to common virus-based illnesses, such as the common cold and influenza. Low vitamin C levels also impede the production of adrenaline, resulting in lethargy. Obtain as much vitamin C as possible from your plant food intake; plant material brings additional nutrients and co-agents that enhance the utilization and effectiveness of the vitamin C. It's worth keeping your vitamin C levels boosted with moderate supplementation.

Vitamin D can be synthesized in the skin, as part of a response to UV in sunlight. Because it can be made in the human body, it's no longer regarded as a true vitamin but as a hormone. However, most people still call it a vitamin. Either way, it's important. Vitamin D plays a key role in cell repair, antioxidation, thyroid functioning and in balancing immune reactions, which guards against Crohn's disease and inflammatory bowel disease. Food sources of vitamin D include milk products, eggs, liver and oily fish. Ideally, if people eat a wide selection of foods containing vitamin D, and spend some time outside, then they should have enough in their system. Still, vitamin D3 deficiency is common, even among people who are exposed to sunlight every day. You are likely to be one of the people whose lifestyle, metabolism and skin sensitivity work together to keep your vitamin D levels low. If so, vitamin D supplements are necessary. My advice: Have your vitamin D levels checked, and take supplements if necessary. Vitamin D supplementation is much better than risking skin cancer by overexposing the skin to UVB rays.

Vitamin E is a group of eight related compounds; they're all effective antioxidants that can help combat free radicals and reduce the chance of Alzheimer's. Vitamin E supports skin health, helps protect the nervous system, protects against heart disease and stroke, and may protect against Alzheimer's. Vitamin E is naturally available in seeds, nuts, fruits and leafy green vegetables.[269]

Vitamin H (Biotin): Another name for vitamin B7.

Vitamin K is a group of vitamins that the body uses to build bones and manage coagulation of the blood. Adequate intake of vitamin K helps to avoid osteoporosis and heart disease. Vitamin K1 is available in green leafy vegetables, avocados and grapes. Because vitamin K is fat-soluble, the addition of oil (salad dressing) can increase absorption.

APPENDIX C2: VITAMIN-LIKE NUTRIENTS

There are a few nutrient substances that do not easily fall into any of the main categories of nutrients. These are often described as "vitamin-like" because of their role as antioxidants or coenzymes, but they are synthesized within the body—so, strictly speaking, they're not vitamins.

Choline performs a wide range of valuable functions in the body related to chemical messaging, cell integrity and synthesis of other nutrients. Your body can make some choline itself but not enough, so supplement with food; choline is one of the constituents of lecithin, a fatty substance found in a wide variety of plants and animals.

CoQ10 (also called coenzyme Q10 or ubiquinone) is an antioxidant and coenzyme that helps to reduce and repair cell damage, supports cell functioning, and plays a role in a number of metabolic processes. Every part of your body needs CoQ10, and its presence (or absence) affects every cell. CoQ10 plays a role in recovery from cardiovascular illness, and slows the progress of neurological diseases. Low levels of CoQ10 are associated with cognitive decline, diabetes and cancer. Your body makes CoQ10 itself, and also absorbs it from meat, fish, whole grains, and some fruits and vegetables. It is common for CoQ10 levels to decrease with age, so you should use CoQ10 supplements if your micronutrient blood test shows that your level is too low.

Inositol is a nutrient that works to support cell functioning, chemical messaging, gene expression, immune system health, cell membrane health, insulin utilization and much more. Your body can absorb inositol from many natural plant and animal foods, including fruit, grains, beans and nuts. Your body can make additional inositol from glucose especially from foods containing lecithin. Inositol was once designated vitamin B8, but because the body can make its own inositol, it is no longer formally classified as a vitamin.

Lycopene is a carotenoid phytochemical that is common in tomatoes as well as some other red or orange fruits. It has been suggested that it has an antioxidant benefit for skin, prostate and heart health, but the evidence not conclusive.

Vitamin D can be synthesized in the skin, as part of a response to UV in sunlight. Because it can be made in the human body, it's no longer regarded as a true vitamin but as a hormone. However, most people still call it a vitamin and so, for now, I've included it in the list of true vitamins.

APPENDIX D: MINERALS AND TRACE MINERALS

Calcium is good for bones and, in the correct quantity, it's one of the minerals (along with magnesium) that helps to control blood pressure. Calcium occurs naturally in dark green leafy vegetables and in dairy products. Anyone who does not eat dairy products may have difficulty consuming the recommended minimum daily amount, which is 1,000 milligrams for most adults, and 1,200 milligrams for women age 50 and older, and men 70 and older. Calcium supplements are available as calcium citrate and calcium carbonate; the citrate version is generally easier to absorb. Adequate levels of vitamin D are required to absorb either type fully. If you need to supplement calcium, it's convenient to use tablets that combine calcium, magnesium, plus vitamin D. And don't forget to exercise; calcium plus exercise builds strong bones. Too much calcium, that is more than three or four times the daily dose, can seriously interfere with your sodium levels and cause a wide range of adverse reactions, including headaches, thirst and fatigue (all symptoms of dehydration).

Chloride in the body comes from sodium chloride (common salt) and potassium chloride. Chloride ions, which are negatively charged, work with positively charged sodium and potassium ions to provide a balanced electrolyte system that conducts electrical signals throughout the body. Supplies of electrolytes are needed to maintain stability in the system, or else dehydration may occur. Normal food contains quite a lot of salt, so no need to reach for the table salt. In the event of dehydration (for example, following extra-strenuous exercise), you may need to drink a properly balanced mix of rehydration salts to fix the problem.

Chromium is required in very small amounts as an agent that is involved in the conversion of food inputs (carbs, fat, and proteins) into energy for use by body cells.

Cobalt: See vitamin B12.

Copper works along with iron to form red blood cells and is essential for immune system and nervous system health. It also is involved in collagen production, so adequate copper supports the health of skin and joints. Copper, along with tyrosine and vitamin C, is instrumental in the creation of adrenaline, which is needed for mental alertness and a sense of happy well-being. Copper deficiency can contribute to anemia, thyroid problems and neurodegeneration, but too much copper can cause damage to the brain and nervous system. Healthy humans with a balanced food plan are rarely deficient in copper. Good food sources of copper include nuts, dark leafy greens, yeast products, beans, whole grains, oysters and organ meats.

Fluoride in natural trace quantities (in the form of calcium fluoride or sodium fluoride) is absorbed into the body much the same way as calcium chloride or sodium chloride. The portion that is absorbed ends up in bones and teeth, and the fluoride embedded in teeth reduces dental decay. The portion that is not absorbed is excreted. The fluoride added to public water supplies is in the form of hydrofluorosilicic acid, which supplies the same fluoride ion but in a different molecular package. This has been the topic of raging controversy for decades.

Iodine is essential for good thyroid health. Poor thyroid functioning has been associated with skin conditions such as alopecia and (speculatively) vitiligo. Iodine is a natural component of fish and shellfish, kelp and seaweed, dairy products, eggs and meat. Iodine can be found in some plant-based foods, but the amount depends on the iodine content of the soil in which the plants are grown. Some table salts are supplemented with iodine and iodine tablets also are available. Most omnivores will have enough iodine as part of a normal healthy diet; vegans may have to take supplements. If you have concerns about your thyroid condition, see a doctor before taking iodine supplements.

Iron, a key component in your red blood cells, is instrumental in transporting oxygen from your lungs to all the cells in your body. Healthy people can obtain sufficient iron from food sources, like green leafy vegetables (spinach, kale), beans, lentils, nuts and seeds, meat, liver, shellfish and fish. To help absorb iron efficiently, consume lots of vitamin C foods too. Iron deficiency is a major problem worldwide. Although healthy people generally can find enough iron in food, there is a range of problems that can push a human body toward iron deficiency (anemia). In those cases, iron supplementation may be part of the remedy.

Lithium, in the form of lithium carbonate, is a naturally occurring trace mineral that appears in tiny quantities in drinking water, and in most fruits and vegetables. The amount in your food depends on the amount of lithium in the soil where the plants grow. Lithium in trace amounts is good for brain functioning and nervous system health—and may protect against Alzheimer's and other neurodegenerative diseases. Medically, lithium is used in much higher concentrations for certain psychiatric disorders. In even higher doses, lithium is toxic.

Magnesium is involved in many body processes, including building bone mass and muscle, making DNA, healthy nerve functioning, and managing blood-sugar levels. A shortage of magnesium can lead to fatigue, migraines, gum disease, anxiety and muscle weakness. Foods that contain magnesium include dark green leafy vegetables (chard, spinach), pumpkin seeds, yogurt, almonds and beans. Adequate magnesium is essential for health, but it may be difficult to obtain sufficient amounts just from food. Alcohol, sodas and refined sugars tend to deplete magnesium. Obese people often do not absorb enough magnesium. Heavy exercise that induces sweat causes a loss of magnesium (as well as other minerals)—so, for an active adult, some supplementation is needed. Although too much magnesium can cause dehydration-like symptoms and an irregular heartbeat, supplementation of around 400 milligrams per day should be safe for most adults.

Manganese is a mineral needed by the body in very small amounts. It's found throughout the body, in bones and major organs. Low intake of manganese can result in a variety of symptoms from general weakness to bone disease and seizures. Normal healthy adults should have no difficulty deriving sufficient manganese from a healthy mixed diet. It's available in nuts, seeds and whole grains. Obtaining manganese just from food, without supplementation, is recommended because too much manganese can cause neurological disorders.

Methionine is an amino acid, important for protein creation, cell building, and healthy cell functioning. The most plentiful sources of methionine are meat, fish, eggs, poultry and dairy products. Plant products that contain methionine include sesame seeds, Brazil nuts, walnuts and whole grains. Omnivores following *Age Later* guidelines certainly will consume enough methionine, perhaps more than enough. Vegans will naturally ingest less methionine than omnivores, but there is no evidence that this is a problem. Indeed, there is some evidence that a low methionine diet may increase life expectancy. Too much methionine can be unsafe.

Molybdenum acts as a cofactor to activate enzymes that perform essential maintenance roles in the body, including preventing the accumulation of sulfites, and breaking down cell debris and toxins (such as aldehydes and alcohol) so they can be excreted as waste. Molybdenum is plentiful in many foods; the body only requires small amounts, so molybdenum supplementation is rarely needed.

Nickel supports iron and zinc absorption and also is involved in the production of adrenaline. Nickel deficiency slows body growth and decreases red blood cell production, causing anemia. Nickel in trace amounts is available in many plants, especially beans, lentils, nuts and whole grains. Seafood (mussels and oysters) and chocolate also contain nickel. Some people are allergic to nickel and must avoid these foods. In higher doses, nickel can be toxic.

Phosphorus plays a role in energy storage and conversion. It's an essential part of your bone structure and is one of only four chemical elements found in DNA. Adequate intake of phosphorus is essential for strong bones and teeth, as well as correct functioning of your metabolism. The most ready sources of phosphorus are dairy products (milk, cheese, yogurt). Fish is rich in phosphorus, and beef, turkey and chicken are good too. Non-animal sources of phosphorus are beans, lentils, seeds and nuts and whole grains. Note that plant-based phosphorus is in phytate form, which is less easily absorbed. Adequate vitamin D intake helps to improve phosphorus absorption from plant sources.

Potassium along with sodium, provides positive ions that support the operation of the body's nervous system. It is vital for the normal operation for many of the body's major organs, including the heart and kidneys. Potassium occurs naturally in many foods, especially bananas, citrus fruits, milk, nuts, avocados, and leafy green vegetables. While sodium tends to increase blood pressure, potassium tends to reduce it, so eat more bananas.

Rubidium is a highly reactive metallic element that can sometimes replace phosphorus in the human body in small quantities (since, chemically, it's very similar). That said, it appears to have no specific function of its own. There has been some research into the use of rubidium chloride as a treatment for depression, but there is no strong evidence that such supplementation has value.

Selenium is an essential mineral that is known to be important in trace amounts for thyroid health. It also has antioxidant properties, so it might have some other roles in protecting against inflammatory diseases. However, more clinical research is needed in this area. Foods that generally are rich in selenium are Brazil nuts, some meats, halibut, oysters, brown rice and other grains, and eggs. Note that the selenium content in products can vary widely depending on their source.

Silicon is a mineral that is now known to be important for bone formation. There are indications that silicon from food can be instrumental in protecting against loss of bone mass as we age. Silicon is abundant in nature, mostly in the form of silicon dioxide (silica): It's a component of most rocks and sand, yet it is only required in the human body in trace amounts. Fortunately silicon is readily available in many plant foods: oatmeal, whole grains, bananas, mangoes, green beans, spinach and other leafy green vegetables, beets and other root vegetables. Once again, a vegetable-rich diet should provide sufficient silicon for a healthy adult. Research interest in silicon has grown with recent findings that we can absorb it from plants and use it in the formation and maintenance of bones and the integumentary system (skin, hair and nails).

Sodium is a trace element in food, in the form of sodium chloride. Both sodium and chloride are vital for health, in small quantities. In the body, sodium is an electrolyte that supports the operation of your nervous system and your heart. For balanced nutrition, cut out added salt; your food intake should provide enough. Too little sodium causes symptoms of dehydration and ultimately can be life-threatening. Too much sodium causes high blood pressure and increases the risk of strokes and heart disease.

Vanadium is a trace mineral in the human body, but its value to humans is uncertain. It may be there as a result of eating plants and animals that contain the mineral; vanadium compounds are water soluble and widely distributed in the soil. Vanadium compounds in concentrated quantities are generally toxic to humans and other mammals. In nature, vanadium has become concentrated in some sea creatures (sea squirts and their close relatives) and in some fungi, where the vanadium compounds may act to repel predators. There is some suggestion that vanadium can reduce blood-sugar levels in diabetic patients. Vanadium may be more common in our food than ever as a result of mineral mining and petroleum extraction; even if it's of value, it's doubtful we need supplements. Foods that contain vanadium include mushrooms, shellfish and grains. Most plants contain vanadium in trace quantities.

Zinc deficiency can contribute to skin problems, as zinc assists in the process of building collagen. You can add enough zinc to your diet simply by following the *Age Later* food guidelines, in which case supplements aren't necessary. While it's important to consume enough zinc, that doesn't mean the more the better. Too much zinc intake can cause iron deficiency and gastric problems. Natural foods that contain zinc include oatmeal, cashews, almonds, kidney beans, chickpeas (garbanzo beans), seafood (oysters, lobster, crab) and most fresh meats.

APPENDIX E: HIGH-NUTRIENT FOODS

These are some of my favorite nutrient-rich foods. On their own, they don't constitute a full meal, but incorporate them wherever possible.

Include walnuts, almonds or Brazil nuts in your morning muesli or oatmeal. Try cinnamon or turmeric in your smoothies. Include spices or aromatic herbs in every evening meal. And if you must have a between-meal snack, consider one of these foods rather than a commercial snack.

Almonds are rich in minerals and antioxidants, especially polyphenols and vitamin E. Eat a few almonds every day instead of supplement pills for vitamin E, manganese, magnesium, copper, riboflavin and phosphorus.[270]

Blueberries: All readily available berries are nutritious; they're loaded with antioxidants. Blueberries are near the top of the list.

Brazil nuts: Use Brazil nuts as a supplement instead of pills to boost your intake of calcium, copper, magnesium, selenium and thiamine.[271] Brazil nuts are our richest source of selenium; four or five nuts per day will deliver most of your daily selenium requirement.

Carrots are a rich source of beta-carotene, which, in turn, provides vitamin A. Eating carrots and other strongly colored fruits and vegetables daily can meet your vitamin A needs.

Cinnamon contains powerful antioxidants and helps lower blood-sugar and cholesterol levels—plus, it fights inflammation.[272] If you're at risk of heart disease or other inflammatory diseases, it might be beneficial to take up to a half-teaspoon of cinnamon per day as a supplement (mixed into a drink or smoothie). Use the Ceylon cinnamon (Cinnamomum zeylanicum) and not the cassia version.[273]

Curry powder is a mixture of turmeric, cumin, cayenne, coriander and sometimes cinnamon and allspice. A good quality curry powder can be used in small quantities to enliven and add nutrients to almost any vegetable dish (and in larger quantities to make a real curry).

Fermented foods: Fermentation of food by the action of enzymes or bacteria produces some remarkable changes. Often, new and valuable nutrients are synthesized in the process: omega-3 fatty acids, vitamin B and useful enzymes. When not subjected to further cooking, the fermentation agents add to your friendly stomach bacteria. In other words, fermented foods are natural and useful probiotics. Almost any food is capable of being fermented, but some taste better than others. Most countries in the world have created fermented foods of one sort or another. Milk becomes yogurt, kefir, buttermilk and a host of products around the world. Cabbage becomes sauerkraut and kimchi. Beans are transformed by fermentation into tofu, soy sauce, bean curd, bean paste and much more. Lots of meat and fish products are fermented too. Some pickles undergo a fermentation. Tea leaves are subjected to different degrees of enzymatic oxidation during the drying process. Cocoa beans are fermented before they become chocolate, which is one of the reasons that unsweetened chocolate is a nutritious food.

Flaxseed (also known as linseed) has been recognized as a healthy food for centuries. It contains high levels of omega-3 fatty acids, lignins (which have an antioxidant effect), soluble fiber and insoluble fiber.

Garlic can help your immune system fight against everyday illness (coughs and colds), reduce blood pressure and lower LDL levels ("bad" cholesterol). Its antioxidant properties help fight inflammatory diseases. Garlic contains allicin, lots of trace minerals (manganese and selenium), vitamin B6 and vitamin C. Garlic also contains fiber, which is converted into butyrates—that's food for your good bacteria.[274]

Gelatin helps the body build collagen. Taking collagen itself requires the body to break down the collagen into components and rebuild it again, so consuming gelatin is a traditional alternative. Gelatin is made by boiling down collagen from animal sources. This makes gelatin a convenient and energy-efficient source of the chemicals needed for building collagen in the human body for non-vegetarians.

Ginger is high in antioxidants and long has been known to aid digestion and reduce nausea. Ginger root can be consumed fresh or dried, in a tea or as a spice in food. It is known to reduce inflammation, and there is evidence that regular consumption can lower the risk of colorectal cancer.[275]

Ginkgo is made from the leaves of the ginkgo biloba tree and has a long history of use in traditional medicine. It improves blood flow to the brain and limbs, and it's credited with alleviating many circulation-linked diseases (especially problems of the nervous system)—as well as boosting cognitive function.

Ginseng is made from the roots of various members of the Panax genus. It has been used for centuries as a general tonic, mild stimulant and energizer. There has been very little modern research on the effectiveness of this traditional remedy, but millions of regular users worldwide are convinced that it works. It can be taken as a tea, or as an extract in pill form.

Green tea is rich in antioxidants and has been shown to combat oxidative stress throughout the body, especially in the brain. Regular consumption of green tea can reduce blood cholesterol levels, reduce blood pressure and lower blood-sugar levels.[276]

Linseed: See flax seeds.

Nuts and seeds: All nuts and seeds contain a range of amino acids, minerals and fatty acids that are essential to cell health.[277] Nuts and seeds are a convenient way of getting lots of nourishment in one small package. I encourage you to add nuts and seeds to your daily food plan. You have plenty of choices: almonds, Brazil nuts, chia seeds, flax seeds, hazelnuts, pecans, pumpkin seeds, sesame seeds and walnuts.

Peppers: Bell, birds-eye, cherry, cayenne, habanero, jalapeño, serrano, srirachi (and others) are all high in antioxidants and therefore fight inflammatory diseases.

Rosemary is an anti-inflammatory that also quiets allergies.

Sage is a traditional preventative for almost all common disorders. Recent research indicates that sage may reduce symptoms related to neuropsychological disorders.[278]

Turmeric is high in curcumin, a powerful antioxidant and anti-inflammatory. The spice has been used for hundreds of years as a remedy for a variety of ailments. Today, it is recognized as helping to reduce the risk of inflammation-related diseases, including diabetes, arthritis, acne and psoriasis. Turmeric is available in tablets, but it's easier to keep a jar on hand and add it to different recipes (not just Asian dishes)—and even to smoothies.

Walnuts are a great source of amino acids, minerals and other nutrients. They're also at the top of the list for polyphenol antioxidants. Use walnuts as a supplement instead of pills to boost your intake of these minerals: copper, iron, magnesium, manganese and phosphorus. Around six walnuts will give you 25 percent of your daily quota of manganese. Everyone can benefit by supplementing their morning muesli with a helping of walnuts and their full range of protein-building components, including lysine and methionine, plus omega-3 fatty acids and minerals. I recommend walnuts for everyone, not just vegetarians.[279]

Yogurt is a good source of calcium, magnesium, potassium, vitamin B2 and protein for non-vegans. It also contains a population of live bacteria that boost your stomach flora, acting as a natural probiotic. Always make sure the yogurt you buy contains multiple strains of live bacteria, no added sugar and no artificial flavoring. Many people who cannot consume other milk products because of lactose-intolerance find they can eat yogurt and other cultured milk products such as buttermilk and kefir.

Appendix F: Gluten and Lectin

Gluten

In recent years, we have seen more and more people convinced (by intensive marketing campaigns) that they are sensitive to gluten. Certainly, there are people with celiac disease (an estimated 1 percent of the population of the United States) who suffer when they eat food that contains gluten, and they must follow a gluten-free diet. Extensive research in recent years has revealed that there are genetic markers for celiac disease, and clinical tests have identified antibodies associated with the condition.

Reported sensitivity or allergy to gluten in individuals who do not have celiac disease is now called "non-celiac gluten sensitivity" (NCGS).[280] I'm skeptical about this condition, because there is no convincing evidence that this is a genuine widespread problem. Most people who follow a gluten-free regimen have not been diagnosed with NCGS. In fact, diagnosis of NCGS is more along the lines of a trial-and-error approach. The range of symptoms attributed to NCGS is wide, from digestive disorders to eczema to forgetfulness. All of these symptoms may be caused by other conditions (for example, poor stomach microbiota health or excessive mental stress),[281] and unless those have been considered and excluded, going gluten-free may not be effective. Moreover, it may cause harm by reducing intake of nutrients and fiber.

My guess is that the majority of people who eat only gluten-free foods are doing it unnecessarily. I suggest any non-celiac who has digestive issues, instead of experimenting with excluding gluten, should first follow the *Age Later* food guidelines, especially when it comes to focusing on fresh vegetables and fruit, and eliminating refined sugar and white flour.

Lectins

Another novel condition (possibly a fad) is lectin intolerance. I recognize that high levels of lectin consumption are bad for everyone, and it's true that some plant foods naturally contain high levels of lectin. This includes some grains, beans, lentils, peas, tomatoes and eggplants. In fact, there are no naturally occurring foods that do not contain some lectins, and low levels of lectin are easily tolerated. There is some research that some lectins in small quantities can be beneficial.[282]

Some people avoid all beans, peas and lentils because, when uncooked or undercooked, they contain high levels of lectins, proteins that are known to cause stomach irritation and digestive problems.[283] Small amounts of lectins do not seem to cause a problem for most people.

The mechanism for lectin toxicity is still not fully understood, but it's known that lectin can pass through the gut unaffected by digestive enzymes and can bind to cells in the stomach lining, interfering with cell maintenance. Since just about every animal and plant food source contains some lectins, it's not easy to avoid that substance completely.

Dried beans are mature seeds: The maturing and natural drying process increases the levels of lectin in the seeds. On the other hand, fresh, immature beans and bean sprouts have much lower levels of lectins. It makes sense to remove most of the lectins from both dried and fresh beans. You can do this easily by properly cooking them, or by choosing fermented bean products instead.

Those foods that are high in lectins are traditionally cooked thoroughly, and with good reason. Proper cooking dramatically reduces lectins to a low level that humans can handle without problems.

Fear of lectins is not a good reason for denying yourself useful foods.

GLOSSARY

The glossary provides brief details of some of the more technical terms used in the book and other terms where clarification may be needed. This glossary does not include information about specific substances such as vitamins, minerals and proteins, which are listed separately in the Appendices.

Addiction	Addiction is compulsive use of drugs or other substances and may also be applied to some mental habits, such as compulsive gambling or game playing. Physical dependence is often but not always associated with addiction.
Adrenaline	A hormone generated by the adrenal gland in response to stress. Adrenaline boosts heart rate, blood circulation and respiration, preparing the body for action.
Advanced Glycation End products (AGEs)	A wide range of chemicals produced as a result of the bonding of sugars with fats and proteins (glycation). In the human body, certain AGE have been linked to age-related diseases. AGE can be ingested in foods, and can also be created within the body.
Aesthetician	A trained and certified specialist in the care of skin, hair and nails.
AGE	See advanced glycation end products
Alcohol	Ethyl alcohol is the intoxicating ingredient in wine, beer, liquor and other fermented drinks.
Alcoholism	An addiction to alcohol.
Allergy	A severe or damaging immune system reaction to exposure to a food or substance in the environment.
Antibacterial	A substance that kills bacteria, used in some cleaning products.
Antibiotic	A medicine designed to stop or slow the growth of targeted microorganisms (bacteria) within the body. Antibiotics are not effective against viral infections.
Antioxidants	In the body, antioxidants are nutrients that act to reduce the oxidizing effects of free radicals, thereby helping to prevent cell damage.

Antiviral	A medicine designed to stop or slow the growth of specific viruses within the body.
Apoptosis	A body process for the programmed death of body cells when they become unneeded or damaged.
Appendix	In the body, a branch of the intestine at the junction of the small intestine and large intestine. It is thought to play a role in immune system health.
Archaea	An ancient type of single-celled organism, similar in some way to bacteria, but archaea have no cell nucleus. They are widely present in nature, including in the human microbiome.
Artificial sweeteners	A substance that provides sweetness, like sugar, but with no nutritional value.
ATP	Adenosine Triphosphate, a source of energy used by body cells for many purposes, including building proteins.
Bacteria (singular: bacterium).	Bacteria are single-celled organisms widely present in nature. Some are essential to human well-being. Others can cause illnesses in humans.
Base pair	The information inside DNA is coded chemically using just four chemicals (or bases): adenine (A), guanine (G), cytosine (C) and thymine (T). A base pair consists of either a combination of A+T or of C+G. The sequence of base pairs in our DNA forms a code that can be replicated in new cells, and in new individuals.
Bio-electronics	The use of electronic products to directly influence biological processes in the body, often by stimulating or blocking nerve signals.
Body Mass Index (BMI)	Body Mass Index is a standard way of measuring a person's weight relative to healthy standards, thus giving a rough indication of body fat content. BMI is measured by the formula W/H*H where W is the person's weight in kilograms and H is their height in meters. The NIH publishes an easy-to-use BMI calculator. BMI is an accepted standard measurement method in most countries. BMI is not the only way of measuring (or estimating) body fat. Several others are widely used, for example the Waist to Hip Ratio (WHR).
Body Mass Index Categories	BMI categories are defined in the U.S. and most other countries as: BMI less than 18.5 = Underweight BMI between 18.5 and 24.9 = Normal BMI between 25 and 29.9 = Overweight BMI 30 or more = Obesity.

Calorie	A measure of the energy content of foods.
Capillaries	Tiny blood vessels; the smallest blood vessels in the body
Carbohydrates	Carbohydrates are chemical compounds containing carbon, hydrogen and oxygen. Foods containing large amounts of these compounds, in the form of sugars, starches and cellulose, are also called carbohydrates, and these are a source of energy for the body.
Cardiac arrest	Cardiac arrest is a result of a malfunction of the electrical signals reaching the heart. This causes irregular heartbeat (or stoppage) and disrupts the blood flow to the brain, lungs and other vital organs.
Cells	A cell is a microscopic component of an organism. In any complex organism (such as a human body), cells of many different types form all of the tissues and perform vital functions.
Cellulose	A carbohydrate found in the cell walls of plants.
Chromosome	Chromosomes contain the genetic material that defines certain characteristics of living creatures. Humans have 23 pairs of thread-like chromosomes inside each cell nucleus. Each chromosome is a bundled up, loose-ended thread of DNA. (See also genes and DNA).
Cleanser (skin care)	A skin cleanser is used instead of soap. Non-soap cleansers allow the skin to retain more natural oils and are less likely to cause dryness and provoke allergic reactions.
Cognition	Thought processes associated with building knowledge, understanding and mental skills.
Collagen	Collagen is a strong and flexible protein that is contained in connective tissue in the human body. Along with elastin, collagen gives skin its elasticity, and joints their spring and resilience.
Connective tissue	In the human body connective tissue holds our body organs, muscles and bones together.
Corneocytes	Dead skin cells in the outermost layers of skin. The dead cells help to make the skin resistant against damage and infection.
Cosmetic surgery	Cosmetic surgery aims to enhance appearance through surgical methods.
Cytoplasm	The content of a cell enclosed within the outer membrane—but outside the nucleus.

Dependence	See physical dependence.
Dermis	A layer of skin tissue that connects the upper layers of skin to the body tissues below, such as muscle and fat.
Diabetes	Diabetes mellitus is a range of conditions related to production of the hormone insulin, which plays a role in converting food to energy. If the body produces no insulin, sugar in the bloodstream can't be converted to energy. This is typical of Type 1 diabetes. In some cases the body produces insulin but is unable to use it because of insulin resistance, which is common in Type 2 diabetes. There are other forms of diabetes, but Type 2 and Type 1 together account for the majority of cases.
Diabetes: Type 1	Type 1 diabetes often appears early in life and may be associated with a genetic pre-disposition. The pancreas fails to produce sufficient insulin, and the symptoms can be alleviated with insulin injections. There is no cure, as yet.
Diabetes: Type 2	The most common type of diabetes is Type 2 diabetes, in which both insulin resistance and failure to produce enough insulin both play a role. Type 2 diabetes is predominantly caused by diet and lifestyle.
DNA	DNA is deoxyribonucleic acid. DNA is the material that contains genetic codes in humans and other organisms, including all animals and plants. In humans, DNA is present in all body cells (apart from blood cells). Most human DNA is located in the cell nucleus (nuclear DNA) in the form of chromosomes. A small amount of DNA is contained in our mitochondria.
Double helix	The structure of DNA is often described as a double helix. Two strands of sugar-phosphate are connected by base pairs to form a long spiral ladder.
Electrolytes	Ions in body fluids that are vital to normal body functioning. Too much or too little of these substances can be dangerous. Electrolytes include bicarbonate, calcium magnesium, potassium, sodium ions.
Enzyme	Enzymes are proteins that act to support or speed up chemical reactions in living organisms. The human body relies on many different types of enzymes for healthy survival.
Elastin	Elastin is a spring-like protein that is one of the components of the connective tissues in the body. It stretches and (when young and healthy) quickly springs back to its original shape.
Epidermis	The skin's epidermis consists of layers of living tissue within the skin lying below the surface cells.
Exfoliate, Exfoliation	Exfoliation is a scrubbing or chemical process that removes the outermost layer of dead skin cells. Exfoliation improves skin health and appearance.

Extrinsic aging	Extrinsic aging is caused by external factors, and is not primarily genetically determined. External factors include everything in our environment: the effects of sun and wind, pollutants in air, water and food, and what we ingest (food, drink, drugs, smoke). Extrinsic aging affects all body cells, but the term is most often used in the context of skin aging, as the damage to our skin is visible to everyone.
Free radical	When a covalent bond in a molecule is split apart as a result of some chemical process, one or more of the products may be potentially highly reactive. Conversion of food to energy in the body creates such reactive components: free radicals. In excess, they can react with the fabric of human cells and cause damage,
Fungus (plural: fungi)	Organisms that reproduce using spores, including mushrooms, molds and yeasts.
Gene	A gene is the basic unit of heredity. Each gene is a section of a chromosome that defines one or more heritable characteristics, which are coded in specific sequences of DNA base pairs.
Gene expression	Gene expression is the process in which the coding in genes results in physical development or changes in the body. The degree of expression can be influenced by external factors such as nutrition and environment.
Gene therapy	Gene therapy is a method of treating or preventing disease by directly changing genes. This may involve implanting healthy genes to replace mutated genes, deactivating specific genes or inserting new genes.
Genetic engineering	Genetic engineering involves the direct chemical modification of genetic coding in genes. The modified genes can be implanted in living cells as part of a program of gene therapy, or to breed plants and animals with improved characteristics.
Germ	"Germ" is a general purpose word that has been applied to many different types of organisms, from the young sprouts of plants, to a virus or bacterium that initiates a disease.
Glycation	Glycation occurs when a sugar molecule bonds with a protein or fat. It is the first step in the process of creating advanced glycation end products.
Heart attack	A heart attack occurs when the blood supply to the heart is impeded resulting in a lack of oxygen to the heart muscles. The physical damage to the heart causes chest pain, breathlessness and other symptoms. A heart attack is not the same as cardiac arrest, but it can cause cardiac arrest.
Heart inflammation	See Myocarditis.

HGP (Human Genome Project)	The Human Genome Project (HGP), initiated in 1990, was a collaborative effort to map the entire structure of genes in the human body, by determining the exact sequence of billions of base pairs on every strand of human DNA.
HMP (Human Microbiome Project)	The Human Microbiome Project (HMP) was initiated in 2008 by the U.S. National Institutes of Health (NIH) to improve understanding of the microbial flora involved in human health and disease.
HRV (Heart Rate Variability)	Heart Rate Variability is a measure of how well your heart keeps pace with your body's needs. In an active body, your heartbeat rate should always respond quickly to changing needs, going faster as soon as you work hard, getting slower quickly when you're resting. A high HRV measure shows that your heart is coping well.
Human microbiome	The collection of microbes that live in and on human beings; the genetic makeup of those microbes.
Hydration	Hydration is the process of adding moisture. The human body is mostly water, and maintaining adequate levels of water in body cells is vital for health.
Immune system	The human immune system provides defense against diseases by attacking pathogens. It consists of a large number of organs and processes, including many types of white blood cells (leukocytes) located in various lymphoid organs.
Inflammation	Inflammation in the body is part of a normal immune system response as protective agents gather around damaged or diseased cells. Inflammation can become a problem when it becomes chronic or excessive, as this signals that the immune system may be overreacting or targeting body cells unnecessarily.
Integumentary system	The integumentary system protects the inside of the body from the outside environment and includes human skin, nails and hair. Some animals have additional integumentary components: scales, feathers, claws and hooves.
Intrinsic aging	Intrinsic aging is a degenerative process that takes place over time at a rate determined largely by genetic factors. It is sometimes referred to as chronological aging. See also extrinsic aging.
Meditation	Meditation is a mental discipline that aims to provide mental clarity and awareness. The practice also can relax the body physically and reduce psychological stress.
Meiosis	A multistage event in the sexual reproduction process which results in sex cells (eggs or sperm) containing a selection of genetic material (DNA), which then are available for the egg fertilization stage.
Microbe	A general term for microscopic organisms, including bacteria, viruses, protozoa and archaea. Some microscopic fungi and algae also may be described as microbes.

Microbiome	In general, a microbiome is the collection of microbes in a defined environment.
Microbiota	The collection of microbes in a specific location.
Micro-organisms	Microscopic organisms. See microbe.
Mindfulness	Mindfulness is a mental discipline of being fully aware and accepting of one's thoughts and sensations in the present moment. Though mindfulness originated as a meditative technique, psychologists increasingly recognize it as a beneficial practice.
Mitochondrion	An organelle inside each body cell that works to maintain correct functioning of the cell.
Mitochondrial DNA	Mitochondria DNA is located inside each mitochondrion in every human cell.
Mitosis	As one step in the process of cell division, mitosis involves division of a cell nucleus resulting in two nuclei each containing a copy of the DNA contained in the original cell. The mitosis stage comes after DNA replication and before complete cell division (cytokinesis)
Moisturizer (skin care)	A skin-care product that supplies moisture to the skin and helps to retain moisture.
mtDNA	Mitochondrial DNA.
Mutation	In genes, a change in DNA that arises randomly or due to damage. Specifically a mutation causes a change in the sequence of base pairs within a gene.
Myocardial infarction	A heart attack.
Myocarditis	Inflammation of the heart muscle responsible for pumping blood.
Nucleus (cell)	In the center of a human cell, enclosed in its own membrane, is a core region that contains the cells nuclear genetic material, in the form of DNA arranged in chromosomes
Obesity	The U.S. National Institutes of Health defines obesity as having a body mass index (BMI) of 30 and above.

Organelle	A functionally specialized component within a cell.
Pathogen	A microorganism that initiates a disease or disorder in humans. Pathogens include disease-causing bacteria, viruses, prions and fungi.
Physical dependence	Physical dependence on a substance (drug, alcohol, tobacco) occurs when the chemistry of the body and the drug interact to both increase tolerance to the effects of the substance, and create physical and mental pain or stress during withdrawal. Physical dependence is often associated with addiction, but it is possible to be addicted without being dependent on an ingested substance; it's also possible to be dependent on a substance without being addicted.
Plastic surgery	Plastic surgery generally focuses on the repair and reconstruction of disorders and damage using surgical methods. The aim is to improve both function and appearance.
Processed (food)	Processed foods are products that are designed for a long shelf life, easy transportation, and quick and convenient preparation in the home, at modest cost. Generally the processes and added ingredients used to achieve these objectives result in a product that is lower in nutrients and higher in damaging substances than we need as humans to live and thrive.
Procrastination	Avoidance of doing a necessary task.
Psychology	The science of the human mind, cognition and behavior.
Public Health and Public Sanitation	Public Health is all about maintaining a healthy environment for everyone. That includes sanitation (clean water supplies, effective sewage and waste treatment and disposal), health education, and disease and accident prevention measures.
Serum (skin care)	A skin-care serum is a liquid skin treatment that contains nutrients and anti-aging agents. Compared to traditional creams and lotions, serum products omit thickeners and heavy moisturizers, so that the concentrated active ingredients are not prevented from penetrating the skin.
SMAS	Superficial muscular aponeurotic system (SMAS) is an area of muscles in the face underlying the skin.
SPF	Sun Protection Factor (SPF) provides a guide to the effectiveness of sunscreen products. The higher the SPF, the greater the protection. SPF30 means that it (in theory) increases the time you can spend in the sun by 30 times. The SPF number is measured under lab conditions and assumes the user has applied it exactly according to directions and re-applies it frequently.

Stem cells	Stem cells have the potential to take on a range of different functions as they grow and divide, according to genetic instructions or environmental influences.
Stratum corneum	The stratum corneum is the outermost layer of the skin that acts as a barrier to help retain moisture and prevent pathogens
Stroke	A stroke is a type of brain damage caused by a disruption in the supply of oxygen and nutrients to brain cells.
Sub-cutaneous tissue	Subcutaneous tissue is sometimes called the hypodermis. It is the innermost layer of skin and contains fat, blood vessels, nerves and connective tissue.
Superficial muscular aponeurotic system	See SMAS.
Telomere	Telomeres are the end sections of each strand of nuclear DNA. They do not contain genetic data so when a DNA strand shortens (with replication) the telomere protects the data in the main length of the strand.
Telomere shortening	Telomeres become shorter with each DNA strand replication. After multiple replications, the telomeres do not fully protect the genes, which is why telomere shortening is linked to a wide range of age-related diseases.
Toxins	Toxins are poisonous or damaging substances derived from or created by plants or animals. They can be present in foods, or created within the body from ingested substances. (The term is often used for substances like lead or arsenic.)
Ultra-violet radiation	Ultraviolet is a section of the non-visible light spectrum. UVA, UVB, UVC are different wavelengths of ultraviolet, each of which has a range of different impacts on human skin cells.
Virus	A virus is a tiny organism that infects the cells of living organisms. When a virus penetrates, it is able to replicate very quickly and interfere with normal cell functioning. Cell death and/or replication helps to spread the virus within the body.
Vitamins	Vitamins are organic compounds (not minerals) that are essential in small quantities for human health. Vitamins cannot be created by human body organs, and so they must be ingested in food, or in food supplements.
Waist-to-Hip Ratio (WHR)	Waist-to-Hip Ratio is a simple measurement that provides a scale that approximates body fat content. The ratio is waist measurement divided by hip measurement. The World Health Organisation considers that obesity is represented by a WHR of above 0.9 for males or above 0.85 for females. See also: Body Mass Ratio.

INDEX

REFERENCES

This reference list provides additional information and references to sources and further reading. Some of the web links provided are quite long and complicated, so to make this information more accessible, I've provided a list of links on my website, agelaterbook.com, where you can simply click the links to reach the sources.

I recognize that the Internet is always changing, and so over time some of the links in your copy of the book will expire. So as a service to readers, we will do our best to keep the web version up to date so you always have access to useful further reading.

1 Radiation from terrestrial sources, such as naturally occurring radon, have health implications. Radon is the second-largest cause of lung cancer in the United States, after smoking, and kills more people than drunk driving. If your home has not been radon tested in recent years, you should probably arrange a test. (**epa.gov/radon/citizens-guide-radon-guide-protecting-yourself-and-your-family-radon**) Radiation in the form of galactic cosmic rays and nuclear particles from the sun are of much less significance for people on Earth, as we are protected to some extent by the atmosphere, the sun's magnetic field and the Earth's magnetic field. (**swpc.noaa.gov/phenomena/galactic-cosmic-rays**)

2 CDC overweight statistics: IHME: **healthdata.org/news-release/vast-majority-american-adults-are-overweight-or-obese-and-weight-growing-problem-among**

3 Mediaeval life expectancy: **news.bbc.co.uk/2/hi/health/241864.stm**

4 Life expectancy USA 1900: **cdc.gov/nchs/data/hus/2010/022.pdf**

5 Stephen Paget: **nature.com/milestones/milecancer/full/milecancer01.html?foxtrotcallback=true and ncbi.nlm.nih.gov/pubmed/17191105**

6 An example of confirmation of the "soil and seed" model: **ncbi.nlm.nih.gov/pubmed/7388794?dopt=Abstract&holding=npg**

7 Metastatic cancer: **cancer.gov/types/metastatic-cancer**

8 You can read more about the meiosis process here: **nature.com/scitable/definition/meiosis-88**

9 Red blood cells do not contain a nucleus or organelles, so they do not carry any DNA. An adult human typically has around 20 trillion or more blood cells, so they easily outnumber the other cells in the body.

10 How many cells in the human body? (2013) **ncbi.nlm.nih.gov/pubmed/23829164**

11 We obtain 23 chromosomes from our mother and 23 from our father. So, that means we have two sets of instructions, in 23 pairs of chromosomes. Because chromosomes come in pairs (one in each pair from the mother, one from the father) there are always two possibilities for hereditary features. Usually the outcome depends on which genes are dominant (or, to put it another way, which genes fail to be expressed). Most of the chromosomes (22 pairs) carry genes that define or predispose the human to have certain physical characteristics. The 23rd pair defines the sex of the recipient. Sex chromosomes are coded X and Y, and females have two X sex chromosomes (XX); males have one X and one Y sex chromosome (XY).

12 DNA cannot be seen clearly through an optical microscope. The structure of DNA was discovered using X-ray crystallography, and modern electron microscopes can now reveal a lot of the structure. **newscientist.com/article/dn22545-dna-imaged-with-electron-microscope-for-the-first-time**

13 Those four chemicals (bases) in the rungs of DNA (represented by code letters A, B, G and T) are adenine (A), cytosine (C), guanine (G), and thymine (T).

14 The pairs of chemicals are either A-T or C-G.

15 Each DNA strand also contains a lot of other chemical rungs that don't define genes. Some of that material is possibly no more than a legacy from our prehistory and may be of no importance. But some may be relevant; really, we don't yet know. Researchers are finding clues that may implicate non-coding material in inhibiting or promoting certain diseases. I don't want to speculate, but this is a line of inquiry that may bear fruit at some point in the near future.

16 ATP is adenosine triphosphate.

17 Mitochondrial waste products include free radicals and other reactive oxygen species (ROS).

18 Sugar and neural mitochondrial health: **news.yale.edu/2016/02/25/sugar-rush-shrinks-brain-cell-powerhouse**

19 Revised estimates for human and bacteria cells in the body: **ncbi.nlm.nih.gov/pmc/articles/PMC4991899**

20 **sciencemag.org/news/2016/07/microbes-our-guts-have-been-us-millions-years**

21 Bacteria that synthesize vitamins: **now.tufts.edu/articles/microbiome**

22 The Human Microbiome Project: **commonfund.nih.gov/hmp/programhighlights**

23 How the Gut's "Second Brain" Influences Mood and Well-Being: **scientificamerican.com/article/gut-second-brain**

24 Genes associated with late-onset Alzheimer's: **mayoclinic.org/diseases-conditions/alzheimers-disease/in-depth/alzheimers-genes/art-20046552**

25 The Human Genome Project (HGP), initiated in 1990, was a massive collaborative effort to map the entire structure of genes in the human body. The challenge of HGP was to determine the exact sequence of all those billions of base pairs on every strand of DNA. Every human's personal genome is slightly different, which is why we are all slightly different from the day of birth. How different? Around 99.9 percent of our genomes are exactly the same. The impact of HGP has already been huge. The existence of a genome map allows us to identify which tiny changes within genes are correlated with human characteristics and predispositions. With a map, exploration can continue at a faster rate, and is doing so. As a result, we are now acquiring and making use of insights into the role of genes in many aspects of disease, dysfunction and, indeed, aging. **www.genome.gov/11006943/human-genome-project-completion-frequently-asked-questions/**

26 Estimates for the role of genes in aging vary. Most recent estimates put genetic influence in the range of 20 percent to 30 percent (for example, **ncbi.nlm.nih.gov/pmc/articles/PMC4822264**).

27 Genetic changes are not always a bad thing because change is fundamental to the mechanism driving biological evolution. If the gene mutation affects an egg cell or a sperm cell, the change (for good or bad) will be passed on to the offspring. If the offspring survives long enough to breed, then that change will be retained in future generations, whether it is a beneficial change or a serious problem. Most cellular damage does not affect egg cells or sperm cells, so it is not passed on to the next generation. What is a gene mutation/how do mutations occur: **ghr.nlm.nih.gov/primer/mutationsanddisorders/genemutation**

28 In bacteria, each DNA strand forms a circle, and a circle has no loose ends, so the problem of telomere shortening doesn't occur in bacteria.

29 Some cells can regenerate telomeres, given the right conditions, but that's unusual. Research on telomere regeneration is extensive, but we're not there yet.

30 The DNA methylation process its complicated and still not fully understood, but essentially the end result is that certain methyl-based compounds are inserted into the DNA where they have the effect of suppressing the action of the gene sequence with which they are associated. Role of DNA methylation in gene expression: **nature.com/scitable/topicpage/the-role-of-methylation-in-gene-expression-1070**

31 Ibid, and **ncbi.nlm.nih.gov/pmc/articles/PMC2873040**

32 Hypomethalization and cancer: **ncbi.nlm.nih.gov/pmc/articles/PMC2873040**; hypermethalization also has been linked to birth defects in babies: **ncbi.nlm.nih.gov/pubmed/25587870**.

33 Impact on DNA methylation in cancer prevention and therapy by bioactive dietary components: **ncbi.nlm.nih.gov/pmc/articles/PMC2904405**

34 Smoking has a very broad, long-lasting impact on the human genome: **sciencedaily.com/releases/2016/09/160921215106.htm**

35 A DNA methylation biomarker of alcohol consumption: **ncbi.nlm.nih.gov/pubmed/27843151**

36 While oxygen is the most common oxidizing agent, oxygen itself may not be involved in all oxidizing reactions. Oxygen readily accepts electrons, and when it does the substance that it steals an electron from is said to be "oxidized." The oxygen atom itself is said to be "reduced." Consequently, any substance that behaves like oxygen, (specifically that grabs electrons in the same way that oxygen does) is described as an oxidizing agent. This may be archaic terminology, but because it has a long history, and is entirely familiar to chemists, it still persists, confusing though it might be to those who snoozed during chemistry classes.

37 Free radicals and antioxidants: **nccih.nih.gov/health/antioxidants/introduction.htm**

38 AGE and diabetes: **sciencedirect.com/science/article/pii/S1262363609001931**

39 Aging of the skin linked to glycation: **ncbi.nlm.nih.gov/pmc/articles/PMC3583887**

40 TAGE (toxic AGEs) hypothesis in various chronic diseases: **ncbi.nlm.nih.gov/pubmed/15288366**

41 TAGE (toxic AGEs) hypothesis in various chronic diseases: **ncbi.nlm.nih.gov/pubmed/16869341**

42 Tobacco is a source of toxic reactive glycation products: **ncbi.nlm.nih.gov/pmc/articles/PMC28407**

43 Expression of Advanced Glycation End products on Sun-Exposed and Non-Exposed Cutaneous Sites during the Ageing Process in Humans: **journals.plos.org/plosone/article?id=10.1371/journal.pone.0075003**

44 Exercise reduces circulating AGEs: **sciencedirect.com/science/article/pii/S0899900714004420**

45 Benjamin Gardner and Susanne Meisel, (**blogs.ucl.ac.uk/bsh/2012/06/29/busting-the-21-days-habit-formation-myth**) and Lally, P., van Jaarsveld, C. H. M., Potts, H. W. W., & Wardle, J. (2010). How are habits formed: Modeling habit formation in the real world. European Journal of Social Psychology, 40, 998-1009. (**onlinelibrary.wiley.com/doi/10.1002/ejsp.674/abstract**)

46 **nccih.nih.gov/health/pain/chronic.htm**

47 **medlineplus.gov/chronicpain.html**

48 Stephani Sutherland, Rethinking Relief. Scientific American Mind, May/June 2017

49 The science behind procrastination: **psychologicalscience.org/observer/why-wait-the-science-behind-procrastination**

50 Timothy Pychyl: **psychologicalscience.org/observer/why-wait-the-science-behind-procrastination**

51 Tobacco-related mortality: **cdc.gov/tobacco/data_statistics/fact_sheets/health_effects/tobacco_related_mortality/index.htm**

52 Alcohol dependency and early death: **sciencedaily.com/releases/2015/04/150402092057.htm**

53 VOCs exist in many household products and can cause irritation and nausea. In lab tests, some VOCs have caused cancer and nervous system damage. Volatile Organic Compounds (VOCs) in Commonly Used Products: **health.ny.gov/environmental/indoors/voc.htm**

54 Does tobacco smoke contain harmful chemicals? **cancer.gov/about-cancer/causes-prevention/risk/tobacco/cessation-fact-sheet#q1**

55 Smoking has a very broad, long-lasting impact on the human genome: **sciencedaily.com/releases/2016/09/160921215106.htm**

56 **who.int/tobacco/quitting/benefits/en**

57 The health arguments in favor of and against alcohol consumption are laid out well in this Healthline article: **healthline.com/nutrition/alcohol-good-or-bad#section1**

58 What is a standard drink? **niaaa.nih.gov/alcohol-health/overview-alcohol-consumption/what-standard-drink**

59 Habit Reversal Therapy: **psychcentral.com/blog/archives/2012/07/17/the-golden-rule-of-habit-change**

60 Motivational Interviewing: **sciencedaily.com/releases/2015/05/150504101258.htm**

61 Medications to help reduce alcohol consumption: **npr.org/sections/health-shots/2016/09/26/495491533/medications-can-help-people-stop-abusing-alcohol-but-many-dont-know**; medications to help stop smoking: **smokefree.gov/tools-tips/medications-can-help-you-quit**

62 Ways to stop smoking: **smokefree.gov/tools-tips/explore-quit-methods**; tips to reduce alcohol consumption: **rethinkingdrinking.niaaa.nih.gov/Thinking-about-a-change/Strategies-for-cutting-down/Tips-To-Try.aspx**

63 The skin microbiome: **ncbi.nlm.nih.gov/pmc/articles/PMC3535073**

64 The other layers of the epidermis are the stratum granulosum and stratum spinosum, which are essentially transition layers between the living cells in the stratum basale and the dead cells in the stratum corneum. Sometimes, the stratum corneum also is described as part of the epidermis.

65 The upper layer of the dermis (called the papillary) mainly consists of connective tissue binding the dermis to the epidermis layer above. A deeper layer, made of more elastin and collagen, is folded irregularly ("reticulated") where it meets and connects to the subcutaneous fat below.

66 Visible blue light causes inflammation and oxidative stress: **sciencedirect.com/science/article/pii/S0014483515000044**. Blue light at night affects circadian rhythms: **health.harvard.edu/staying-healthy/blue-light-has-a-dark-side**.

67 **skincancer.org/skin-cancer-information/skin-cancer-facts**

68 **cancer.org.au/preventing-cancer/sun-protection/about-skin-cancer.html**

69 The UV subgroup wavelengths ranges are: UVA 320-400nm, UVB 290-320nm, and UVC 100-290mm.

70 UVA radiation damages DNA: **sciencedaily.com/releases/2010/07/100701103415.htm**

71 Vitamin D and the skin: Focus on a complex relationship **ncbi.nlm.nih.gov/pmc/articles/PMC4642156**

72 Vitamin D for Health A Global Perspective: **mayoclinicproceedings.org/article/S0025-6196(13)00404-7/fulltext; ncbi.nlm.nih.gov/pmc/articles/PMC3356951**

73 Retinyl palmitate in sunscreen: **ewg.org/sunscreen/report/the-problem-with-vitamin-a/#.Wp7B-ZP4-Rs**

74 CDC statistics on US physical activity: **cdc.gov/nchs/fastats/exercise.htm**

75 Health risks associated with inactivity: **who.int/gho/ncd/risk_factors/physical_activity_text/en**

76 Regular moderate exercise reduces advanced glycation: **ncbi.nlm.nih.gov/pubmed/19608208t regular**

77 Exercise improves your skin: **psychologytoday.com/blog/shake-your-beauty/200904/improve-your-skin-exercise**

78 Exercise reverses aging? **well.blogs.nytimes.com/2014/04/16/younger-skin-through-exercise**

79 Exercise reduces depression: **mayoclinic.org/diseases-conditions/depression/in-depth/depression-and-exercise/art-20046495**

80 How much exercise per day? **mayoclinic.org/healthy-lifestyle/fitness/expert-answers/exercise/faq-20057916**

81 Constrained Total Energy Expenditure and Metabolic Adaptation to Physical Activity in Adult Humans, Herman Pontzner et al. **cell.com/current-biology/fulltext/S0960-9822(15)01577-8?_returnURL=http%3A%2F**

82 Physical activity and resting metabolic rate: **ncbi.nlm.nih.gov/pubmed/14692598**

83 Exercise and Sleep: **berkeleywellness.com/healthy-mind/sleep/article/exercise-and-sleep**

84 Making Physical Activity a Part of an Older Adult's Life: **cdc.gov/physicalactivity/basics/adding-pa/activities-olderadults.htm**

85 Heart Rate Exercise Zones: **healthyforgood.heart.org/move-more/articles/target-heart-rates#.WfvB7baZOR**

86 Exercise and skin conditions: **webmd.com/skin-problems-and-treatments/acne/features/exercise#1**

87 The Right Way to Stretch Before Exercise: **well.blogs.nytimes.com/2016/01/21/stretching-back-to-the-past**

88 Jumping jacks: **wikihow.com/Perform-Jumping-Jacks**

89 Incidental Physical Activities (IPA): **sciencedaily.com/releases/2011/06/110628113141.htm**

90 Hotel Maids Challenge the Placebo Effect: **npr.org/templates/story/story.php?storyId=17792517**

91 Sex makes you look younger and live longer: **cosmopolitan.com/uk/love-sex/sex/a9538529/health-benefits-of-regular-sex** and **prevention.com/sex/7-things-happen-when-you-stop-having-sex?utm_content=listiclefooter&utm_medium=Outbrain&utm_source=prevention.com**

92 Sitting is bad: **cnn.com/2015/01/21/health/sitting-will-kill-you/index.html**

93 Harvard Business Review: **hbr.org/2015/12/proof-that-positive-work-cultures-are-more-productive**

94 A Global History of Sitting Down: **theatlantic.com/international/archive/2016/08/chairs-history-witold-rybczynski/497657**

95 6,000-Year-Old Knee Joints Suggest Osteoarthritis Isn't Just Wear and Tear: **npr.org/sections/health-shots/2017/08/15/543402095/creaky-knees?sc=tw**

96 Foam roller: **breakingmuscle.com/fitness/what-is-a-foam-roller-how-do-i-use-it-and-why-does-it-hurt**

97 Muscle strength training exercises at home (no equipment, except two exercises need simple dumbbell weights): **cdc.gov/physicalactivity/basics/videos/index.htm**

98 Exercises: **agelaterbook.com**

99 Muscle strengthening at the gym: **cdc.gov/physicalactivity/basics/videos/index.htm#MuscleGym**

100 HIIT, American College of Sports Medicine: **acsm.org/docs/brochures/high-intensity-interval-training.pdf**

101 "Overweight" is defined as having a Body Mass Index of between 25 and 29.9 while "obesity" is defined as being over 30 BMI.

102 OECD (Organisation for Economic Co-operation and Development) Obesity update 2017: **oecd.org/health/health-systems/Obesity-Update-2017**.pdf; WHO Obesity in Southeast Asia **who.int/gho/ncd/risk_factors/obesity_text/en**

103 Waist to Hip ratio: **healthline.com/health/waist-to-hip-ratio**

104 Obese people have less brain tissue: **newsroom.ucla.edu/releases/more-obesity-blues-100147**

105 Science Compared Every Diet, and the Winner Is Real Food: **theatlantic.com/health/archive/2014/03/science-compared-every-diet-and-the-winner-is-real-food/284595**

106 Heart disease on the rise: **news.heart.org/cdc-u-s-deaths-from-heart-disease-cancer-on-the-rise**

107 Paul A. Offit, Pandora's Lab, excerpt in National Geographic, June 2017

108 **npr.org/sections/thesalt/2014/03/28/295332576/why-we-got-fatter-during-the-fat-free-food-boom**

109 Saturated Fats: A Perspective from Lactation and Milk Composition: **ncbi.nlm.nih.gov/pmc/articles/PMC2950926**

110 Saturated fats are not the problem: **annals.org/aim/article/1846638/association-dietary-circulating-supplement-fatty-acids-coronary-risk-systematic-review**

111 CLA trans fats: **cbsnews.com/news/are-all-trans-fats-as-bad-as-we-think**; **ncbi.nlm.nih.gov/pmc/articles/PMC201014**

112 Definition of vitamin: **en.oxforddictionaries.com/definition/vitamin**

113 The human body cannot produce vitamins, but the molecule we call vitamin D is in fact synthesized in the skin. This makes it, strictly speaking a hormone, not a vitamin (**ncbi.nlm.nih.gov/pubmed/2825606**), but traditional usage is now well established. Vitamins A, B1 (thiamine), B7 (biotin), B9 (folic acid), B12, and K all can be synthesized within the human body, but they are synthesized by gut bacteria, not by human organs, so they still count as vitamins. The microflora and nutrition: **ncbi.nlm.nih.gov/books/NBK7670**

114 Soluble and insoluble fiber: **webmd.com/diet/features/insoluble-soluble-fiber**

115 Fiber-Famished Gut Microbes Linked to Poor Health: **scientificamerican.com/article/fiber-famished-gut-microbes-linked-to-poor-health1**

116 Inhibitory actions of selected natural substances on formation of advanced glycation end products and advanced oxidation protein products: **ncbi.nlm.nih.gov/pmc/articles/PMC5041538**

117 Inhibitory actions of selected natural substances on formation of advanced glycation end products and advanced oxidation protein products: **ncbi.nlm.nih.gov/pmc/articles/PMC5041538**

118 Resveratrol inhibits AGEs-induced proliferation and collagen synthesis activity: **ncbi.nlm.nih.gov/pubmed/10903896**

119 Onions, sleep and mood: **medicalnewstoday.com/articles/276714.php**

120 Preventing the common cold with a garlic supplement: **ncbi.nlm.nih.gov/pubmed/11697022**

121 Lectins and digestive problems: **healthline.com/nutrition/dietary-lectins#section2**

122 Soy bad or good? **healthline.com/nutrition/is-soy-bad-for-you-or-good#section1**; soy possible side effects: **ncbi.nlm.nih.gov/pmc/articles/PMC4270274**

123 Lectins and digestive problems: **healthline.com/nutrition/dietary-lectins#section2**

124 **healthline.com/nutrition/11-health-benefits-of-fish**

125 Longevity in Japan: **ncbi.nlm.nih.gov/pmc/articles/PMC5400241** and **independent.co.uk/life-style/health-and-families/health-news/high-life-expectancy-in-japan-partly-down-to-diet-carbohydrates-vegetables-fruit-fish-meat-a6956011.html**

126 Plastic in the oceans: **news.nationalgeographic.com/news/2015/02/150212-ocean-debris-plastic-garbage-patches-science**

127 Fish: Friend or Foe? **hsph.harvard.edu/nutritionsource/fish**

128 For example, here is the healthy fish and sustainability guidance provided by Washington state: **doh.wa.gov/CommunityandEnvironment/Food/Fish/HealthyFishGuide**

129 A more general-purpose source of useful information about both sustainability and pollutants is at: **seafood.edf.org**

130 An example of an encyclopedia of herbs and spices: **harpercollins.com/9780062375230/the-encyclopedia-of-spices-and-herbs**

131 Ruminant-derived trans fats: **dairynutrition.ca/scientific-evidence/experts-summaries/who-report-on-trans-fats-effects-of-industrial-versus-ruminant-trans-fat**

132 Dairy fat and cardiovascular disease: **hsph.harvard.edu/nutritionsource/2016/10/25/dairy-fat-cardiovascular-disease-risk**

133 Could low-fat be worse than whole milk? **theguardian.com/lifeandstyle/2015/oct/09/low-fat-whole-milk-usda-dietary-guidelines**

134 Why butter is good for you: **healthline.com/nutrition/7-reasons-why-butter-is-good-for-you#section3**

135 Eggs and heart health: **health.harvard.edu/heart-health/are-eggs-risky-for-heart-health**

136 Nutritional value of egg whites vs. yolks: **ahealthiermichigan.org/2011/10/11/the-nurtional-value-of-egg-whites-versus-egg-yolks-what-do-you-use**

137 Too much water: **scientificamerican.com/article/strange-but-true-drinking-too-much-water-can-kill**

138 How much water to drink: **mayoclinic.org/healthy-lifestyle/nutrition-and-healthy-eating/in-depth/water/art-20044256**

139 IoM report on water intake: **www8.nationalacademies.org/onpinews/newsitem.aspx?RecordID=10925**

140 Electrolytes: **www.medicalnewstoday.com/articles/153188.php**

141 Planning a healthy vegetarian diet: **mayoclinic.org/healthy-lifestyle/nutrition-and-healthy-eating/in-depth/vegetarian-diet/art-20046446?pg=2**

142 Sugar in Britain: statistics from the book, Sweetness and Power: The Place of Sugar in Modern History, by Sidney Mintz, quoted in **theguardian.com/uk/2007/oct/13/lifeandhealth.britishidentity**

143 USA sugar consumption 2008: **healthline.com/nutrition/how-much-sugar-per-day**

144 **npr.org/sections/health-shots/2017/07/17/537262142/artificial-sweeteners-dont-help-people-lose-weight-review-finds?sc=tw**

145 Sucralose can potentially damage your gut microbiome balance: **ncbi.nlm.nih.gov/pubmed/18800291**

146 Artificial sweeteners: **health.harvard.edu/blog/artificial-sweeteners-sugar-free-but-at-what-cost-201207165030**

147 Advanced Glycation End Products in Foods and a Practical Guide to Their Reduction in the Diet: **ncbi.nlm.nih.gov/pmc/articles/PMC3704564**

148 HCA and PAH: **cancer.gov/about-cancer/causes-prevention/risk/diet/cooked-meats-fact-sheet**

149 Note that nitrates and nitrites, in and of themselves, are probably not harmful, and may even be beneficial (**healthline.com/nutrition/are-nitrates-and-nitrites-harmful**). Nitrates occur naturally in lots of vegetables and can be converted in the body to nitrites (**ncbi.nlm.nih.gov/pubmed/15223073**), which in turn creates nitric oxide, known to help in the control of blood pressure.

150 BPA, Bisphenol A: **scientificamerican.com/article/just-how-harmful-are-bisphenol-a-plastics**

151 While there has been a general reduction in trans fats in food products, trans fats may exist in amounts less than 0.5 percent, even in packages marked as containing 0 percent. Trans fats, zero doesn't mean zero: **npr.org/sections/thesalt/2014/08/28/343971652/trans-fats-linger-stubbornly-in-the-food-supply**

152 The Okinawa Diet and Hara Hachi Bu: **okinawa-diet.com/okinawa_diet/hara_hachi_bu.html**

153 More lycopene available from cooked tomato: **sciencedaily.com/releases/2002/04/020422073341.htm**

154 Soil depletion and nutrition loss: **scientificamerican.com/article/soil-depletion-and-nutrition-loss**

155 Mental health: a state of well-being: **who.int/features/factfiles/mental_health/en**

156 What is homeostasis? **scientificamerican.com/article/what-is-homeostasis**

157 Benefits of mindfulness: **apa.org/monitor/2012/07-08/ce-corner.aspx; Mindfulness interventions: psy.cmu.edu/~creswell/papers**

158 **health.harvard.edu/heart-health/meditation-offers-significant-heart-benefits**

159 Mindfulness a chore? **psychologytoday.com/blog/think-act-be/201612/5-attitudes-behind-the-mindfulness-backlash**

160 MBSR: **positivepsychologyprogram.com/mindfulness-based-stress-reduction-mbsr**

161 MBSR reduction: **ncbi.nlm.nih.gov/pubmed/15256293**

162 **umassmed.edu/cfm/mindfulness-based-programs/mbsr-courses/about-mbsr**

163 **mbct.com**

164 Reviews of mindfulness books: **positivepsychologyprogram.com/mindfulness-books**

165 Online sources for getting started in mindfulness: **mindful.org/meditation/mindfulness-getting-started**;

166 Examples of online Mindfulness courses: **bemindfulonline.com/the-course**; harvardpilgrim.org/portal/page?_pageid=1434,360741&_dad=portal&_schema=PORTAL; audiodharma.org/series/1/talk/1762

167 Mindfulness apps: **mindful.org/free-mindfulness-apps-worthy-of-your-attention**; healthline.com/health/mental-health/top-meditation-iphone-android-apps#intro1

168 Mindful Breathing Practice: **ggia.berkeley.edu/practice/mindful_breathing#**

169 The value of sadness: **psychologytoday.com/blog/compassion-matters/201507/the-value-sadness**

170 Davidson, K.W., Mostofsky, E. & Whang, W. (2010). "Don't worry, be happy: Positive effect and reduced 10-year incident coronary heart disease; The Canadian Nova Scotia Health Survey." European Heart Journal, 31, 1065-1070. **academic.oup.com/eurheartj/article/31/9/1065/590670/Don-t-worry-be-happy-positive-affect-and-reduced**

171 Research shows how stress can lead to heart attacks and stroke: **bhf.org.uk/heart-matters-magazine/news/behind-the-headlines/stress-and-heart-disease**

172 Stress fuels cancer spread by triggering master gene: **medicalnewstoday.com/articles/265254.php**

173 The effects of stress exposure on prefrontal cortex: **ncbi.nlm.nih.gov/pmc/articles/PMC4244027**

174 Psychological stress, through an increase in glucocorticoids, compromises the stratum corneum layer of the epidermis and so can reduce the effectiveness of the barrier function: Denda, M.; Tsuchiya, T.; Elias, P.M.; Feingold, K.R. (2000). "Stress alters cutaneous permeability barrier homeostasis." Am J Physiol Regul Integr Comp Physiol. 278 (2): R367–372. PMID 10666137. **ncbi.nlm.nih.gov/pubmed/10666137**

175 medicalnewstoday.com/articles/317631.php

176 City living and urban upbringing affect neural social stress processing in humans: **nature.com/nature/journal/v474/n7352/full/nature10190.html**

177 Helliwell, J., Layard, R., & Sachs, J. (2017). World Happiness Report 2017, New York; Sustainable Development Solutions Network: **worldhappiness.report/ed/2017**

178 Heart Rate Variability: **datasci.com/solutions/cardiovascular/heart-rate-variability**

179 Cohen, S., Kamarck, T., and Mermelstein, R. (1983). A global measure of perceived stress. Journal of Health and Social Behavior, 24, 386-396.

180 Download PDF of the Perceived Stress Scale form: **google.com/url?sa=t&rct=j&q=&esrc=s&source=web&cd=7&ved=0ahUKEwjp-pbGS29fWAhUJrFQKHdfkAtsQFghYMAY&url=https%3A%2F%2Fdas.nh.gov%2Fwellness%2FDocs%2FPercieved%2520Stress%2520Scale.pdf&usg=AOvVaw3keuc8anKghk_HPvN8dYVF**

181 Two examples of websites for PSS-based stress testing (there are many more): **bemindfulonline.com/test-your-stress and highered.mheducation.com/sites/0073381225/student_view0/chapter4/self-assessment_4_7.html**

182 Sleep statistics: **sleepassociation.org/about-sleep/sleep-statistics**

183 Why lack of sleep is bad for your health: **nhs.uk/Livewell/tiredness-and-fatigue/Pages/lack-of-sleep-health-risks.aspx**

184 While you call it quits for the day, your mind does some serious work: **sleep.org/articles/brain-during-sleep**

185 How sleep deprivation affects your heart: **sleepfoundation.org/sleep-news/how-sleep-deprivation-affects-your-heart**

186 Sleep and immune function: **ncbi.nlm.nih.gov/pmc/articles/PMC3256323**

187 World Sleep Survey: **worldsleepsurvey.com/sleep-score**

188 The Physiology of Sleep—The Cardiovascular System: **sleepdisorders.sleepfoundation.org/chapter-1-normal-sleep/the-physiology-of-sleep-the-cardiovascular-system**

189 Sleep and immune function: **ncbi.nlm.nih.gov/pmc/articles/PMC3256323**

190 **Sleep-stress cycle: apa.org/news/press/releases/stress/2013/sleep.aspx**

191 How to break the stress-sleep cycle: **ahchealthenews.com/2016/11/28/break-vicious-stress-sleep-cycle-2**

192 Sleep deprived: **medicaldaily.com/nearly-third-americans-are-sleep-deprived-240273**

193 The myth of the eight hour sleep: **bbc.com/news/magazine-16964783**

194 Siesta is good for you: **telegraph.co.uk/news/worldnews/europe/spain/9458799/Spanish-scientists-prove-the-siesta-is-good-for-you-and-issue-guidelines-for-a-perfect-nap.html**

195 How many neurons do we have? **ncbi.nlm.nih.gov/pubmed/27187682**. Also, "The search for true numbers of neurons and glial cells in the human brain: A review of 150 years of cell counting." von Bartheld CS1, Bahney J2, Herculano-Houzel S3.

196 **blogs.scientificamerican.com/brainwaves/know-your-neurons-what-is-the-ratio-of-glia-to-neurons-in-the-brain**

197 **blogs.scientificamerican.com/brainwaves/know-your-neurons-meet-the-glia**

198 Glia: **scientificamerican.com/article/without-glia-brain-would-starve**

199 Glial cells: **scientificamerican.com/article/the-root-of-thought-what**

200 The effects of stress exposure on prefrontal cortex: **ncbi.nlm.nih.gov/pmc/articles/PMC4244027**

201 A two-year multidomain intervention of diet, exercise, cognitive training and vascular risk monitoring versus control to prevent cognitive decline in at-risk elderly people (FINGER): a randomized controlled trial. Tia Ngandu and others in Lancet Neurology, Vol 15, No. 5. April 2016.

202 "Experts agree that in the vast majority of cases, Alzheimer's, like other common chronic conditions, probably develops as a result of complex interactions among multiple factors, including age, genetics, environment, lifestyle and coexisting medical conditions." (**alz.org**)

203 Mental strain helps maintain a healthy brain: **health.harvard.edu/blog/mental-strain-helps-maintain-a-healthy-brain-201211055495**

204 "A number of studies indicate that maintaining strong social connections and keeping mentally active as we age might lower the risk of cognitive decline and Alzheimer's." (**alz.org**)

205 "Regular physical exercise may be a beneficial strategy to lower the risk of Alzheimer's and vascular dementia. Exercise may directly benefit brain cells by increasing blood and oxygen flow in the brain." (**alz.org**)

206 The expression "mens sana in corpora sano" (a healthy mind in a healthy body) is attributed to the poet Juvenal around 100 A.D.

207 "Several conditions known to increase the risk of cardiovascular disease—such as high blood pressure, diabetes and high cholesterol—also increase the risk of developing Alzheimer's. Some autopsy studies show that as many as 80 percent of individuals with Alzheimer's disease also have cardiovascular disease." (**alz.org**)

208 "Current evidence suggests that heart-healthy eating may also help protect the brain." (**alz.org**)

209 Serine and neuroprotection: **ncbi.nlm.nih.gov/pmc/articles/PMC5343079**

210 Omega-3 for the brain: **healthline.com/nutrition/omega-3-6-9-overview#section1**

211 Why your brain needs water: **psychologytoday.com/us/blog/you-illuminated/201010/why-your-brain-needs-water**

212 The Gut Microbiome and the Brain: **ncbi.nlm.nih.gov/pmc/articles/PMC4259177**

213 Parkinson's disease "may start in gut": **bbc.com/news/health-38173287**

214 MIND=Mediterranean-DASH Intervention for Neurodegenerative Delay

215 DASH=Dietary Approaches to Stop Hypertension

216 Some biologists argue that the eye and optic nerves count as part of the CNS because they are so close to and partly protected by the brain. Others disagree. This is an academic quibble.

217 NFL CTE survey: **nytimes.com/interactive**

218 **spineuniverse.com/conditions/spinal-cord-injury/airbags-seat-belts-spine-protection**

219 Lead poisoning and health: **who.int/mediacentre/factsheets/fs379/en**

220 Common waterborne contaminants: **wqa.org/learn-about-water/common-contaminants**

221 Gene therapy: **scientificamerican.com/article/experts-gene-therapy; sciencecare.com/blog-gene-therapy-future-medicine**

222 TALEN and CRISPR: **ncbi.nlm.nih.gov/pmc/articles/PMC4207558**

223 SPC: **webmd.com/back-pain/guide/spinal-cord-stimulation**

224 Bioelectronics: **nytimes.com/2014/05/25/magazine/can-the-nervous-system-be-hacked.html; theguardian.com/breakthrough-science/2017/jun/06/the-future-of-medical-technology-bioelectronics-and-the-treatment-of-chronic-conditions**

225 Cancer, evolution research: **scientificamerican.com/article/evolution-research-could-revolutionize-cancer-therapy**

226 **thelocal.de/20171123/life-expectancy-much-lower-in-germany-compared-to-eu-neighbours-study**

227 Liver damage: **ncbi.nlm.nih.gov/pubmed/22701432**

228 Alcohol consumption and cancer risk: **ncbi.nlm.nih.gov/pubmed/21864055**

229 Alcohol use before and during pregnancy implications for the prevention of fetal alcohol spectrum disorders: **ncbi.nlm.nih.gov/pubmed/19027093**

230 Brain damage from alcohol: **ncbi.nlm.nih.gov/pubmed/21487421**

231 Weight gain from alcohol: **ncbi.nlm.nih.gov/pubmed/15483203**

232 Weight gain in relation to history of amount and type of alcohol: **ncbi.nlm.nih.gov/pubmed/12587005**

233 Association of alcohol consumption with selected cardiovascular disease outcomes—a systematic review and meta-analysis: **ncbi.nlm.nih.gov/pubmed/21343207**

234 Links between alcohol abuse and depression: **ncbi.nlm.nih.gov/pubmed/19255375**

235 Alcohol intake and incidence of type 2 diabetes in men: **ncbi.nlm.nih.gov/pubmed/10857962**

236 Alcohol consumption and risk of dementia: **ncbi.nlm.nih.gov/pubmed/12636463**

237 Alcohol and risk of becoming overweight: **ncbi.nlm.nih.gov/pubmed/19255375**

238 Alcohol and cardiovascular health—the razor-sharp double-edged sword: **ncbi.nlm.nih.gov/pubmed/17825708**

239 Relationship between moderate alcohol consumption and adiponectin and insulin sensitivity: **ncbi.nlm.nih.gov/pubmed/15111562**

240 Red wine consumption increases antioxidant status and decreases oxidative stress in the circulation of both young and old humans: **ncbi.nlm.nih.gov/pubmed/17888186**

241 Silicon and bone health: **ncbi.nlm.nih.gov/pmc/articles/PMC2658806**

242 Arginine: **webmd.com/diet/supplement-guide-l-arginine#1**

243 Asparagine and breast cancer: **theguardian.com/science/2018/feb/07/cutting-asparagus-could-prevent-spread-of-breast-cancer-study-shows**

244 Creatine: **aminoacidstudies.org/creatine**

245 Creatine as a supplement: **webmd.com/men/creatine#2-5**

246 Creatine problems: **mayoclinic.org/drugs-supplements/creatine/safety/hrb-20059125**

247 N-acetyl cysteine: **webmd.com/vitamins-supplements/ingredientmono-1018-n-acetyl%20cysteine.aspx?activeingredientid=1018**

248 Glycine: **aminoacidstudies.org/glycine**

249 Glycine uses and risks: **webmd.com/vitamins-and-supplements/glycine-uses-and-risks#1**

250 Lysine: **examine.com/supplements/lysine**

251 Lysine for cold sores: **examine.com/supplements/lysine; peoplespharmacy.com/2016/12/18/can-you-avoid-cold-sores-by-taking-l-lysine**

252 Methionine: **pubchem.ncbi.nlm.nih.gov/compound/L-methionine#section=Top**

253 Serine as neuro-protective: **ncbi.nlm.nih.gov/pmc/articles/PMC5343079**

254 Serine: **nutritional-supplements-health-guide.com/serine.html**

255 Threonine: **webmd.com/vitamins-supplements/ingredientmono-1083-threonine.aspx?activeingredientid=1083&activeingredientname=threonine**

256 Tryptophan: **pubchem.ncbi.nlm.nih.gov/compound/L-tryptophan#section=Top**

257 Tyrosine: **pubchem.ncbi.nlm.nih.gov/compound/6057#section=Top**

258 Valine: **pubchem.ncbi.nlm.nih.gov/compound/L-valine#section=Top**

259 Thiamine: **webmd.com/vitamins-supplements/ingredientmono-965-THIAMINE+VITAMIN+B1.aspx**

260 Riboflavin: **ods.od.nih.gov/factsheets/Riboflavin-HealthProfessional**

261 Niacin: **webmd.com/vitamins-supplements/ingredientmono-924-NIACIN+AND+NIACINAMIDE+VITAMIN+B3.aspx?activeIngredientId=924&activeIngredientName=NIACIN+AND+NIACINAMIDE+(VITAMIN+B3)&source=2**

262 vitamin B6: **ods.od.nih.gov/factsheets/vitaminB6-HealthProfessional**

263 vitamin B6: **mayoclinic.org/drugs-supplements-vitamin-b6/art-20363468**

264 Biotin: **ods.od.nih.gov/factsheets/Biotin-HealthProfessional**

265 **medicalnewstoday.com/articles/219718.php**

266 Benefits and Risks of Folic Acid: **sciencebasedmedicine.org/the-benefits-and-risks-of-folic-acid-supplementation**

267 vitamin B12: **ods.od.nih.gov/factsheets/vitaminB12-HealthProfessional**

268 vitamin B12 supplements for vegans: **vegansociety.com/resources/nutrition-and-health/nutrients/vitamin-b12/what-every-vegan-should-know-about-vitamin-b12**

269 vitamin E: **healthline.com/health/all-about-vitamin-e#ways-to-get-it7**

270 Almonds: **healthline.com/nutrition/9-proven-benefits-of-almonds**

271 Brazil nuts: **bbcgoodfood.com/howto/guide/health-benefits-brazil-nuts**

272 Cinnamon and Chronic Diseases: **ncbi.nlm.nih.gov/pubmed/27771918**

273 Most supermarket cinnamon is the Saigon variety, also called cassia cinnamon; recent research suggests that Ceylon cinnamon is just as good, and less likely to harm your liver. **peoplespharmacy.com/2013/12/30/cinnamon-offers-health-benefits-but-also-carries-serious-risks** An ingredient in cassia cinnamon called coumarin increases the chance of liver damage and might also interact adversely with some painkillers and anticoagulants. Ceylon cinnamon, which is harvested from a different species of tree and contains much less coumarin, provides at least some of the same health benefits without the adverse affects on the liver. It is also possible to buy cassia cinnamon extract where the coumarin has been removed. But don't expect any health benefits from eating cinnamon pastries no matter which type of cinnamon they use. (Too much sugar and white flour.)

274 Garlic: **healthline.com/nutrition/11-proven-health-benefits-of-garlic#section1**

275 Ginger root: **medicalnewstoday.com/articles/265990.php**

276 Green Tea benefits: **healthline.com/nutrition/10-benefits-of-green-tea-extract#section9**

277 Nuts for nutrition: **healthyeating.sfgate.com/nuts-eat-nutrition-1812.html**

278 Salvia for dementia therapy: **ncbi.nlm.nih.gov/pubmed/12895683**

279 Walnuts are the healthiest nut: **bbc.com/news/health-12865291**

280 NGCS: **ncbi.nlm.nih.gov/pmc/articles/PMC4406911**

281 The list of causes of digestive problems is long. In addition to poor gut flora condition and mental stress, we can add lack of exercise, too much alcohol, too much sugar and refined starches, undercooked lectin-containing foods, eating too much at one time, and more. There are many ingredients in wheat (other than gluten) that are known to contribute to the severity of irritable bowel syndrome (IBS), so reducing wheat intake may help some people with IBS.

282 Benefits of lectins: **healthline.com/nutrition/dietary-lectins**. Medical use of lectins: **ncbi.nlm.nih.gov/pubmed/25730388**

283 Lectins and digestive problems: **healthline.com/nutrition/dietary-lectins#section2**

ARCHITECTS OF BABYLON

by

Chris Betts

Grosvenor House
Publishing Limited

This book is published by
Grosvenor House Publishing Ltd
28-30 High Street, Guildford, Surrey, GU1 3HY.
www.grosvenorhousepublishing.co.uk

A CIP record for this book
is available from the British Library

ISBN 978-1-908105-79-0

Architects Of Babylon

"Europe's nations should be guided towards the super state without their peoples knowing what is happening. This can be accomplished by successive steps, each disguised as having an economic purpose, but which will eventually and irreversibly lead to federation."

Jean Monnet - one of the founding Fathers of the European Union

"The end goal is to get everybody chipped, to control the whole society, to have the bankers and the elite people control the world."

Nicholas Rockefeller - Member of the Council on Foreign Relations, World Economic Forum and International Institute for Strategic Studies

"Countless people will hate the New World Order and will die protesting against it!"

H. G. Wells

"We shall have world government whether or not you like it, by conquest or consent."

James Warburg February 17th, 1950.

Foreword

J. Edgar Hoover, one-time Director of the FBI, speaking of the issues raised here, said:

"The individual is handicapped by coming face to face with a conspiracy so monstrous that he cannot believe it exists."

When we look organised evil right in the face we feel stunned. The psychological term is 'Cognitive Dissonance'. Some things are so chilling that many people cannot face them and retreat immediately into denial. In the face of certain horrors we are numbed; 'No! That just can't be!' I recall feeling like that when, as a teenager I discovered the full extent of the Nazi atrocities in the holocaust.

What I will try to communicate is monstrous on a global scale; so monstrous that some will say it's too crazy to take in. I refer to a long term plan, hidden from the ordinary citizen, that has been advancing inexorably over generations. Those within it are striving for its final fruition within the next few years.

The following is intended as a starting point for your own investigations and does not allow the scope to explore all that is involved. I can only hope to alert those who are interested in taking their explorations further.

I have attempted to include some of the historic background to what is being planned and some insight as to how those involved go about achieving their goals. Some feel that in informing people about these issues we should confine ourselves only to the events of the last few years. However, nothing happens in a vacuum and in order to truly understand how we have reached the present state of affairs, we need to at least be aware of the plans certain elitist groups have been pursuing for generations. The 'modern' faces of these groups are banking cartels setting up the scenario for The World Bank, the bloodlines which run the elites of American, British and European politics including the so called royals, the

1

Masonic hierarchy with its manifold links, planning groups such as the Trilateral Commission and the Bilderberger Group, which disseminate the bidding of the puppet masters. Other 'foot soldier' groups such as Common Purpose train and place the pawns in lower positions of influence. However, although many of those involved at lower levels are kept deliberately ignorant of the overarching aims they are pursuing in their daily tasks, they are frequently building on foundations put in place long before they were born.

It is not my intention to cause fear or insecurity but rather to inform 'those who have ears to hear'. What you choose to do with the information is, of course up to you but I trust that the following will stimulate you to research these matters for yourself.

"Go, post a lookout and have him report what he sees. When he sees chariots with teams of horses, riders on donkeys or riders on camels, let him be alert, fully alert." Isaiah 21:6

We are entering a time in history where World Government, long the dream of tyrants, is truly feasible for the first time. We are all being set up for it and soon those who control the powerful World Banking System will trigger the economic crisis from which it will rise.

As Joan Veon has said;

"Jesus Christ was born into World Government. The early Church certainly understood the rules of Rome and worked around and through it without becoming part of it or adding to it. In contrast the end time Church is going into World Government without knowing it or understanding its agenda. Therefore it is blind as to how to stand in the gap." Joan Veon 'The United Nations Straight Jacket'

The Signs Of The Times

"When evening comes you say, 'It will be fair weather for the sky is red.' and in the morning, 'Today will be stormy for the sky is red and overcast.' You know how to interpret the appearance of the sky, but you cannot interpret the signs of the times." (Jesus speaking to the Pharisees and Sadducees).
Matthew 16 verses 2 and 3

Many Christians have felt for a long time, as they read the papers and watch the news, that what they are being fed by the media just doesn't line up with reality.

They know that they are being misled about certain political issues, even military conflicts. The real point is that they are not in a position to uncover the actual level of deception they are being subjected to.

In recent years even folks who might fit the description of Noam Chomsky's character 'Joe Sixpack', have been heard to talk about 'cover-ups' and politicians lying publicly. The fact is the deception is on such a huge scale that, in the words of George H W Bush;

"Sarah, if the American people knew what we have done, they would string us up from the lamp posts."
George H. W. Bush (Daddy Bush) during an interview with Sarah McClendon 1992.

"I have seen professional, award – winning journalists so shell-shocked that they were unable to fathom the truth of what they had just witnessed......when I stepped into that world, I immersed myself in a universe I found so perverse and evil that it has left an indelible mark on my soul. It is the price of involvement."
Daniel Estulin –'The True Story of the Bilderberg Group'

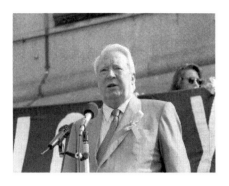

Shuffled into Europe

I spent my younger years in Canada. When my family returned to England I had to re-think dollars, dimes, nickels and cents into pounds, shillings and pence - coinage like 'half a Crown' or a 'florin'. I picked it up, of course, especially after a few clips around the ear from teachers in English school classes where I got arithmetic wrong. They were proud of their identity, these Brits, individual currency and all.

Most of the English relatives I met on our family's return from Canada had endured tough times through the war years and were content to have settled back into the British way of life just as it was. If they'd been to Europe, it had been in uniform and they were happy to be back at home. Most of them had no idea that Britain was being steered by a powerful elite on a pre-determined course into union with Europe.

As time went on I would catch an article or overhear a discussion about certain politicians and their vision of a 'United Europe'. By 1970 the Conservative Manifesto was promising that they would try to negotiate entry to the EC, even though the Gallup polls showed that half of the ordinary citizens asked didn't even want talks on the issue! Although Prime Minister Ted Heath's cabinet was dominated by pro-Europeans, he was presiding over a Conservative party that was deeply ambivalent about the 'Common Market'. Only 19% supported the idea of Britain joining the EC. However,

4

I have long realised that it doesn't matter what the ordinary citizens of any country think or feel!

Late in 1970 a meeting of senior information officers in Whitehall was convened to discuss what could be done to reverse things and get public opinion on track with the European agenda. For nearly two years the MI6 - linked 'Information Research Department' of the Foreign Office funded a covert propaganda operation aimed at ensuring Britain joined the European Community. Invitation – only meetings between senior media figures, pro-European politicians, diplomats and business men were arranged. Held at the Connaught Hotel, these took the form of lavishly expensive breakfasts which were understandably well attended. The lobbying organisation was called the European League for Economic Co-operation.

When Civil Service Head, Sir William Armstrong found out about the events, he went to see Heath and the funding promptly stopped. As a result, the ELEC took over running the breakfast meetings and Alistair McAlpine, later Lord McAlpine, was recruited as treasurer and fund-raiser *extraordinaire*. The whole point of course was to cultivate contacts who could and would use their positions and influence to strengthen support for entry to the EEC. Insiders from Government and the Civil Service sat down with media figures and opposition leaders.

Pro-Europeans from all parties were represented. Roy Jenkins, Roy Hattersley and Gwyn Morgan from the Labour ranks discussed the issues with people such as Michael Ivens, Director of Aims of Industry and Ernest Wistrich, the Director of the European Movement.

The media was represented by people such as Nigel Ryan from 'News at Ten', Ian Trethowen, then Managing Director of BBC Radio, Marshall Stewart from BBC's 'Today' programme. Ideas for pro-European TV and Radio programmes were put forward. 'News at Ten' started a series of five minute specials on the EEC with a strong factual tone as a direct result of the meetings behind closed doors.

Few of the participants appear to have been aware of the source of the funding for these breakfast meetings, though some must have had suspicions.

The process of chipping away at public opinion and influencing the way the ordinary people thought was kept up on all possible fronts.

Norman Reddaway, Under Secretary of State at the British Foreign Office, put together a special unit to propagandise in favour of British entry and counter those who opposed it. They worked closely with pro-European politicians to rebut anti-EEC arguments. The Information Research Department wrote and brokered articles which were placed in the press.

"There was no shortage of MPs who were pleased to see something published under their name in *The Times* and elsewhere," a former insider said.

Up and down Britain dozens of groups with this intent made their best efforts to change attitudes.

On the 15th of February 1971, they got their first victory as the step of making Britain's currency metric was taken.

In January 1973, Heath and his cohorts got their way and Britain was railroaded into the EEC.

In 1975 the heavily propagandised public swayed the way they were required to in a 'referendum'. The meetings referred to went on, latterly at the Dorchester Hotel, right up until that time.

"One matter I really do know about is how to organise a good breakfast" said McAlpine.

(In depth article on this by Paul Lashmar and James Oliver, Sunday Telegraph, 27 April 1997, page 10)

A Common Market

This alignment was talked up as a 'trade agreement'- a 'common market'.

This has been the case with all the subsequent alignments. Although originally portrayed as a development that would equalise trade balances and tariffs, the real agenda had little to do with convenient trade arrangements.

In fact by the time the 'Treaty Establishing The European Community' (Maastricht Treaty) was signed in 1992 the word 'Economic' had been entirely deleted from the treaty. As Jim Marrs has pointed out in his excellent book 'The Rise of the Fourth Reich', the Nazi vision of a unified Europe had become reality.

In the years that followed other pieces of the plan were put into place.

If you were on a salary, you could no longer be paid in cash. Everything became computerised. In the name of convenience, Credit Cards with Personal Identification Numbers were issued and one could pay for everything at a swipe. People got used to it very rapidly.

A gruesome experiment showed that, if you put a frog in a beaker of water and heated the water up slowly, the frog would stay put and boil to death. If, however, you threw the frog into hot water from outside, it would jump straight out to safety. In the same way, the Globalist power brokers are shrewd in the way they introduce their agenda. Getting people used to a concept is the first step.

When that's accomplished you can turn up the heat little by little and they won't protest too much. Those who run the money system actually run the world. They can afford to bide their time and get people used to each new step in their agenda. Occasionally things have to be hurried along but, not often. In the main the general populace are suggestible and can be brought into line with a little propaganda.

Note; British and American intelligence services had traditionally supported Britain's entry in the EEC. The CIA funded the European Movement, the most prominent extra-Government group, seeking to influence public opinion for a European Community. Between 1949 and 1953 the CIA had subsidised the Movement to the tune of $330,000. This was NOT a new idea - it had been planned for a very long time.

I had been brought up with what I started to see as a rather naïve view of politics.

I honestly thought that governments were there to listen to and carry out the will of the people. Here it seemed to be going the other way. Not knowing what scheming had gone on behind the scenes, some were puzzled as to how so many people could seemingly change their dearly held opinions in so short a time.

At this time I had friends with a lot more insight into what was actually happening in the world than I had. I just wasn't listening to their statements, for example, about the American military-industrial complex and its involvement in the Vietnam War. Gradually though, I found myself starting to seriously question the template of the world that I had been given by my parents.

Our whole educational process teaches us that Wars and Revolutions are the accidental results of conflicting forces. At first you cannot believe that there are people who actually set them up and then manage their outcomes for profit. The idea is so utterly shocking, it takes some getting used to.

As Dr Anthony Sutton pointed out, at the cost of his career, wars are created by an elite who control the banks in order to move the chess pieces into the positions they wish them to occupy for maximum profit and control.

War = Big Profit for bankers.

You won't find that in the carefully vetted history books.

For example, when the Second World War broke out, my father, like most of his generation went off to fight Nazism. He saw Hitler as the evil one and England on the side of justice and liberty. As a Tank Gunner/Driver under General Montgomery he watched helplessly as many of his fellows were fried alive in direct hits. Their dying screams stayed with him for the rest of his life. He saw the carnage his gunnery barrages caused when ordered to fire upon towns or villages where the enemy was dug in. He could cut a sniper's nest in half with his heavy guns but, on moving up would find the remains of innocents caught in the fire storm. His own armoured vehicles were hit several times and on one occasion the turret of a tank was blown clean away over his head. He lived through the most incredible near misses and as a result suffered horribly with 'survivor's guilt'. If you had asked him why he was fighting, he would have pointed out that Hitler was a dictator who wanted to enslave ordinary people. People like that had to be stopped. He was 'fighting for his country'. If he had only known that the fuel for the Nazi tanks and the Luftwaffe aircraft as well as the enemy shells directed against him were paid for by Bankers in America, the homeland of his allies. These were financial dictators every bit as evil as Adolf Hitler and his Nazis. It is mind numbing but, in fact they were American members of the same loathsome occult brotherhood that Hitler belonged to.

"The general consensus at the bankers' meetings was that the only way to free Germany from French financial clutches was by revolution – either Communist or National Socialism. Rockefeller argued that the money should go to Hitler. After some negotiation, 10 million dollars was transferred to the Nazis. During subsequent meetings it was explained that Hitler's storm troopers and S.S. were insufficiently equipped and badly needed machine guns, revolvers and carbines. Hitler explained that he had two plans for takeover in Germany. a) Revolution b) Legal Takeover Plan. Hitler is quoted as saying "...revolution costs five hundred million marks. Legal takeover costs two hundred million marks – what will your bankers decide?" Legal takeover thus offered the best deal......After further negotiations Rockefeller and the American banking and oil interests offered an additional $15 million which would help finance the legal takeover. Revolution would be too expensive and destructive. In the months after Hitler took power, in 1933, Warburg delivered yet another payment from Rockefeller and Carter and their associates in banking, industry and oil, i.e. $7 million....."

Antony Sutton – from Warburg's 'Financial Sources of National Socialism'.

One of the players in this vile game of chess was George W Bush's grandfather.

Yes, <u>that</u> George W Bush – the President of the Unites States who, like his father and grandfather before him, was enrolled into Lodge 322, ('Skull and Bones') during his time at Yale University! You might well ask 'How can a man hold a public office, let alone fulfil the role of the American President, while belonging to a secret society?!' The really frightening truth is that it is happening all the time. Hidden from our sight, it has been going on for generations.

In both Britain and America, members of a powerful elite control who is placed in the most senior political positions.

"My senior years I joined 'Skull and Bones'. A secret society – so secret I can't say anything more"......George W Bush in his autobiography 'A Charge to Keep'

At this point, if you were not previously aware of these facts, the chuckle factor will kick in. 'Oh, come on! You cannot be serious! You watch too much TV or, you read too much pulp fiction.'

As J. Edgar Hoover pointed out - the greatest weapon these people possess is that you cannot really bring yourself to believe what they have done and continue to do. Hoover ought to have known, being the director of one of the most evil organisations in American history.

Heads They Win – Tails You Lose!

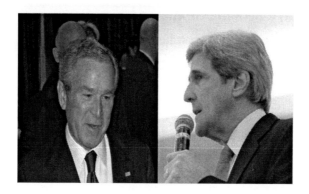

No matter which way Americans voted in the Bush/Carey 'election', they were set up to have a member of the 'Skull & Bones' Lodge from Yale as their President! In public these two men debate as if their policies differ. In fact they both belong to the same 'brotherhood' – Lodge 322. 'The Order' at Yale University.

"My senior years I joined 'Skull and Bones'. A secret society – so secret I can't say anything more"......George W Bush in his autobiography 'A Charge to Keep'

Looking Back to Shape The Future

The Babylon Connection...

Lately in Presidential speeches references have been made to ushering in a 'New World Order'. Most interpret this as a reference to a bold new plan for ridding the world of evil and making us all safe and prosperous. Not so.

For generations there have existed elite groups who trace their origins back through ancient bloodlines. These people bring their offspring up in the belief that their destiny is to rule. Those on the lower levels in their grand, pyramidal scheme of things are referred to as 'sheep' or 'cattle'. To rule one must have the right heritage.

What we know as Fascism today adheres to the 'philosopher-king' belief that only one class – by birth, education or social standing – is capable of understanding what is best for the whole community and putting it into practice. This idea of a ruthless hierarchy of superior beings, born and 'bred to rule' is embedded in the ancient most pristine form of satanism. Its roots are in the Sumero-Akkadian Babylonian Mystery religion which is practised today all over the world.

All very interesting, but what has that got to do with us today? After all, most ordinary people don't believe in witches or the devil these days, do they?

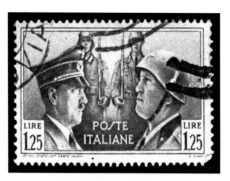

Mussolini and Hitler

Well, *you* might not believe in witchcraft, human sacrifice or satanism, but that doesn't alter the fact that these things are actually going on all around you. It might not be a pleasant thought, but these practices have thrived in the homes, temples and lodges of highborn adepts for generations. Over generations, their carefully reared children have infiltrated the very fabric of the society you live in and adherents occupy the highest positions in Banking and Government all over the world. Luciferian dynasties hold and control the finances of the entire world. In turn their children will be tutored and prepared in order to take up their roles in the next generation. One of the factors that many ordinary folks find most difficult to grasp in all this is the passing of the baton from generation to generation. The Gospel of Matthew was 'right on the money'…..

"Again, the devil took Him to a very high mountain and showed Him all the Kingdoms of the World and their splendour. "All this I will give you" he said, "if you will bow down and worship me." (Matthew 4: 8.)

We know that Jesus refused him. There are many who have had the same kind of offer and accepted it!

America – New World to Birth
A New World Order

As we trace things through, America must be given special consideration because, from its inception, it has been steered on the course required of it by the occult societies which birthed it. As a nation it was, from the beginning, to fulfil the role of the 'New World' of the Rosicrucian and Masonic Lodges and be the instrument through which the 'New World Order' would come. Whereas the ordinary person saw a new nation, the occultist hierarchy saw the New Atlantis rising!

But, wait a minute, surely America was founded as a Christian nation, wasn't it !?

Well, its true that many early settlers were Bible believing Christians.

Most were dissenters from the Anglican Church. They had come to the 'New World' wanting nothing more than the freedom to live and worship in peace.

However, at the same time as Christianity was establishing its beachhead in America, so were the Rosicrucians, among many other Secret Societies.

Their agenda was <u>very</u> different to the Puritan Christians.

So where is the evidence of Occult societies in the founding of the U.S.A.?

Well let's get that out of the way before we go any further. Take a few minutes and consider the following;

1. The Great Seal of the United States of America.
2. The Dollar Bill.
3. Washington D.C.
4. The Beliefs of the visible 'Founders' of America
5. The Constitution

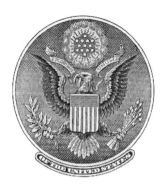

1. The Great Seal of the USA.

When you think of the States, you probably think of an Eagle as its emblem.

The designer of The Great Seal was a Freemason called Charles Thompson.

It's actually a powerful, high Masonic symbol – the Phoenix. It was intended to illustrate the words 'E Pluribus Unum' *(Out of Many – One)*. This rich symbolism traces back to ancient Egypt and the Phoenix was shown rising from the flames and ashes. On the original Seal of 1782, the neck of the bird was much longer and the distinctive tuft of feathers on the upper, back part of the head was noticeable. The beak bore little resemblance to an Eagle's, its body was thinner and its wings were shorter. So many people saw it as the representation of a turkey, that in 1841 the Seal was amended and given more the appearance of a bald eagle. It's been toned down all right but, comparing the two, anyone familiar with symbolism sees that the 'eagle' is a conventionalised Phoenix.

As leading Masonic scholar Manly P Hall himself points out;

'European mysticism was not dead at the time the United States was founded. The hand of the Mysteries controlled in the establishment of the new government, for the hand of the Mysteries may still be seen on the Great Seal of The United States Of America. Careful analysis of the Seal discloses a mass of Occult and Masonic symbols, chief among them the

1 5

so-called American Eagle – a bird which Benjamin Franklin declared to be unworthy to be chosen as the symbol of a great, powerful and progressive people.....in a coloured sketch submitted as a design for the Great Seal by William Barton in 1782, an actual Phoenix appears sitting upon a nest of flames.....'
(Manly P.Hall 'The Secret Teachings of All Ages' XC.)

The mythical Phoenix was regarded as sacred to the Sun, and the length of its life (500 to 1000 years) was taken as the standard for measuring the motion of heavenly bodies. It was also a measure for cycles in time used in the Ancient Mystery Religions to designate the periods of existence. The Phoenix was re-born from its dead parent and remained the single one of its kind. Modern Freemasons realise the special Masonic significance of the Phoenix, for the bird is described as using sprigs of acacia in the manufacture of its nest. Acacia is regarded as a symbol for purity, regeneration and immortality. Perfect imagery for a new nation that was to be born out of an old one.

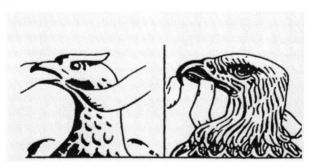

Phoenix of Original Draft for Seal is now taken for the Eagle. Note tuft of Feathers at back of head in Original Drawings.

The Phoenix (the mythological Persian roc) is also the name of a Southern constellation and so the symbol has both astronomical and astrological significance.

Mediaeval Hermetists regarded the Phoenix as a symbol of the accomplishment of alchemical transmutation – a process equivalent to human regeneration.

Further, it is the name of one of the secret alchemical formulae.

Even what is taken for a Pelican in Rosicrucian imagery is, in fact a representation of the Phoenix. Careful examination shows that the characteristic, ungainly lower part of the bird's beak is missing and the head is far more like an Eagle's than a Pelican.

In the rites of the Mystery religions, it was customary to refer to initiates as 'Phoenixes' or, 'men who had been born again', for, just as physical birth gave man consciousness in the physical world, so the neophyte, after nine degrees in the womb of the Mysteries, was 'born into a consciousness of the spiritual world'.

"If you mean – have I been 'born again' – then, yes, I'm a Christian" – George Bush

The Seal is riddled with 'opposite' occult symbolism from the alchemical tradition, stemming from the Egyptian Therapeutate (medicine). War and peace, darkness and light, male and female, good and evil are all evident. The bird clutches in its right talon a branch bearing 13 leaves and 13 berries – 'Peace' and in its left a sheaf of 13 arrows –'War'. Above it is the motto 'E Pluribus Unum' (out of many – one). Mark that intention well! The motto also contains 13 letters.

Much is made of the fact that there were 13 original American colonies.

The number 13 has far more occult significance than just that. The Sacred Emblem of the Ancient Initiates, composed of 13 stars appears above the Phoenix.

2. The Dollar Bill

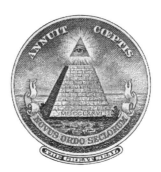

Hidden on the obverse of the Seal for years before being transferred onto the Dollar Bill in 1933, is another potent set of symbols. An un-finished pyramid is topped with the all-seeing 'Eye of Horus'. According to Ancient Egyptian Religion, Horus was the son of Isis and Osiris, and disputed the leadership of the gods with Seth who had tried to destroy him in infancy. He became more and more important and his identity evolved over the whole of Egyptian history. In effect he became the main god of Ancient Egyptian religion and the patron deity of the Pharoahs.

'He was the god of time, hours and days and this narrow span of time recognised as mortal existence.' Manly P Hall – The Secret Teachings of All Ages XLVII

Freemasons describe the symbol as 'The Eye of Providence'. However, other occult scholars recognise it as the Eye of Lucifer. The pyramid is constructed of 72 stones arranged in 13 layers. Above it is written 'Annuit Coeptus' – 13 letters again.

Gaillard Hunt described this as an allusion to line 625 in the Aeneid by Virgil;

'Jupiter omnipotes, audacibus annue coeptus' – All powerful Jupiter, favour my daring undertakings.' Thompson changed the imperative annue to annuit, the third person singular form of the same verb. In the motto 'annuit coeptus' the subject of the verb must be supplied and the translator must choose the tense. In his brochure of 1892 Hunt suggests that the missing subject was in fact 'the Eye', translating the motto '(The Eye of) Providence is favourable to – or has favoured our undertakings.' Beneath it written 'Novus Ordo Seclorum' – Translated 'A New Order of Centuries' begins anew – more recently 'A New Order of Ages' or 'New World Order'. The word seclorum is where we get our word 'secular' from so you could say it is announcing the 'new secular or godless order'.

Let's skip the eloquent smoke and mirrors – in ordinary language it means;

'Announcing the Birth of the New Secular World Order'!

"America was not created to be one great power among many. It was created to be the Novus Ordo Seclorum' – A New Order for the Age. Our nation has come to a defining moment. A time when our choices will be hardened into history"

(Presidential Candidate Jack Kemp while running for Office.)

There's still more. There is a date at the base of the pyramid – 1776. May the 1st, 1776 was the date of the inauguration of the Order of Illuminati.

May the 1st has tremendous significance throughout occult societies. It is the date for initiation into Orders – e.g. George W Bush was 'tapped' into Lodge 322 'Skull and Bones' at Yale on the 1st of May 1968.

3. Washington D.C.

The entire layout of Washington D.C. and its architecture are Masonic.

There are symbols everywhere. You might have gathered by now that the people I am writing about delight in hiding their origins and intentions 'in plain sight'.

At the very highest level they take delight in 'misleading the dumb cattle' - ordinary people who are considered too stupid to comprehend what is in front of them.

The laying of the original cornerstone took place in an occult ceremony involving George Washington (a Freemason). Two hundred years later in a ceremony commemorating this event, Senator Strom Thermond (a 33rd Degree Mason) spread cement on a reproduction of the original Capital Cornerstone.

On the back was clearly visible the Masonic symbol of Square and Compass.

If you think Washington D.C. is a nightmare to drive around it's because the entire street layout was designed to Masonic patterns by a French Freemason, Pierre L'enfant. Like the pyramids of Egypt, the entire city was built in alignment with the stars. Esoteric symbols abound. One of the occult intentions was probably that America be empowered by the gods of the ancient world.

We could go on but suffice it to say that all the icons of America have pagan origins. If it is a nation founded on Christian thinking as so many dear folk fiercely assert, then where, in all its imagery, are there any representations of Jesus and His Apostles, Old Testament prophets or even angels? They are not there.

But, look at a Washington street map! Take a good look at the symbols that _are_ there.

The Washington Obelisk - an obelisk dedicated to the Egyptian Sun God. Elsewhere, even the most well known symbol, The Statue of Liberty is not what she appears to most people. Her stature inspired by the 'Colossus of Rhodes', one of the wonders of the Ancient World, is combined with the image of Semiramis, Goddess of Ancient Babylon.

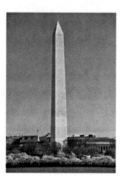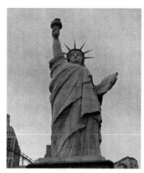

4. The Beliefs of the Founders of America.

In February 2000, CBS News.Com posted an article entitled 'Our Godless Constitution';

'Our nation was not founded on Christian principles but on enlightenment ones. God only entered the picture as a very minor player and Jesus Christ was conspicuously absent......' *Brook Allen. CBS News.Com.*

All of the above clues should give a fair indication of what beliefs the Founders of America held. The Founding Fathers of America had broken with traditional religious thought. They followed enlightenment thought and were influenced by writers such as Locke, Rousseau, and Voltaire as well as the scientific reasoning of Newton. None of the Founding Fathers practiced Christian orthodoxy.

They supported the freedom to exercise any faith, but for themselves, they were deists. Washington, Franklin, Hancock, Hamilton, La Fayette and many others accepted Freemasonry.

The Constitution reflects the founders view of a secular Government.

Historian Robert Middlekauff observes;

"The idea that the Constitution expressed a moral view seems absurd.

There were no genuine evangelicals in the Convention and there were;

"no heated declarations of Christian piety..."

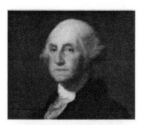

George Washington

Mason Weems wrote a book on Washington which portrayed him as a devout Christian. However, Washington's own diaries show that he hardly ever attended Church. Not once does the Name of Jesus appear throughout the thousands of letters he wrote.

He was initiated into Freemasonry at the Fredericksburg Lodge on 4th November 1752. Later, in 1799, he became a Master Mason and he remained a Freemason until he died.

After his death, his friend Dr. Abercrombie was pushed for answers about Washington's religious views.

In a reply to a Dr. Wilson he was unequivocal; '*Sir, Washington was a Deist*'.

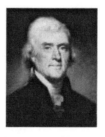

Thomas Jefferson

In many of his letters, Thomas Jefferson denounced what he saw as the superstitions of Christianity. He believed neither in spiritual souls or angels and certainly not miracles. He did not believe in the Divinity of Christ or any of His miracles.

In a letter to Peter Carr dated 10th August 1787, he wrote; "*Question with boldness even the existence of God.*" What he did believe in were materialism, reason and science. *"You say you are a Calvinist"*, he wrote to Ezra Stiles *"I am not. I am of a sect by myself as far as I know."*

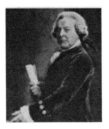

John Adams

John Adams simlarly denied Christian doctrine;

"I almost shudder at the thought of alluding to the most fatal example of the abuses of grief which the history of mankind has preserved – the Cross. Consider what calamities that engine of grief has produced." (John Adams in a letter to Thomas Jefferson).

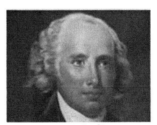

James Madison

James Madison, known by many as the 'Father of the Constitution', wrote in 1785;

"During almost fifteen centuries has the legal establishment of Christianity been on trial. What have been its fruits? More or less in all places, pride and indolence in the clergy, ignorance and servility in the laity; in both superstition, bigotry and persecution...."

(James Madison from Memorial and Remonstrance against Religious Assessments)

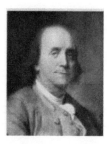

Benjamin Franklin

Having been brought up by Christian parents, Franklin had not come to believe.

A kind of 'shuttle diplomat' between France, England and America, like Francis Bacon, he was deeply involved in espionage. In Britain one of his underground haunts was the famous 'Hellfire Club' where he conferred with its founder, the colourful Francis Dashwood. Much time was spent in carousing and as the Satanic side of affairs became more prominent the club literally met underground.

Many hold that the club was a key centre for those involved in international espionage.

"...Some books on Deism fell into my hands....it happened they wrought an effect on me quite contrary to what was intended by them; for the arguments of the Deists, which were quoted to be refuted, appeared to me much stronger than the refutations; in short, I soon became a thorough Deist."
(Benjamin Franklin – Autobiography)

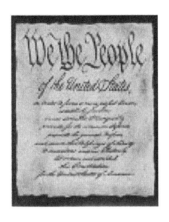

5. The United States Constitution

The United States Constitution itself gives the best evidence that America was not grounded on Christianity. If the Founders had set out to frame a Christian republic they would hardly have left out their Christian intentions from the law of the land.

Actually, there is no mention of Christianity anywhere in the Constitution.

There is not one reference to God, Jesus or even a Supreme Being.

In fact there are only two references to religion and these are worded in exclusionary fashion;

The First Amendment's states;

"Congress shall make no law respecting an establishment of religion...."

Article VI, Section 3; "...no religious test shall ever be required as a qualification to any office or public trust under the United States."

Christians who wish to think of an America based on Christianity often present the Declaration of Independence as their argument. They do this because this document mentions God. But, take a close look and you see that the God in the Declaration is not the God of Christianity. It runs; *"..the Laws of Nature and of Nature's God..."*

This falls nicely into line with Masonic or Deist outlook but it can't be used to support the case for Christianity.

There is another crucial point frequently overlooked in this argument. This document does not represent the law of the land as it came before the Constitution. Although an important historical document setting out rebellious intentions against Great Britain, it has no legal gravity. It looks forward to a future Government upheld by citizens instead of a religious Monarchy.

Those at the birth of America founded a government on Enlightenment thinking. They paid no heed to political beliefs about Christianity.

Finally, The Treaty of Tripoli, an instrument of the Constitution, clearly states the non-Christian foundation which had been laid.

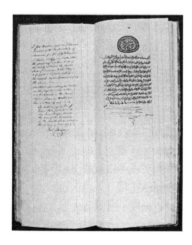

Some Players and Their Parts

'All the world's a stage and all the men and women merely players; they have their exits and their entrances; and one man in his time plays many parts'
(As You Like It – Shakespeare).

It is important to identify some key people and the parts they have had in creating the present shape of the world we think we know.............

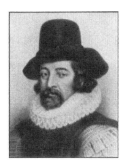

Francis Bacon, Lord Verulam and Viscount St. Albans was born in 1561. The son of the Lord Keeper of Britain's Great seal, Bacon was highly educated and became a lawyer and Member of Parliament. He served as England's Grand Chancellor during the reign of King James the 1st.

A genius intellect, most correctly think of him as a key figure in the development of modern scientific method. So much has been written about his public life, achievements and disgraces that we need hardly go over the ground. It is the other side of Bacon's life which concerns us.

He was relentless in his scientific explorations and had no time for the endless debates which took place at the universities of his time. While some of the academics of the day were given to a speculative approach, Bacon saw how ineffective this route was. While others argued as to how many teeth a horse had, he believed in marching out to the fields, finding a horse and pulling its mouth open to count them. Though this sounds a fairly common sense approach now, science in his time had stagnated to an abysmal level.

Bacon was just as relentless in his secret life. Deeply into the occult, much of his activity was cloaked in secrecy and he was a key figure in international espionage.

"The founder of (English) Freemasonry....the guiding light of the Rosicrucian Order, the members of which kept the torch of true universal knowledge, the Secret Doctrine of the Ages, alive in the dark night of the Middle Ages."

Marie Bauer Hall on Sir Francis Bacon

The Rose and Cross

He was Head of the secret Rosicrucian Order in England and deeply involved with the Knights Templar traditions which had gone underground into the Secret Lodges.

Taking its name from its primary symbols, the Order of Rose and Cross, like Masonry traces its religious practices back to the ancient Mystery religions.

Their present headquarters in San Jose', California, centres around an Egyptian museum. Their order is overshadowed by the chief of Secret Societies, Freemasonry. Nevertheless they were first of the Secret Societies to open a door in America, establishing the Ephrata Cloister on the East Coast in the 1600s.

Long before Columbus, the existence of America was known to the secret societies.

Those born into the elite bloodlines or initiated into their geo-political aims become aware that the steering of world events is planned methodically and, when needful, implemented incrementally. The largest objectives are passed down through generations of the dynasty.

Those same secret societies that were midwives at the birth of the new American nation are, in their modern forms, still forcing nations to conform to their objectives right now. They do this through the immense wealth and influence they have come to control. The scope of their hidden power is beyond what most ordinary people can imagine in their wildest dreams.

They were the nurses in America's infancy, carefully guiding it's first tentative steps along a pre-ordained path. America was seen by them as a key player in the outworking of the grand, Globalist scheme.

The land was to be colonised and a country born with a gigantic historical purpose. Its destiny was to fulfil the role of the New Atlantis. (see Bacon 'New Atlantis')

As head of the Rosicrucian Order in England, Francis Bacon sent emissaries to America to put in place the first foundations of the Great Plan. He wanted to carefully guide the establishment of the esoteric empire he and his fellow initiates envisaged.

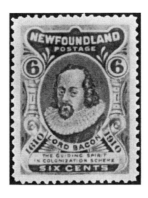

A 1930 Newfoundland stamp has the inscription 'Lord Bacon, The Guiding Spirit in the Colonization Scheme.'

Among his many other achievements, Francis Bacon was the first to formalise the Ancient Mystery Teachings into a system now recognisable as Modern Freemasonry.

Until his time Masonry was largely taken up with the craft, each country having its own form. The skilled stonemasons who built cathedrals all over Europe guarded their secrets fiercely, leaving esoteric riddles in the stone they carved.

There was nothing too brotherly on an international scale. The ancient secrets were held in different lodges all over the world. Bacon was hugely responsible for its coalescence into the international form in which it entered the New World.

While the Rosicrucians were careful to deliberately preserve their anonymity, Masonry went on to ascend to the very heights of power in America.

Bacon's insatiable thirst for knowledge drove him deeper and deeper into occult practices. Working with a medium who summoned up forbidden spirits, he exposed himself to more and more dangerous levels of exploration....

"When you enter the land the Lord your God is giving to you, do not learn to imitate the detestable ways of the nations there. Let no one be found among you who sacrifices his son or

daughter in the fire, who practices divination or sorcery, interprets omens, engages in witchcraft, or casts spells, or who is a medium or spiritist, or who consults the dead. Anyone who does these things is detestable to the Lord and, because of these detestable practices, the Lord your God will drive out those nations before you." Deuteronomy 18 verses 9 to 13

Bacon felt that if the beings summoned in the secret ceremonies could offer knowledge, he would take the risk with his immortal soul. There were terrifying incidents and demonic manifestations. In his cipher writings he reveals how a 'heavenly voice' gave him the inspiration for his life's work. The voice inspired him towards secrecy and imitation of 'the work of God';

"The divine majesty takes delight in to hide his work......according to the innocent play of children. Surely for thee to follow the example of the most high god cannot be censured......therefore put away popular applause and after the manner of Solomon, the king, compose a history of thy time and fold it into enigmatical writings and cunning mixtures of the theatre..." Francis Bacon's instructions from the 'heavenly voice'.

Although he was known as a writer and lawyer and involved in the affairs of court, for the rest of his life Francis Bacon tried to carry out what he believed was his calling. On the one hand he continued to take an unseen role in the shaping of the 'New World'. On the other hand, he threw himself into writing a series of theatrical works that would help to educate the English people and rescue the English Language. At the time, English was a mongrel mixture with little of the sophistication required to compete with French as a language of diplomacy.

He was determined to rescue and reform the tongue. His time at the French Court had made him envious of the French and the eloquence with which their language could accommodate poetry, science and the manners of High Court along with great theatre and literature.

The ancient plan that drove him required a language fit to serve an empire that would one day dominate the world.

Because of the commission he had received from the 'heavenly voice' he published nothing under his own name from that time, but rather used the name of 'Shak-speare'. The 'e' was added much later. Shak-spear was a synonym for the god and goddess Apollo & Pallas Athena. Both were known as the 'shakers of the spear'. They shook their weapons in the eyes of the 'dragon of ignorance' in classical tradition. The spear represented a ray of light or wisdom.

Apollo and Athena are the muses behind the other nine muses said to inspire all writers throughout the ages.

"The Universe is not only queerer than we imagine, it is queerer than we can imagine"
JBS Haldane

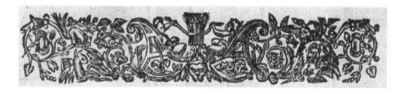

Bacon incorporated a double 'A' headpiece into the pages of the Shakespearian folio representing Athena and Apollo. Of the two, Athena seemed to most fire Bacon's imagination. Some speculate that he felt he had heard Athena herself commissioning him in his work.

The Stratford actor, Shakespeare, credited with the work, could not possibly have been the real author. Barely literate enough to make his mark, no correspondence seems to exist between him and his contemporaries. A man of very limited social circles with no experience of the International Courts of Italy, Spain or France, he couldn't possibly have possessed the insights, experience or legal expertise to have produced the works credited to him. The fact was that Bacon didn't care about public acknowledgement for the work. His writing was deliberately carried out in secret as per his instructions 'from beyond'. As far as he was concerned, he was on a mission to uplift and inform the English. As long as the works were out there and reaching the intended audience he was satisfied.

*(Among others, see Manly P Hall – The Secret Teachings –
on Shak-spear/Bacon)*

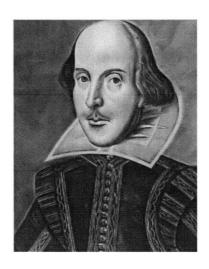

Note the visible masque line from collar to ear in this familiar image.

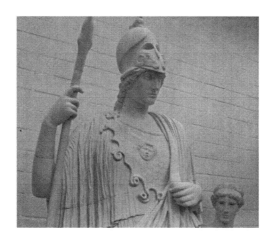

The Knights Of The Helmet

Some question how Bacon managed the volume of output among his other endeavours. This is to thoroughly underestimate his genius and organisation.

One of the masques of court that Francis Bacon produced was entitled 'The Knights of the Helmet'. This became the name of the unseen team he set in place to achieve his goals.

Again the reference is to the same deities. Athena's helmet conferred invisibility. As a man of means, he set up a writing group along the same lines as a Renaissance artist's studio. Some were cipher experts, many were poets and writers.

A number of these people he employed personally, the rest were glad to contribute to this exciting project voluntarily. In the same way as a Renaissance artist would paint in the head of a figure and leave a student to finish the robes in the style of his master, so Bacon would proceed with his writings. A man way ahead of his time, even then he had his own private printing press to get the end products out to the public.

The Inspiration for Bacon - The New world Order

Where does the inspiration to fashion a New World Order originate?

For Francis Bacon and many of his group, one of the most absorbing obsessions was Atlantis. Later in his life he wrote 'The New Atlantis'.

The story of lost Atlantis has been the inspiration for many films, TV series and adventure books. Because it occupies this sort of trivial place in our present Western culture, it is hard for people to treat it seriously; it's a joke or an old wives' tale. For serious students of the occult and Ancient Mysteries however, it's far from a joke.

Adolf Hitler was involved in the deepest levels of the occult through his membership of The Order 'Skull and Bones'. While in power, he sent official scientific expeditions to investigate various sites for evidence of the remains of the lost continent of Atlantis.

In the Critias and Timaeus, Plato puts in the mouth of the character Critias a description of travels made by Solon, 'the wisest of seven wise men'.

At a time of unrest, he embarks on a journey to seek answers to the social problems in Greece. He tells of a conversation with an Egyptian priest. Solon finds that he and his countrymen are actually ignorant of antiquity. The priest tells Solon that compared to the Egyptians, the Greeks are merely children in their understanding, as they have no really ancient knowledge. He discovers that there is ancient knowledge that he knows nothing about;

'Oh, Solon, Solon, you Greeks are all children and there's no such thing as an old Greek.' 'What do you mean by that?' inquired Solon. 'You are young in mind' came the reply: 'you have no belief rooted in old tradition and no knowledge hoary with age......'

He goes on to describe an amazing, rich and well ordered civilisation called Atlantis. For many scholars, it is a myth representing the perfect civilisation. For others, it is a description of actual, historic events. There are two or three views held by serious scholars as to exactly where its submerged ruins lie. The religious and mystical side of the knowledge referred to is the ancient satanic craft claimed by the secret societies. There is much detail about the organisation of the Atlantean civilisation and how its eventual arrogance and intent to make war brought its downfall. Amidst earthquakes and floods of extraordinary violence, the description tells of the entire landmass of Atlantis being swallowed into the sea.

In his introduction to his translation of the Timaeus, Thomas Taylor quotes from a history of Ethiopia by Marcellus. It contains a reference to Atlantis;

"For they relate that in their time were seven islands in the Atlantic Sea, sacred to Proserpine; and besides these three others of immense magnitude; one of which was sacred to Pluto, another to Ammon, and another, which is in the middle of these, and is of thousand stadia, to Neptune."

Although generally regarded as mythical, for Masonic scholars, those of privileged birth and students of the occult, it is much more than an invention of Plato.

It really doesn't matter whether you or I take the Atlantean story seriously.

The important thing is that the writings of Plato and the shape of the hierarchy of Atlantis inform the occult belief system of those lineages who wish to impose a one world government.

Atlantis was said to be a three-tiered society.

At the top were the <u>Golden</u> ones - the Elite. This class ruled absolutely by virtue of birth and bloodline.

Below them were a class characterised by <u>Silver</u>. This class included Civil Servants and the Military who were there to protect the exalted ones from those in the lower reaches of society.

At the bottom were the ignorant drone class – basically slaves. The <u>Bronze</u> Class! They would only ever be educated to the level required to serve their masters absolutely.

Possibly due to his own sexual preferences, Plato did not include families as part of this ideal society. Children were bred for their role in society and then raised and educated by the state.

Ask yourself – does this 'Ideal Society' appeal to you? It will only appeal to you if you see yourself as a member of the Golden Elite. This is how those engaged on re-creating it see themselves. They believe that they are the only ones fit to rule and that they should be totally served by the slave rabble beneath them.

The ancient 'blue blood' belief system held that, within this hierarchy, there were seven root races in Atlantis. Only one of these survived its destruction.

These were the ARYAN race. These survivors are said to have escaped the flood and gone to Tibet from whence they migrated to Scandinavia and became known as the 'blue eyed blonde' royal lines. Many then settled in England.

'Star Wars' portrays a version of the Atlantean belief system. There's 'The Force' which could be used for either good or evil. This 'force' could be harnessed to power technology and the flying machines of Atlantis and other mechanical gizmos ran on it. This 'Force' is 'Thule' – ring any bells?

Those who claim 'Blue Blood' heritage back to the Atlanteans genuinely believe that this Aryan 'Thule' runs in their blood. Hence the importance of bloodline preservation. Marrying your relatives preserves this occult power. Its trace is referred to as 'Vril'. This is why there has been so much 'in-breeding' among those who see themselves as 'elite' groups over the generations.

This belief system gives rise to the belief in 'The Divine Right of Kings'. Why should they be the ones to rule? Because they believe themselves to be divine and have the Divine right to rule. Their belief system is that the exalted ones actually become gods. Remember the opening of the book of Genesis? Satan was bent on convincing both man and woman that God was only forbidding certain things so as to prevent their progress to becoming godlike themselves. This is the exact lie that those from satanist bloodlines are brought up to believe.

The obsession with and involvement in the deep Occult is shared by most members of these elites. This needs to be kept in mind when studying individuals and societies involved in bringing about 'The New World Order'.

In reality the horrors of World War II were largely the results of in-fighting between secret occultist brotherhoods made up of powerful business interests and royal bloodlines. I am concerned that anyone who begins to study these things is made aware of the crucial occult elements early on in their investigations. It cannot be stressed too much. Winston Churchill (himself a Druid) was insistent that the occultism of the Nazi Party should not under any circumstances be revealed to the public during The War Trials of Nuremberg. Trevor Ravenscroft who worked closely with Dr Walter Johannes Stein, a confidential advisor to Churchill, records that

Churchill felt that another three decades at least should be allowed to pass before the extent of the black magic ingredients in Nazi ritual and practice should be made known generally. Airey Neave, one of the Nuremberg prosecutors, felt the occult aspects of Nazi belief were so contrary to the ordinary western mindset that many people might be persuaded that the accused were quite mad and may let them off execution with a plea of insanity.

"For our struggle is not against flesh and blood, but against the rulers, against the authorities, against the powers of this dark world and against the spiritual forces of evil in the heavenly realms." Ephesians 6: v 12

Mme. H.P. Blavatsky – Founder of the Theosophical Society

Adolf Hitler read from Mme Blavatsky's writings on these topics almost daily. He was intent on raising a pure 'Aryan' race and his fascination with tracing the lineages back led to him despatching expeditions to find the remains of Atlantis. He wanted also to rid the planet of what he thought of as 'mongrel' races.

"Under the evil insinuations of their demon Thevetat, the Atlantis-race became a nation of wicked magicians. In consequence of this, war was declared, the story of which would be too long to narrate; its substance may be found in the disfigured allegories of the race of Cain, the giants and that of Noah and his righteous family.

The conflict came to an end by the submersion of the Atlantis; which finds its imitation in the stories of the Babylonian and Mosaic flood...'and all flesh died ... and everyman'. All except Xisuthrus and Noah who are substantially identical with the Great Father of the Thlinkithians in the Popol Vuh, or the sacred book of the Guatemaleans, which also tells of his escaping in a large boat..." (H.P. Blavatsky) See 'Isis Unveiled'.

Several underwater expeditions believe they have
located the ruins of Atlantis

*"Was the religious, philosophic and scientific knowledge
possessed by the priestcrafts of antiquity secured from Atlantis,
whose submergence obliterated every vestige of its part in the
drama of world progress?.....both the cross and the serpent were
Atlantean emblems of divine wisdom. The divine (Atlantean)
progenitors of the Mayas and the Quiches of Central America
coexisted within the green and azure radiance of Gucumatz, the
'plumed' serpent. The six, sky-born sages came into manifestation
as centres of light bound together or synthesised by the seventh -
and chief- of their order the 'feathered' snake. (see the Popol
Vuh) The title of 'winged' or 'plumed' snake was applied to
Quetzalcoatl, or Kukulcan, the Central American initiate. The
centre of the Atlantean Wisdom-religion was presumably a great
pyramidal temple standing on the brow of a plateau rising in the
midst of the City of Golden Gates. From here the Initiate-Priests
of the Sacred Feather went forth, carrying the keys of Universal
Wisdom to the uttermost parts of the earth.*

*The mythologies of many nations contain accounts of gods
who 'came out of the sea.' Certain shamans among the American
Indians tell of holy men dressed in birds' feathers and wampum,
who rose out of the blue waters and instructed them in arts and
crafts. Among the legends of the Chaldeans is that of Oannes, a
partly amphibious creature who came out of the sea and taught the
savage peoples along the shore to read and write, till the soil,
cultivate herbs for healing, study the stars, establish rational forms
of government and become conversant with the Sacred Mysteries....*

*May it not have been that these demigods of a fabulous age
who, Esdras-like came out of the sea were Atlantean priests?"*

(Manly P Hall – The Secret Teachings of All Ages XXXIV)

43

The Knights Templar

Pioneers of The World Banking System

The idea that a New Atlantis would emerge was a cherished dream of Occult scholars which seemed to be presenting itself as the lands of America were first explored.

Long before Amerigo Vespucci or Christopher Columbus 'discovered' these lands, they were known to the Secret Societies. The Knights Templar was one such group which had already travelled there and brought back knowledge from their voyages.

The Templars played an important role in advancing both World Systems of Banking and knowledge about the land of America. Their role as a Secret Society was a factor in their eventual conflict with the French King and Catholic Church.

Godfroi de Bouillon led the First Crusade and following a long and bloody struggle, his forces finally took Jerusalem in 1099. The Latin Kingdom of Jerusalem was founded.

He refused the crown of Jerusalem and settled for the title 'Defender of The Holy Sepulchre'. His time in this office was short. His only official act was re-approving the charter of an abbey on Mount Sion before he died on July 18th 1100.

Following the taking of Jerusalem, pilgrims began to flock to the Holy Land from all over the world. In their religious fervour they often risked their lives to see the sacred sites.

"Muslims lurked by day and night in caves in the mountains between Jaffa and Jerusalem, ready to ambush Christians journeying to and from the coast."

(Karen Ralls –The Knights of the Quest).

As the pilgrimages increased, so did the banditry. Tourists were easy targets.

The situation became worse and worse until, in 1119, Saracens killed three hundred pilgrims and took sixty prisoners. The leaders of Christendom decided that a response must be made and the idea of an order that married military expertise with a religious way of life was brought into being. The same year 1119, the 'Order of the Poor Knights of Christ and the Temple of Solomon' emerged.

Their original mission was to protect Pilgrims to the Holy Land.

At the outset, the Order was a family affair as several of the original Knights were from old Bergundian and Flemish families, based around Troyes in Champaigne, part of old Bergundy. There were originally only nine knights employed on this matter. King Baldwin II gave them exclusive accommodation in his palace close to what is known today as the Dome of the Rock. The palace was called the al-Aqsa Mosque; crusaders had earlier called it Solomon's Temple. The site had an extensive tunnel system beneath it. Speculation about the Templars finding secrets or treasure chests of golden scrolls here has fuelled the plots for dozens of books.

There is even a myth about them finding the Ark of the Covenant there. What we <u>do</u> know is that they became very successful and staggeringly rich.

The original nine Knights included the scions of several noble families.

Hugh de Payns a vassal of Hughes I, Count of Champagne as was Andre' de Montbard, the uncle of Bernard of Clairvaux (later canonise as St Bernard).

Godfroide St. Omer of Picardy was a son of Hugh de St. Omer.

The ruling family of Flanders was represented by Payen de Montdidier and Achambaud de St.-Amand. The others were Godfroi, Geoffroi Bisol, Gondemar and Rossal.

As the order grew and saw service, they won recognition as being fiercely capable in battle. This was to shock many who felt that 'priests in arms' didn't line up with Christian doctrine.

The Templars regarded the Saracen leader, Saladin with great respect and certain Muslim chroniclers refer to the Templars with mutual respect.

However, the Templars were more than just spiritual special forces for Christ. They proved themselves able diplomats, became trusted advisors to popes and kings to the extent that they undertook guardianship of royal treasuries. They were proven maritime experts, property developers, caretakers of large estates and vast numbers of livestock. On top of this they excelled in business, trading and running markets and fairs. They went on to become one of the wealthiest, most powerful organizations the West had ever seen. During the twelfth and thirteenth centuries, the order had acquired extensive properties, not only in the West, but in Palestine and Syria. Large numbers of Commanderies and Preceptories were established throughout Europe and the Latin East. People from kings to aristocrats and fallen soldiers donated or bequeathed the Templar Order money, farms, mills, ports, monasteries and churches to support them in their crusades.

Their rise to prominence and power was unlike almost anything that had gone before. Within ten years or so of the founding of the Order they had ownership of lands in just about every part of western Europe and far beyond. As their reputation grew so did the number of men who presented themselves as recruits to join the Templar Order.

In 1112, when Bernard de Fontaine (St. Bernard) arrived at Citeaux he had with him thirty or so nobles from the houses of Tonnerre, Montbard and Bergundy . Some were his relatives. He was twenty two years old at the time and his relatives considerably older. Yet they all agreed to give up everything and join him in the austere Cistercian Order. For some this meant leaving their wives and their children. It is said that he was a magnetic personality and this sort of incident is put down to his persuasive powers. What could have motivated these thirty nobles to drop everything and become 'instant Cistercians' when they had never considered this sort of life before? As Karen Ralls points out, Faith can certainly be a strong motivator. But all thirty? And all at once?

Bernard was also instrumental in getting Papal recognition for the Templar Order at the Council of Troyes in 1129. The Templar Order was closely associated with the Cistercians, especially in Northern France. Both had connections with Troyes. There were a number of key family associations and it is speculated that, even at this stage, something must have been going on behind the scenes of the Order – perhaps directed from Champagne that involved the First Crusade, Godfroi de Bouillon and the old Bergundian nobility, The Cistercians, Troyes and the original nine Knights Templar. Many suspect that, from the start, there was much more to the Templars than has ever been brought to light.

The true extent of Templar wealth can only be speculated. Imagine a huge modern, multi-national corporation. The Templar Empire began to take on this kind of form. There were tremendous stores of gold and money in their treasuries and they lent vast sums to Popes, prominent merchants and Kings.

The First Travellers' Cheques

Travel was deadly dangerous in the 12th Century. Entire villages and towns were controlled by bandits who would kill for even a meagre sum of cash. It was suicidal to be seen with money in transit. The Templars solved this by a system of promissory notes. If a merchant from England was doing business in France, he deposited the required sum of cash at the Templar establishment in his own town. On arrival in France he presented proof of his identity and a note written carefully in cipher. He was then issued the cash for the transaction he wished to conclude.

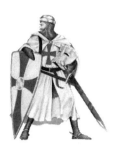

It would be presented in the local currency and he would be charged a handling fee. The fee was not large and the assurance of safe transit well worth the charge. No robber was interested in coded notes he couldn't cash.

It was forbidden by the Church to charge interest or usury. The method of a 'handling fee' allowed the Templars to profit without appearing to extract usury. They developed a whole banking system, loaning money with provisions for making up any depreciation in coinage value during the time span of the loan.

What had started out as a simple service to pilgrim travellers spiralled into a gargantuan financial empire. They were known to be trustworthy to deal with and so princes and peasants alike used their services.

Lending to Popes and Kings can be a risky business. As the Templar wealth and influence continued to expand, those who owed them money cast envious eyes on their holdings.

Ever wondered why people call Friday the 13th unlucky? It comes from the downfall of the Templar Order. On the morning of Friday the 13th of October 1307, in the early hours of the morning every known member of the Knights Templar in France was arrested. The charge was suspicion of heresy and the orders came direct from King Phillip IV in collusion with Pope Clement V.

The fact was that The King was up to his eyes in debt to the Templar Bankers. Having them all done away with was one way of cancelling the debt.

Heresy was a very serious charge.

The hunt was on and Templars went on being rounded up wherever they were found. Among a long list, they were accused of;

- Worshipping cats
- Spitting on the Cross
- Denying Christ
- Sodomy
- Obscene kissing at their reception into the Order
- Being sworn to secrecy about the Order
- Venerating an idol
- Illegal acquisition of property
- Perjury
- Holding secret chapters at night
- Not believing in the mass

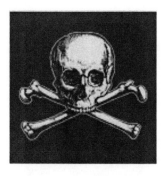

The Templar Ships often sailed under the sign of the Skull and Bones. The same terrifying insignia has been employed for centuries by other pirates.
The badge of the Hitler's S.S. is also the insignia of the 'Skull and Bones' Lodge 322 – the Yale University Secret Society whose members include President George Bush, his father, his grandfather and a great many others prominent in U.S. politics. This secret society was founded as a counterpart to Hitler's home Lodge in Germany.

The Templars captured were subjected to the most disgusting forms of torture under the Inquisitors. Confessions were forced out of starved and abused prisoners.

In the middle of a power struggle between the King and Pope over whose jurisdiction was valid, many were left rotting in prison. Some were burned alive at the stake. Their Order was abolished.

However, the best laid plans of scheming Popes and Kings don't always have total success. A great number of Knights Templar escaped. Estimates vary depending on the source. However, it is widely held that a considerable fleet escaped from France.

The Order had of course become international and there would have been many survivors outside France. The Brotherhood would have had word of Phillip's 'secret' plan with the Pope.

One place they knew they'd be safe was in Scotland.

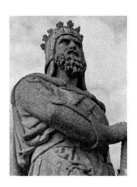

Robert the Bruce

Robert the Bruce, in defiance of England, had crowned himself King of Scotland.

In an age when most ordinary people lived in fear of the dictates of the Roman Catholic Church, the Pope had excommunicated King and Country of Scotland.

That meant that Scotland was viewed as a renegade nation. The arrival of the fugitive Templars meant that it gained a renegade army. It is believed that these Knights played a decisive role in Scotland's struggle for independence. The Templars were given refuge under the Sinclair clan. The alliance had historic significance. Many of the Templar Knights, like the Sinclairs, were of Norman blood and traced back their ancestry through five hundred years to the Norwegian Vikings. They shared the blood of seafaring adventurers.

These new arrivals must have awakened some of the dormant Viking in Henry Sinclair. He mounted an exploratory voyage by the clan in 1398.

Their destination? The Americas!

They left evidence of their arrival on Oak Island and New Ross in Nova Scotia, in Westford and Fall River in Massachusetts, at Lake Mephramagog in Vermont and in the harbour of Newport in Rhode Island.

Their impact on the North American inhabitants spread widely. There is evidence that Henry Sinclair even founded a colony as a refuge for those whose thinking didn't line up with rigid religious doctrines. The Sinclair fleet (the remnant of the Templar fleet) made several voyages to the New World. Not all were successful. Famine and ill fortune meant that some stayed and married into the native population. Those who returned brought with them hard evidence of their travels.

The stones of the Roslyn Chapel in Edinburgh, the Sinclair family home, were put in place a full fifty years before Columbus reached the Americas. Yet, in these same stones are carved images of American Maize and Aloe!

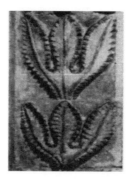

The Templars brought back evidence of their extensive travels. These images of American Maize along with images of Aloe were carved into the stones of Roslyn Chapel many years before the 'Official' discovery of America.

Sinclair's daughter Elizabeth married John Drummond, scion of another of Scotland's wealthiest families. Their son, also a John, was made of the same stuff as his grandfather. He too had the seaman's spirit and travelled to the Portuguese islands of Madeira. Explorers were taken aback to find the flag of the re-formed Templar Order flying as boldly as ever in Madeira. The Portuguese, in contrast to the rest of Europe, allowed the Templars to resurrect their Order under a different name. Here they were known as The Knights of Christ. The Grand Master of The Knights of Christ was Henry - called 'The Navigator'. The mission of his men was to open the highways of the sea.

When John and Elizabeth Drummond arrived in Madeira, the islands were governed by a small group of Italian families from the same city where Christopher Columbus was born. Columbus had joined the Knights of Christ. One of these families was the Perestrellos.

According to Steven Sora, by 1450 the Perestrello family had intermarried with the Drummond-Sinclair family. Felipa Perestrillo was born that year. Columbus and Felipa met at a Lisbon Church and were soon married. Columbus's new Mother–in-Law gave him the maps and charts from her late husband's explorations. As a chart dealer and would-be explorer, Columbus became privy to a body of knowledge unknown to any one person in the world.

(see Steven Sora - Lost Colony of the Templars)

Despite the Pope, the Templars maintained a wealthy international web.

The names changed and members migrated into other Orders but the influence had been established and the roots went deep.

As they sought refuge underground in the Lodges of the Secret Societies, they took with them the expertise that spawned much of the modern banking system. They also transmitted their knowledge of the 'New World' to these other occult societies. The Knights Templar had a profound effect on the development of Modern Freemasonry.

And the Heresies? Well, they <u>had</u> become a Secret Order.

During their time in the Holy Land they had exasperated many strict Roman Catholics by employing Muslim scribes and Interpreters. They not only admired the Muslims as adversaries, they started to syncretise their beliefs with Islamic and Jewish Occult practice. Those with enquiring minds studied the Gnostic and mystic aspects of the Eastern religions.

The Masonic World Network

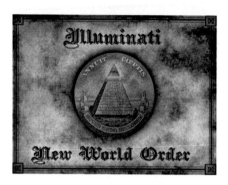

Originally trade guilds for the Masons who built the great cathedrals, the purposes of the Masonic Lodges changed as the need for the craft diminished.

The Reformation had filled forward thinking people with notions of a new, enlightened age. Science was moving to the centre of the stage and it was felt by many that Man's ingenuity and intellect would create a world with no need for God.

A new age was being ushered in and a vast, secret and international network was just ripe for exploitation. It has been likened to a peasant's cottage which could easily be redeveloped as a luxury weekend home for the well-to-do.

Many in the aristocracy transferred lighted candles from the altars of established Churches to the new Masonic Lodges as people with no stonecutting skills were admitted. People with a lot of money and an interest in the occult were admitted in large numbers.

Many of those who joined were interested in building something, but it wasn't a new cathedral!

The Puppet Masters

Down the years, the high temples of Masonry have preserved many occult practices and beliefs that they trace back to the Babylonian and Egyptian Mystery rites.

Babylon was identified with rebellion against God and her most profane customs have been kept alive by the adepts. The same spirit that possessed the Babylonians in their sinful rites of rebellion was, and is presently, celebrated and studied in many of the underground lodges.

I am not speaking about your average businessman who is asked to join the local Masonic lodge and rises maybe to the 3rd Degree. What is espoused at that level is pretty foul – but for the most part, it is jovial and new initiates are deliberately kept ignorant of what it is really all about. There is a great accent on precedent. After all, if Thomas Jefferson and George Washington were Masons it's good enough for someone like you, isn't it? If it's a secret Society, then there's probably a good reason. Who are you to question these ancient rites?

The Masonic Masters view low ranking adherents as 'sheep'. Higher up the Pyramid, however, Initiates preserve and practice the ancient luciferian religion.

In the higher Masonic orders, there is adherence to occult and ritual practice that would turn the stomach of anyone not brought up to it. The generational bloodlines rear their offspring to take their places in the hierarchy and advance the plan for Global government. They are taught that they are bred to rule the planet and have a part to play in bringing about the satanic kingdom.

Although born and brought up to carry forward the generational plan to rule, these children often get their grounding in rituals and hierarchy within the Masonic system. It is often part of their required education. These lodges have been the hatching ground for some of the most incredible schemes in history.

At the highest level, the practice of incestuous relationships is encouraged. It follows that a great deal of study is required to trace specific individuals' backgrounds.

The ceremonies are preserved in the forms of the Mystery religions which stretch back to Egypt and include blood sacrifice and sexual rites. The children of these unions will carry different names from the principle bloodline. In the Rothschild lineage for example, one has to take account of names such as Bauer (their original name), Bower, Sassoon and so forth. Those legitimate children are expected to marry within the bloodline. Of the eighteen marriages made by Mayer Amschel Rothschild himself, for instance, sixteen were between first cousins.

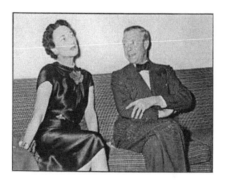

Bloodlines are crucial in these circles. For example, most people believe that the Duke of Windsor abdicated the throne of England because he wanted to marry a divorcee. The real story is somewhat different. He was a Nazi sympathiser as were many of his ilk and had sponsored a Naval man called Simpson into the English equivalent of the German 'Black Sun' which was a Thule group called 'Children of the Sun'. While participating in a 'Children of the Sun' orgy with Simpson at the Coronado Hotel in Santiago he was passed Simpson's wife, Wallis as one of the available women to be bedded.

He obviously enjoyed the experience immensely as things later got serious between the two. The real reason that he had to abdicate was that the powerful Cecil family, an established force behind the British throne since around 1600, objected to him sullying what they saw as the Merovingian bloodline with an 'American cur' by marriage, even if she was good in bed.

The Rothschilds viewed the whole thing slightly differently and thought he should be allowed to get on with it. There was a heated disagreement.

It was resolved by the Cecil family who got Winston Churchill to 'go pack his bags' and give him his marching orders. He duly abdicated the Throne and the happy couple then cleared off. Where? To stay at a Rothschild mansion and have a cruise and honeymoon also paid for by the House of Rothschild.

The Final Pieces of Modern Masonry – The Emergence of the Illuminati.

On 1ˢᵗ of May 1776, the final component in the development of Modern Freemasonry was put in place. Already it was shot through with Ancient Mystery Religion, Fertility Cults, Islamic mysticism, Alchemy, Templary and Rosicrucianism; all parts of the doorway to witchcraft.

Things were sealed when satanist elitists infiltrated the Masonic Lodges of Bavaria in 1777. The front man for this was Dr Adam Weishaupt (1748 – 1830), a professor of Canon Law at Ingolstadt University. Weishaupt did not create the Illuminati, they chose him as a figurehead. The House of Rothschild who were part of a Jewish banking cult known as the tugenbund, commissioned him to centralize the power base of The Mystery Religions into The Illuminati or 'Enlightened Ones' - an amalgamation of Occultic Bloodlines, Elite Secret Societies and High Masonic Fraternities.

The creators were financiers and the origins of some of their fortunes dated back to the bankers during the times of the Templar Knights who financed the early kings in Europe. These same banking dynasties still control the finances of the world today.

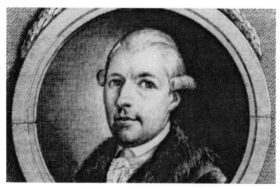

Adam Weishaupt 1748 - 1830

59

May 1st, sacred on the calendar of witchcraft, was chosen for the foundation of the Order of 'Ancient and Illumined Seers of Bavaria'. The following year Weishaupt was initiated into Freemasonry in Munich at the Lodge Theodore of Good Counsel. He played upon the egotism that is rife in Masonry and skilfully created an Order within an Order. The cunning was literally devilish. A Secret Society was concealed within the folds of a Secret Society. By 1779 Weishaupt's 'insinuators' had complete control of the Lodge and it had become part of the Order of Illuminati.

In July 1780 Baron von Knigge was initiated into the Order. A prominent Strict Observance Freemason, he was connected to the court of Hesse-Cassel. He recruited many prominent members and restructured the Order. It grew rapidly in numbers and influence. He and Weishaupt had a bitter disagreement and he later left the Order, but not before he had served his purpose.

The Congress of Wilhelmsbad

In 1782 The Congress of Wilhelmsbad was convened. This congress was of pivotal importance in the formation of an official coalition between secret societies.

'*At Wilhelmsbad near the city of Hanau in Hess-Cassel, was held the most important Masonic Congress of the Eighteenth Century. It was convoked by Ferdinand, Duke of Brunswick, Grand Master of the Lodge of Strict Observance…there were delegates from Upper and Lower Germany, from Holland, Russia, Italy, France and Austria; and the Order of Illuminati was represented by the Baron von Knigge. It is not surprising therefore that the most heterogeneous opinions were expressed.*'

(Albert G Mackey- Revised Encyclopedia of Freemasonry)

At the Congress at Wilhelmsbad the alliance between Illuminism and Freemasonry was sealed. What passed at this terrible Congress will never be known to the outside world, for even men who had been drawn unwittingly into the movement, and now heard for the first time the <u>real designs</u> of the leaders, were under oath to reveal nothing.......the Compte de Virieu, a member of the Martiniste Lodge at Lyons, returning from the Congress's could not conceal his alarm, and when questioned on the 'tragic secrets' he had brought back with him, replied:

'I will not confide them to you. I can only tell you that all this is very much more serious than you think. The conspiracy which is being woven is so well thought out that that it will be, so to speak, impossible for the monarchy and Church to escape from it.'

From this time onwards, according to his biographer, M Costa de Beauregard, 'the Compte de Virieu could only speak of Freemasonry with horror.'

The Bavarian Illuminati were set up for political intriguing. Their agenda then, as now, was to gradually tear down national borders and to overthrow governments and church in order to instigate their own government. The plan was, and still is, far-sighted and overarching. <u>Its Goal – Universal Revolution leading to World Government</u>. From earliest days it based its strategy on total allegiance to the Order, ruthless enforcement and superbly well organised espionage.

"If a writer publishes anything that attracts notice, and is in itself just, but does not accord with our plan, we must endeavour to win him over or decry him."

Adam Weishaupt - Founder of the Illuminati

The nearest thing you can imagine to the World Order the modern Illuminati are striving to set up in our time is Hitler's Third Reich. Many current adherents call their aim the 'Fourth Reich'.

"Do you realise sufficiently what it means to rule – to rule in a secret society? Not only over the lesser or more important of the populace, but over the best of men, over men of all ranks, nations and religions.......men distributed over all parts of the world? ......And finally, do you know what secret societies are?

What a place they occupy in the great kingdom of the world's events? Do you think they are unimportant, transitory appearances?"

Adam Weishaupt – Founder of the Illuminati

Weishaupt was educated by Jesuits and brought with him the mental disciplines he had been taught as a youngster. Illuminism incorporated an incredibly powerful mixture of Masonic secrets, Islamic mysticism and the scientific use of Almamout Hashish to produce an 'illumined' state of mind. This was the drug used by the Assassins. The connection with the Bavarian Seers with a 16th century Muslim cult called the Roshaniya would also have given Weishaupt his insight into Hashish.

Note; While on the Crusades the Knights Templar had encountered the deadly Assassins (Nizari Ismailis, a religio – political Islamic group that is still around). They were the Muslim equivalent of the Templars, trained as holy warriors. There are plenty of stories about the relationship between the Assassins and the Templars. The world explorer Marco Polo put together a collection of writings on them. The phrase about the 'Old Man of the Mountain' refers to the Syrian Chief of the Assassins.

The Law Of Fives – Weishaupt, Drugs and Sorcery

1st Book of Samuel – Chapter 5 verses 1 to 5

"After the Philistines had captured the ark of God, they took it from Ebenezer to Ashdod. Then they carried the ark into Dagon's temple and set it beside Dagon. When the people of Ashdod rose early the next day, there was Dagon, fallen on his face on the ground before the ark of the Lord! They took Dagon and put him back in his place. But the following morning when they rose, there was Dagon, fallen on his face on the ground before the ark of the

Lord! His head and hands had been broken off and were lying on the threshold; only his body remained. That is why to this day neither the priests of Dagon nor any others who enter Dagon's temple at Ashdod step on the threshold...."

One of the most powerful images in Illuminist sorcery is the sign of Dagon, ancient god of the Philistines. The hand is thrust palm forward with all the five digits extended. Remind you of anything?

Weishaupt taught that everything occurs in fives. Human history extends in a cycle of five stages and those who understand these can manipulate history to their own ends.

The stages are;

- Chaos
- Discord
- Confusion
- Bureaucracy
- Aftermath

Illuminism gave an impetus to the geo-political ambitions of Freemasonry on a scale not seen since the empire of the Knights Templar. It had always been involved in the dark side of political manoeuvring but now it took wings. As Weishaupt's teaching on the use of the Law of Fives, Drugs and Occult Practices came in, the large-scale evil of the Modern movement was unleashed. The final melding of Statecraft and Sorcery created the monster now bestriding the world stage.

Without this deadly chemistry, the satanist revival of the 20th Century could not have ignited in the way that it did. Just about every leading witch, occultist and satanist of our time has invariably been a high-ranking Mason.

Some examples;

- Dr Wynn Westcott; member of the Societas Rosicruciana in Anglia was a founding member of the Hermetic Order of the Golden Dawn. Their members introduced Tantric sex magic rituals to the West as a form of worship.

- Aleister Crowley; founded the anti-Christ religion Thelema. A master satanist who advocated child sacrifice in his published work 'Magick in Theory and Practice'. He used children in perverted sexual rituals and held several Masonic titles; Crowley was a 33rd Degree (highest) in the Ancient and Accepted Rite, a 96th degree (second highest) in the Ancient and Primitive Rite. <u>An occultic teacher to many in British royal circles.</u>
- Dr Gerard Encausse; Masterful author, exponent of the Tarot, leader of the occult Martinistes group.
- C. W. Leadbetter; Theosophist, mentor of the failed avatar or New Age 'Christ', Krishnamurti and prelate in the occult Liberal Catholic Church.

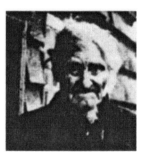

- George Pickingill; Witch, sorcerer, leader of the Pickingill covens.

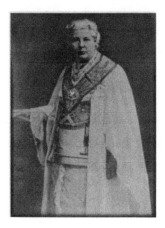

Annie Besant seen here in full regalia.
Yes, that's right – a Senior Mason!

- Annie Besant; (Yes - Highly placed female Masons!) Leader of the occult Theosophical society and Co-Masonic Hierarch.
- Gerald B. Gardner; Member of Crowley's depraved 'Ordo Templi Orientis'.Founder and practitioner of modern witchcraft or 'wicca.'
- Alex Sanders; Self-styled 'King of the Witches' based in London - one of the most influential leaders of wicca after Gardner.

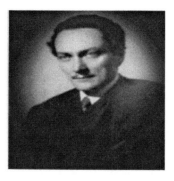

- Manly P.Hall; Rosicrucian adept and author of manuals on Freemasonry. Regarded as one of Masonry's finest 20th century minds.

The list could go on but all these sorcerers, witches and sacrificial satanists were welcomed into Freemasonry at the highest ranks. All levels of Masonry attract occultists and wiccans but the Illuminati, Ancient Rites and Supreme Council are the most infested enclaves.

Whose Light?

Illumination has long been the goal of occultists including those in Freemasonry.

The new candidate desires and is promised 'light' or 'illumination'.

As he progresses through the rituals he is supposed to become more and more 'enlightened'. What he is not told is that the 'light' he is slowly being exposed to is the light of Lucifer. The name Lucifer is not from the Hebrew Bible. It comes via the King James Version of the Bible through the Old English and Latin (Vulgate).

It is a rendering of the Hebrew word 'helel'. The Latin means 'Light bearing one' from 'lux' (light) and ferre (to bear).

As possessors of his light The Seers of Bavaria became known as 'The Illuminati'.

The unfinished Pyramid is a significant satanic icon. It is actually a metaphor for the cruel and controlling hierarchy that reigns above Masonry and even controls Governments. Yes – Governments!

The Illuminati

Families preserving an Illuminati bloodline often use the lodges of Masonry to indoctrinate their children into the symbolism and structure. Even though these offspring would take over key offices and positions because of their bloodlines, the Lodges provide a good 'training ground'.

Illuminati are referred to as 'Masters of the Temple'. Collectively they are known by several other names, but whatever form this may take, they are an elite cadre of 'Over-Masons'. Their understanding of the deep occult and satanic statecraft is often far above that of even 33rd Degree Masons.

There are many highly organised occult groups operating in the world today.

The modern adherents of Illuminism through their Banking Control networks and hierarchical positioning are the main thrust behind Globalisation and the introduction of a New World Order. But it is not the kind of New World Order that most people have in their minds when they hear that phrase.

Other Players who have Influenced the thinking of those behind the NWO..

Other pivotal figures in the history of our time were born as Adam Weishaupt was beginning an academic career.

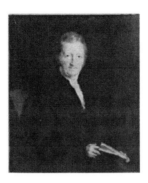

<u>The British economist Thomas Robert Malthus</u> was born in 1766. He was a major influence on Darwinism, Population Control and what became the Eugenics movement. He held that war, disease and famine were mechanisms to protect the earth against over population. Many people use the phrase 'Malthusian Catastrophe' without understanding its origins. As part of the Illuminati goal to de-populate the earth, Malthus advocated starving the unwanted masses to death.

Many of the powerful architects behind the New World Order are adherents of the Malthusian viewpoint; nature provides an excess population for which poverty and starvation are natural outcomes. In getting the population down to figures which are compatible with their plans, let the 'useless eating heads' starve. This can be hastened along by various means and present versions of this are referred to in high political circles as 'The Food Weapon'. Henry Kissinger is one of the better known advocates of this approach to the de-population goals of World Government.

The Georgia Guidestones

What is happening in Africa today is one of several deliberately prolonged Malthusian catastrophes engineered by those behind the New World Order. If you want to see some of their stated aims literally 'written in stone', take a look at The Georgia Guidestones. Their construction was arranged in 1979 by someone going by the name of 'R. C. Christian'. *(This cover name was probably a reference to The Rosicrucian Order).* Erected in Georgia, America they are made of granite and stand nineteen feet tall. The Ten Points recorded upon them are written in twelve languages, Sanskrit, Babylonian Cuneiform, Egyptian Hieroglyphs, Classical Greek, English, Russian, Hebrew, Arabic, Hindi, Chinese, Spanish and Swahili.

They have at their heart the aims of a Global Government, World Court, World Religion and the maintenance of the human population at under 500,000,000. The master race wish the remaining reduced populace to be maintained fit and healthy through 'guidance of reproduction' (in other words forced sterilisation and the elimination of 'useless eaters etc.) *See notes on New Age beliefs.*

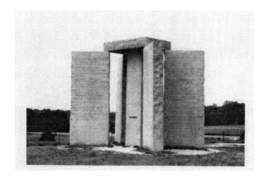

The Georgia Guidestones

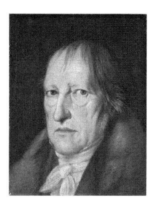

Georg Friedrich Hegel was born four years later in 1770. Hegel's thinking was 'revolutionary' in more than one sense and the practical application of his philosophy would form the basis for Communism, National Socialism and Globalism. Many present conflicts in the world are 'managed' through the use of Hegelian Dialectic.

"For Hegelians, the State is almighty and seen as the 'march of God on earth', indeed a State religion. Progress in the Hegelian State is through contrived conflict; the clash of opposites makes for progress. If you can control the opposites, you dominate the nature of the outcome."

Antony C Sutton 'America's Secret Establishment: An introduction to the Order of Skull & Bones.'

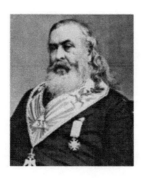

Albert Pike (1809-1891) – The Palladium Rite, The Ku Klux Klan and The Mafia

Soon after the Illuminists had infiltrated Freemasonry in the 18th Century, another extraordinary man appeared and quickly came to prominence. Albert Pike became a Mason in 1850 and rose through the ranks of the Order in meteoric fashion. Historian, lawyer and Brigadier-General in the Confederate Army, Pike became Grand Commander of the Southern Jurisdiction of the United States in 1859. He gave Scottish Rite Masonry its modern form and hated Christianity, showing his contempt for it at every opportunity.

One of his titles was 'Sovereign Pontiff of Lucifer'. He saw Lucifer as the true God in common with witches and pagans today.

Pike followed the Mystery religion of Baal. He acknowledged Lucifer as the true god and Adonai (the Biblical God) as the 'god of evil'.

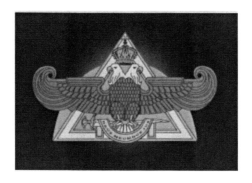

<u>Palladiun</u> *from GreekPalladius, from Pallas, Pallas Athena.*

1. Greek Mythology – Of or characteristic of Athena (see section on Francis Bacon)
2. Characterised by Study or Wisdom

Palladism

By the late 1800s Freemasonry had grown difficult to govern. It manifested in differing sects and lacked unity.

In 1870 Pike and Guiseppe Mazzini agreed to create a supreme, universal rite of Masonry over-arching all other rites. There was a major re-structuring of Illuminised Freemasonry.

"The blind Force of the people is a force that must be economised and also managed. It must be regulated by Intellect (a reference to the high adepts of the Masonic mysteries). When all these Forces are combined and guided by the Intellect and regulated by the rule of right and of justice, the great revolution prepared for by the ages will begin to march. It is because force is ill-regulated that revolutions prove failures."

Albert Pike – Morals and Dogma

Pike was foremost among 19th century adepts in preparing the way for the great revolution of which he spoke.

He was instrumental in the creation of the Ku Klux Klan, a secretive terrorist society in the South of the United States. To say no Negroes were admitted is the least of it. The Klan took delight in keeping anyone with a dark skin where they felt he belonged – right down at the bottom of the pile.

Lynchings, castrations, sacrifices and burnings were carried out by the Klan who saw the white skinned race as superior. As with other forms of political control in Masonry, the idiot 'cattle' carried out the crime under the direction of their Satan worshipping masters.

Pike was in contact with Giuseppe Mazzini the Italian revolutionary leader and the worldwide director of Illuminized Freemasonry from 1834 to 1872. Mazzini positioned Pike as head of the Illuminati's activities in the United States.

On 20 September 1870, the constitution creating the new governing super-rite was signed and put into effect by Albert Pike and Guiseppe Mazzini.

(Miller, Occult Theocracy, p.215).

Power was divided between Pike (Scottish Rite) who had authority as Sovereign Pontiff of Universal Freemasonry while Mazzini (Memphis Misraim Rite) retained executive authority as Sovereign Chief of Political Action.

The new super-rite was called The New and Reformed Palladian Rite.

The operational centres for the *Supreme* or *Palladian Rite* were located in Charleston, Rome, and Berlin. Pike and Mazzini also set up four Grand Central Directories for information gathering in their political and propaganda efforts. These were, The Grand Central Directories for North America in Washington, for South America at Montevideo, for Europe at Naples, and for Asia and Oceania at Calcutta.

Although the plan was to recruit adepts from other rites, initially they recruited from initiates of Ancient and Accepted

Scottish Rite and Memphis and Misraim Rite, men who were already addicted to occultism. Because of their Masonic rank and international contacts these men were accepted in any of the rites and thus were well placed to hand pick other adepts for Palladism. As this process took place, Palladian Lodges, known as Triangles were established around recruits the leaders saw as solid. The least ranking men were long serving Freemasons.

The Holy See of the Dogma for the whole Masonic world was set up at Charleston, the sacred city of the Palladium. Pike, who rejoiced in the title of Sovereign Pontiff of Lucifer, was the president of the Supreme Dogmatic Directory.

This was composed of ten of the highest grade initiates who formed the Supreme Grand College of Emeritus Masons. The Sovereign Executive Directory of High Masonry was established at Rome under Mazzini himself.

Here one can see the immense power of this additional layer to the emerging modern web of international intelligence.

Palladism centralised all the High Masonic bodies in the world under one head – Lucifer! Pike and Mazzini were his human agents. The Palladiun Rite represented the very pinnacle of the Pyramid of Power. Its religious coat of Manichaean neo-gnosticism teaches that Lucifer is the 'god of light and goodness' and struggles with Adonai 'god of darkness and evil'.

He was really only unveiling the true identity of 'TGAOTU'. The Great Architect Of The Universe is the way he is sold to brethren of lower degrees.

Pike states that Masonry is the universal religion and that senior Masons take a conscious decision to mislead and deceive those in lower degrees.

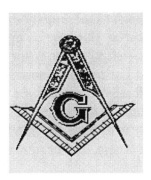

Blue Lodge

"The Blue Degrees are but the outer court or portico of the Temple. Part of the symbols are displayed there to the initiate, but he is intentionally mis-led by false interpretations....The True interpretation is reserved for the Princes of Masonry"
(Albert Pike - 'Morals and Dogma')

The Luciferian doctrine is 'implicit' in the lower degrees and only becomes 'explicit' in the highest degrees. The highest of the high was the Palladium: an international alliance to bring together Grand Lodges, the Grand Orient, the ninety-seven degrees of Memphis and Mizraim (the Ancient and Primitive Rite) and the Scottish Rite (the Ancient and Accepted Rite).

The traditional Palladium imprecation is;

"Glory and love for Lucifer! Hatred! Hatred! Hatred!

To God Accursed! Accursed! Accursed!"

Palladism connected Adam Weishaupt's devilish vision for humanity with Freemasonry, making a truly deadly mixture.

Candidates are taken through – you guessed it – A Five Step Plan!

1. Adoption; The initiate is brought into the fellowship of Lucifer. He is guided into swearing an oath and being yoked to the temple of Lucifer. Ultimately he is led into making a pact with Lucifer.

2. Illumination; Through use of drugs and occult techniques of the seers, the so- called 'third eye' is opened. This 'eye', or the Ajna chakra, is felt to be the point of contact between human beings and Lucifer consciousness. It is supposed to be located in the forehead between the two visible eyes. To 'open' the eye a little is to experience psychic powers. To open it completely is to have the mind flooded with pure Luciferic Consciousness. Hence the symbol of the 'All Seeing Eye'.

3. Conversation; This involves communicating with the 'mighty dead'. Spiritualism plays a large part in the Palladism. Mediumship is actively encouraged. Conversation with the sages of history is a vital part of the procedure.

4. Congress; Initiates are led into literally being 'married' to these dead. A medium of the appropriate gender is possessed by the 'dead spirit'. Yes, we are referring to demons. A sacrilegious 'wedding' is then fully consummated. It is believed that the magical 'virtue' of the spirit then flows from the possessed medium into the initiate through sexual congress.

5. Union; At this stage the soul of the initiate is completely eclipsed by the evil spirit. This is known as 'perfect possession' and can take years of inviting demons to come and 'own' the person.

Mazzini, who later rose to such prominence, had became a 33rd Degree Mason while at Genoa University and joined a secret organisation known as the Carbonari.

Their stated aim was; "that of Voltaire and the French Revolution – the complete annihilation of Catholicism and ultimately all Christianity.

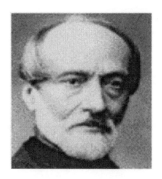

Guiseppe Mazzini

Mazzini formed a Sicilian society known as Oblonica (I Reckon with a Dagger). With the same level of cunning Weishaupt possessed, he went on to form an Order within that Order. He called this inner Order – The Mafia.

It is an acronym;

Mazzini Autorizza Furti, Incendi, Avvelenamenti.

Mazzini Authorises Thefts, Arson and Poisoning! Cute title, isn't it? It is also known by another name, 'Il Mano Nigro' – 'The Black Hand'. Here is the influence of the Illuminati. Mafia crimes were often 'trademarked' with the sign of Dagon – palm facing forward with all digits extended.

Prince Hall Masonry

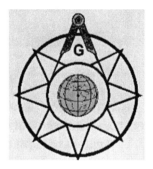

Later, Negroes seeking power, prestige and a piece of the action, went ahead and formed their own Prince Hall form of Masonry, colluding in the same evil institution that had so wickedly mistreated them.

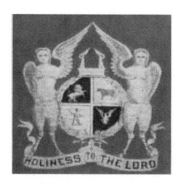

Royal Arch Masonry

The Royal Arch degree is the climax of craft Masonry. It is described as 'the root and marrow of Freemasonry' and is the complete story of Jewish history during some of its darkest times. In the 7th degree, the deity's name is revealed.

Only to those Master Masons who elect to be exalted to the Holy Royal Arch degree of Masonry is the 'lost name' of their supreme being revealed. Up until now they are told about TGAOTU, The Great Architect Of The Universe.

At this point they lose their freedom to believe in a generic word for God according to their own leanings. Now they must subscribe to the idolatrous, unholy, counterfeit trinity of Freemasonry...

Composed of three deities; Jah-Bul-On.

1. Jah from Jahweh – The Old Testament or Jewish Tanakh name for God.
2. Bul – from Baal, the Canaanite fertility god associated with licentious rites and imitative magic.
3. On – from Osiris, the ancient Egyptian god of the underworld.

The 16th Century demonologist, John Weir identifies Baal as a demon.

Freemasonry contradicts the first three of the Ten Commandments and denies that '

Christ is King of Kings and Lord of Lords'.

"Jahbulon is a mongrel word, in part composed of the name of an accursed and beastly heathen god whose name has been for more than two thousand years an appellation of the Devil."
(see Stephen Knight – 'The Brotherhood')

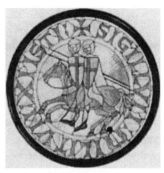

The Order Knights Templar is conferred on
the Order of the Temple.

Founded in the 12th century and older than Craft Masonry in
its present form, it defines the eleven rituals and laws governing
state and local level organisations. The state level is called a
Grand Commandery of Knights Templar.

This represents members of a state or an area of equivalent
size.

The local level is called a Commandery of Knights Templar.

Women, Negroes and the poor are all excluded.

As seen earlier, the Templars represented the first wide-scale
attempt to mobilise the forces of Occultism with the aim of
World control.

The Masonic symbols remain unchanged.

Their mixture of Islamic mysticism and Gnosticism
stemmed from their time in Palestine. The customs of the
Assassins, Phallicism, sodomy as a rite, venerating Baphomet,
the idol of the Luciferians, all became associated with the
Templars.

From their beginnings as defenders of pilgrims to the Holy
Land, they rapidly degenerated into Luciferians who loved
money as well.

As has been stated, the Masonic Network is worldwide.
Although most people are oblivious to the aims and objectives
of their hierarchy, this network exerts unseen influence upon all
the important aspects of political life.

In Britain people have a fascination for the processions and ceremonies that take place without understanding any of the real significance.

Behind the costumes and parades, Queen Elizabeth II is the 'Grand Patroness of Freemasonry'. Her husband Phillip was initiated into Freemasonry Dec 5th 1952.

Queen Elizabeth II presides over the Knights of St John, which is the British, protestant wing of the Knights of Malta. She presides also over The Knights Of The Garter, an order of aristocratic Illuminati knights. The Queen personally replaces members of the Order of the Garter as they die.

Prince Charles tries to appear all things to all men, but was educated at his father's old school, Gordonstoun, an Illuminati education centre where the headmaster was Kurt Hahn, founder of the Hitler Youth Movement. Charles is a member of the Order of The Garter.

They believe that they are members of the 13th Illuminati bloodline – 'The Merovingian', and hold that their blood tracks back to Jesus Himself. The family name was changed to Windsor from Sax-Coburg-Gota.

The red carpet rolled out before these people is symbolic of the bloodline that they hold to be so important.

The British royal family play a large part in International Freemasonry, lending an air of establishment and respectability to what is really a loathsome occultist network. The Queen's cousin, The Duke of Kent, is the present Grand Master of the United Grand Lodge of England and thus the head of British Freemasonry with all its wordwide links.

British statesmen and politicians of all hues need to be 'on the level' or 'on the square' behind the scenes in order to climb to any level of real significance in public. Thus, the illusion goes on and on. In Britain, like America, people still think that voting is a process untampered with and that they actually elect their governments.

Winston Churchill among his Order of Druids

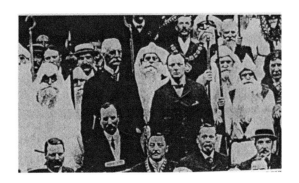

"Another Illuminati invention was Communism. This has been so thoroughly documented in several credible works that I don't know why I have to state it here except for the fact that there are still people who haven't taken the time to study it out. James H Billington's book 'Fire In The Minds Of Men' – a very scholarly work and 'Occult Theocracy' are some good starting points to study this."
    F. Springmeier – 'Bloodlines of the Illuminati'

"It is not my intention to doubt that the doctrine of the Illuminati and the principles of Jacobinism had not spread in the United States. On the contrary, no one is more satisfied of this fact than I am."
    George Washington

The Nature of the Present Illuminati Network

The Illuminati power base has always been in Europe. Their hierarchy all over the globe look to their rulers or 'lords' in Europe. There are thirteen in number.

Each ruler represents an area of Europe under his sway and each one represents an ancient dynastic bloodline. For example, the Hapsburg bloodline (Merovingian) is still active in Europe, although hidden, as well as the Rothschild and Battenburg bloodlines. In many modern European countries the immensely wealthy heirs of these lines are secretly the 'power behind the throne' if not the actual rulers themselves. For example, the Cecil family behind the British Throne. In America, members of ruling councils are always those who can trace direct descent back to the ruling cabal in Europe, whether legitimate or illegitimate. From the lowest to the highest levels, the group operates by instilling intense fear to control members. Often this is done through fear of death. Those who have been through the progressive levels of 'training' will have an intense fear of dying due to the 'Death and Resurrection' experiences they will have been subjected to. This control through terror is commenced at a very early age through systematic abuse (SRA – Satanic Ritual Abuse) and one can only weep at the accounts given by survivors. The MK Ultra programme sponsored by the CIA drew upon these evil practices and integrated many of them into their programming of children to create 'the mindslave' class. Researching these programmes is not for the faint hearted – some of it is literally sickening to wade through.

However, if you wish to understand just how corrupt the people who run governments actually are then read Cathy

O'Brien's account of her hellish existence at the hands of her own family, then former President Gerald Ford, Canadian Premiere Pierre Trudeau, Ronald Reagan, Bill and Hilary Clinton, Dick Cheney and many other prominent names. *('The Tranceformation of America' and 'For Reasons of National Security'- O'Brien and Phillips)*

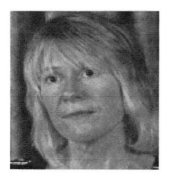

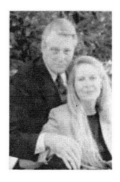

Cathy O'Brien   Cathy with her rescuer
                                 Mark Phillips

Warnings from The Past

'Those who do not learn from history are condemned to re-live it'.

Hegel

The story of the Knights Templar is a warning from the past.

Among Hegel's writings is the phrase that 'those who do not learn from history are condemned to re-live it'. The Templars methodically set up a network which straddled the known world. They sailed under the sign of the 'Skull and Crossbones". Originally a group dedicated to what they saw as God's work, their agenda gradually changed until they sought dominion.

They laid firm foundations for their successors. Eventually they reached the point where they would, and did, deal with the devil if there was a profit to be made.

However;

- They didn't have the assistance of computerised banking systems.
- They didn't have satellite spyware.
- They didn't possess high technology weaponry.
- They weren't dealing with an almost homogenous world culture.
- They didn't have instantaneous communication.
- They didn't have everyone signed up and within their monetary system.
- They did not possess the manipulative power of mass media and mindwashing.

They were tripped and fell hard, but their modern, high-tech successors have learned from every single one of their mistakes.

In place throughout the world right now is a network so terrifying it makes the Templar control of finances look puny. However, like their Templar predecessors, many of its highly placed representatives still sail under the same insignia – the skull and bones.

But, specifically, how have some of these banking dynasties managed to take such control of the banking system of the world? Let's take one of the most prominent examples - that of the Rothschild dynasty. Among others, Frederic Morton and Fritz Springmeier have done in-depth research into the rise of this manipulative, inbred bloodline. Their progress is representative of the constant struggle for dominance among the elite dynasties. The dominance of certain lines changes over time as they vie for supremacy. These bloodlines strive not only to dominate national economies and Governments, but also to gain place over one another.

The Red Shield (Rothschild)

During the latter part of the eighteenth century Europe was a disparate collection of warring kingdoms, duchies and states. Life for the average serf was bleak indeed. The quality of his existence depended on the disposition of his landowning masters.

Mayer Amschel Bauer was born in Frankfurt-On-The-Main in Germany in 1743. His father was Moses Amschel Bauer, a goldsmith and a lender of money. When he wearied of the itinerant life, he settled to open a counting house on Judenstrasse. Over the door he hung a large red shield; the emblem of the revolutionary Jews in Europe.

The young Mayer Amschel Bauer showed a remarkable aptitude for the business and was rapidly becoming efficient when his father died. Mayer took work in the Oppenheimer bank in Hanover where his natural talents quickly gained him advancement as a junior partner.

Back in Frankfurt he purchased the business his father had set up. Realising the significance of the red shield emblem above the door, he changed his name to Rothschild (Redshield).

Recalling his time with Oppenheimer when he had performed errands for General von Estorff, in 1760 he again sought out the military man who was then attached to the Court of Prince William of Hanau. With great cunning he played on the General's interest in rare coins and offered him examples at irresistibly reduced prices. This was his inroad and he was soon accepted into the inner Court. By this means he was introduced to the Prince himself who was also interested in buying some of his rarest coins and medals.

Here was the shape of things to come as he began to deal with other Princes. He was quick to exploit these contacts by appealing to their vanity and fawning on them for their patronage.

Obsequious requests were sent ....

"It has been my particular high and good fortune to serve your lofty princely serenity at various times and to your most gracious satisfaction. I stand ready to exert all my energies and my entire fortune to serve your lofty princely serenity whenever in future it shall please you to command me. An especially powerful incentive to this end would be given me if your lofty princely serenity were to distinguish me with an appointment as one of your Highness' Court Factors.

I am making bold to beg for this with the more confidence in the assurance that by so doing I am not giving any trouble; while for my part such a distinction would lift up my commercial standing and be of help to me in many other ways that I feel certain thereby to make my own way and fortune here in the city of Frankfurt."

On September 21, 1769, Rothschild put up a sign showing the arms of Hess-Hanau in front of his shop. The Gold lettering read:

"M. A. Rothschild, by appointment Court Factor to his Serene Highness, Prince William of Hanau ."

In 1770 Rothschild married and his wife, Gutele Schnaper bore him five sons and five daughters. His sons were Amschul, Salomon, Nathan, Kalmann and Jacob.

Rothschild became an agent for William of Hanau. This cruel noble, who was related to the other royal bloodlines of Europe, traded in human traffic as well as cash, renting out mercenary troops to who ever paid the required fee. Among his regular 'customers' was Britain. They rented troops to keep the American colonies under their thumb. Rothschild must have risen to a position of great trust, for when it was necessary for William to flee to Denmark amidst political turmoil, he left the mercenary army's payroll with him for safekeeping. The money was sent to London with Nathan to start a bank there.

On his death William left a fortune amounting to around $200,000,000.

(Note; The late Commander William Carr, an Intelligence Officer with The Royal Canadian Navy had worldwide contacts in Intelligence. His information reveals that the founder of the House of Rothschild drew up plans for the creation of the Illuminati and then entrusted Adam Weishaupt with its organization and development.)

Sir Walter Scott also recorded in his 'Life of Napoleon that the French Revolution was planned by the Illuminati and financed by the European moneychangers. Significantly, this book is not now listed in any current reference work under Scott's name. It appears to have disappeared from view.

Morton points out that it is difficult for the average person to "comprehend Rothschild nor even the reason why he, having so much, wanted to conquer more." All five brothers shared the same appetite for secrecy and conquest. The Rothschilds held no friendships above business and made no real alliances. They simply used those they associated with and discarded them when they served no further use.

When in 1806 Napoleon declared his intent to 'remove the house of Hess-Cassel from rulership and strike it from the list of powers', Rothschild wasn't the slightest disturbed. He merely saw the passing of one opportunity from which he had benefited seguing into another in Napoleon. Financing Napoleon gave him free access to the French markets at all times. A few years later when England and France were blockading each others' coasts, the Rothschild merchant vessels were allowed through. They were financing both sides!

The Rothschild financial influence was felt via the establishment of five Rothschild banks in five different countries. New money channels opened up and a new system of credits and debits emerged to replace the unwieldy shipping of gold bullion.

A major step was taken with Nathan Rothschild's new technique for floating loans internationally, in that he did away with the payment of dividends in varying currencies and made foreign bonds payable in pounds sterling.

The Battle of Waterloo
Rothschild Control of The Bank
of England

The growth of an empire like The Rothschilds depended upon a spy network of immense complexity. Their agents were active in all the capitals and trading centres of Europe. Their efficiency was legendary and they missed nothing that was of importance to their employers. This spy system had started out as a network between the brothers who sent messages to each other through a network of couriers. As the web developed in its speed and efficiency, it gave The Rothschilds an espionage capability even better than those of the National Governments of the countries where they were based. No expense was spared in manpower, equipment, coaches or shipping. It was vital to the Rothschild operation to have the edge on speed of information transfer to their headquarters.

The future of the European Continent depended upon the outcome of the Battle of Waterloo. If Napoleon's Grande Army won the conflict, then France would be the master of all Europe. If he could be stopped then England would hold the balance of power and could greatly expand its sphere of influence.

Historian John Reeves, a Rothschild partisan, reveals in his book 'The Rothschilds, Financial Rulers of the Nations', that one cause of his [Nathan's] success was the secrecy with which he shrouded, and the tortuous policy with which he misled, those who watched him the keenest.

Fortunes were to be made or lost depending on the outcome of this clash of titans and in London The Stock Exchange was alive with speculation.

The currency at the time was Consuls and if England lost then their value would crash to unprecedented depths. If Britain was victorious, the value of the consul would soar.

At the site of the battle Nathan Rothschild had his best agents placed both sides of the line and as the two armies closed in combat they scrutinized the fighting. Other Rothschild agents stood by to carry news of the outcome to a command post nearby. On the afternoon of June 15th 1815 a Rothschild agent boarded a specially chartered boat and made hurriedly for the English coast. He carried a top secret report on the outcome of the Battle of Waterloo. In the light of dawn he was met by Nathan Rothschild at Folkestone. Nathan quickly scanned the report and set out at speed for the London Stock Exchange.

COUP OF COUPS

On arrival, Nathan took up his customary position beside the famous "Rothschild Pillar." As usual, he showed no emotion and began to issue signals to his agents who began to dump consuls on the market. As their numbers built, their value began to slip downwards at an increasing rate. Rothschild leaned on his pillar and, showing no change of expression, continued to sell and sell.

The value of Consuls fell and kept on falling. The whispers went around; "Rothschild knows something – look at what he's doing. He must know that Wellington has been defeated at Waterloo." The rush was on to dump Consuls which dealers now thought to be worthless. The value of Consuls kept spiralling downwards and after several hours were selling for the equivalent of around five cents on the dollar. At this stage Rothschild's signals started to change subtly. Only the trained Rothschild agents knew what these changes meant and dozens of them went to the order desks and bought up every consul available for just a "song"! It took a while for news of the battle's outcome to arrive through more conventional channels.

The news was that England, not France was now the dominant force in Europe. It only took moments for the English Consul to explode back to far above its original value. As the consequences of Waterloo sank into public consciousness, the value of Consuls climbed further and further.

Napoleon had met defeat at Waterloo. Nathan Rothschild had bought control of the British economy. The vast fortune he already had was multiplied twenty times over.

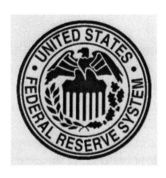

The Federal Reserve

In the United States of America people are led to think that the Federal Reserve is a Government institution. This is a deliberate deception. The Federal Reserve was so named to make folks think that it was their Government's treasury. It is actually a front for a collection of private banks and is run purely for the profit of its members.

Founded in 1913 – It is not Federal and it has doubtful reserves!

How did such a state of affairs come about?! Once again we see the hand of the same elitist interests at work. From the very founding of The United States, the Bankers angled for control of the currency.

Shrewdly, the early American colonies printed and issued into circulation small amounts of paper money. It was called Colonial Script.

Benjamin Franklin explained;

...."We make it in proper proportion to the demands of trade and industry to make the products pass easily from the producers to the consumers.... In this manner, creating for ourselves our own paper money, we control its purchasing power and we have no interest to pay to no one."

Elsewhere this colonial prosperity was viewed with horror by the banking elite. The Bank of England urged the English Parliament to issue The Currency Act of 1764 which prohibited the printing of currency. The colonies were forced to take Bank of England notes. Benjamin Franklin among others held that this outlawing of debt free money was the root cause of the economic depression and unemployment which triggered The American Revolution.

The very idea of a central bank run by professional bankers had always been rightly resisted by the men of real vision in the foundation of this new country. On the other hand, men such as Alexander Hamilton pushed for just such an institution. There was much heated debate between Thomas Jefferson and Hamilton around this issue. In 1781, prior to the drafting of the Constitution, The Bank Of North America was set up by Continental Congressman Robert Morris. He favoured a central Bank model and wanted to copy The Bank of England. *It lasted a mere three years before it was discontinued due to internal fraud and inflation which was caused by creating baseless 'fiat currency'.*

Alexander Hamilton, who had been a former aide to Robert Morris, went on to become Secretary To The Treasury and in 1791 once again attempted to set up The First Bank of The United States.

Thomas Jefferson was rightly and strongly opposed. He understood the way that a Central Bank could exert control on a nation. He had observed European developments and pointed out forcibly;

"The other nations of Europe have tried and trodden every path of force and folly in fruitless quest of the same object, yet we still expect to find in juggling tricks and banking dreams that money can be made out of nothing! I sincerely believe that banking establishments are more dangerous than standing armies; and that the principle of spending money to be paid by posterity, under the name of funding, is but swindling futurity on a large scale. Already they have raised up a money aristocracy…the issuing power should be taken from the banks and restored to the people to whom it properly belongs."

Jefferson held that a Central Bank was unconstitutional.

He wasn't alone in his views on Central Banks

John Adams wrote in 1811;

"Our whole banking system I ever abhorred, I continue to abhor and I shall die abhorring.....every bank of discount, every bank by which interest is to be paid or profits of any kind made by the lender is downright corruption. It is taxation for the public for the benefit and profit of individuals."

As writer and researcher Jim Marrs points out, The First Bank Of The United States, modelled as it was on The Bank of England, carefully went about cultivating links between banking interests and government.

20% of the Bank's capital was obtained through the Federal Government and the remaining 80% was pledged by private investors.

Their foreign investors included the House of Rothschild.

Gustavus Myers writes, "The law records show that the Rothschilds were the power in the Old Bank of The United States".

As always, the grasping elite of European Bankers along with their new toadies and associates in America were looking to gain control of the American money supply. These parasites caused inflation through their introduction of fractional reserve notes. The merchants of money prospered at the expense of the ordinary citizen.

A word of explanation is needed about this term 'fractional reserve'. In simplest terms a person with $10 could logically loan $10. Fractional reserve banking is a situation whereby bankers loan multiple times what they actually have in 'reserve'. They just go on printing currency which has no actual base to back it up. It is literally 'not worth the paper it is printed on'. The bankers merely trust that they won't be called on the amount they say they've guaranteed!

The First Bank of The United States 20 year charter came up for renewal in 1811 and was defeated by one vote in both the Senate and House.

What followed is often glossed over but it is a significant chapter in the development of America. The costs of the War of 1812 and the reigning financial chaos persuaded Congress to issue a 20 Year Charter to - you've guessed it –The Second Bank Of The United States. This was granted in 1816.

Enter President Andrew Jackson. In 1836 he stood against the congressional bill which sought to extend this charter. Like Jefferson and Adams his veto was based on his view that the bank was;

"A curse to a republic; inasmuch as it is calculated to raise around the administration a moneyed aristocracy dangerous to the liberties of the country."

In 1835 a man called Richard Lawrence tried to murder President Jackson. His pistols misfired. When questioned he claimed he was 'in touch with the powers in Europe." Jackson withdrew government funds from the bank, which he likened to 'a den of vipers'. The vipers struck back as the bank's president, Nicholas Biddle who was an agent of Jacob Rothschild in Paris, curtailed credit on a national scale. There was economic panic. Jackson faced the bankers' infiltration and influence in the senate as his veto was annulled by 24 – 19 votes. However, despite the opposition, by the end of his two terms in office, Jackson successfully managed to wipe out the national debt!

Jackson saw the bankers' corruption for what it was – a direct attempt to blackmail the Government into renewing their charter. His warning to the American people was prophetic in view of the events since 1913!

"The bold efforts the present bank had made to control the Government, the distress it had wantonly produced...are but premonitions of the fate that awaits the American people should they be deluded into a perpetuation of this institution, or another like it."

In the years that followed other attempts were made to set up another Central Bank. None of these were successful but the bankers went on plotting and scheming in secret to wrestle control of the prize –The currency of America.

In 1908, The Government was seeking reform in the face of several financial panics. Many researchers hold that these very panics were carefully engineered to set the stage for public acceptance of these 'reforms'.

Author Eustace Mullins was the biographer of Ezra Pound. Pound encouraged Mullins to research the background to the 'Fed' in 1948. Mullins concluded;

"A study of the panics of 1873, 1893 and 1907 indicates that these panics were the result of the international bankers' operations in London."

Under intense pressure from constituents in view of the panic, Congress finally passed the 'Aldrich-Vreeland Bill' in 1908. This authorised national banks to issue emergency currency 'Script'. It also authorised the setting up of the National Monetary Commission to recommend ways of making the U.S. economy more stable.

Many saw the Commission for the sham that it really was – No official meetings were held for nearly two years during which time Aldrich skipped around Europe in the company of senior bankers from England, France and Germany.

The Secret Seven, Jekyll Island and The Creation of 'The Federal Reserve'

On the night of November 22nd 1910, seven men set out for a secretive meeting at JP Morgan's retreat on Jeckyll Island off the coast of Georgia.

JP Morgan was a close associate of The Rothschilds so we see the same banking dynasties working to subvert the American banking system just as they had done the Bank Of England.

These men were conspirators on behalf of vast financial fortunes. It has been speculated that, between them they represented around a quarter of the wealth of the entire world.

As I have stated before, part of the success of associations such as the Rothschilds lies in their commitment to secrecy and top class espionage. To this end, Morgan relieved the regular servants on the island prior to the meeting. Those attending used only their first names and on November the 22nd, 1910 the newly employed servants had no idea of the identities of the men they were waiting on.

Those men were;

- Frank Vanderlip, - who represented William Rockefeller and Jacob Schiff's investment firm of Kuhn, Loeb & Company,
- Abraham Piatt Andrew – Assistant Secretary U.S. Treasury
- Henry P Davidson – Senior Partner JP Morgan Company
- Charles D Norton – President First National Bank of New York(a Morgan dominated bank)
- Benjamin Strong – A JP Morgan associate
- Paul Mortiz Warburg – Partner Kuhn, Loeb & Company
- Nelson W. Aldrich – Chairman of the National Monetary Commission. Although not a banker himself, he was an associate to banker JP Morgan and John D Rockefeller Junior's Father-in –law!

Warburg was also a representative of the European Rothschilds, brother to Max Warburg, Chief of MM Warburg Company, Banking consortium in Germany and The Netherlands.

For a week these men met to formulate a restructuring of the banking system.

The National Monetary Commission's 'final report' was put forward by the secret seven 'duck hunters' who had gathered on Jeckyll Island!

Their conclusion – not one central bank, but several. No one was to use the word 'Central' or the word 'Bank'.

Moreover, the whole arrangement was to have the appearance of an official agency. Too many people saw through this proposal –'The Aldrich Plan'. Congressman Charles Lindbergh warned, "The Aldrich plan is The Wall Street Plan". This attempt never got beyond committee. The banking conspirators made strenuous efforts to propagate their plans using massive leaflet drops running to hundreds of thousands and organising bogus letter writing campaigns.

A further obstacle had to be tackled. The president at the time was Howard Taft who was on record in opposition to plans for a Central Bank.

Woodrow Wilson, on the other hand had become the Bankers' choice for President. An academic and President of Princeton University, his former classmates had included Cleveland Dodge and Cyrus McCormack who were both Directors of Rockefeller's National City Bank of New York.

Author Ferdinand Lundberg writes;

"For twenty years before his nomination, Wilson had moved in the shadow of Wall Street."

He had become Governor of New Jersey, his nomination secured by a figure who became his constant companion and advisor, Edward Mandell House. House was a close associate of both Warburg and Morgan. This man, practically sitting on

Wilson's shoulder, had the support of The Schiffs, Khans, Warburgs, Rockefellers and Morgans. Incestuous isn't it?

With this calibre of moneyed conspirators in the game, manoeuvres were made to get the Bankers' required outcome in the election. Teddy Roosevelt was persuaded to run as a third party candidate, heavily financed by contributors close to JP Morgan. Roosevelt pulled votes away from Taft who had stated his opposition to The Federal Reserve Act. Wilson, who was 'in their pocket' and had stated he would sign the Federal Reserve Act', won by a narrow margin.

On December 23rd 1913, when everyone's attention was predictably elsewhere and when most congressmen had gone home for Christmas, Wilson sat down and signed The Federal Reserve Act.

Congressman Lindbergh ...." *When the President signs this act, the invisible government by the money power will be legitimised. The new law will create inflation whenever the trusts want inflation. From now on depressions will be scientifically created.*"

The Fed quickly appointed its own insiders.....Morgan banker Benjamin Strong became first Governor of The New York Federal Reserve Bank, the first Governor of The Fed's board of Directors was Paul Warburg who had planned many of the details. He went on to become Chairman of The Federal Reserve!

THE FED is not part of the U.S. Government in any way.

It is a Private Organisation, owned by its member Banks, which in turn are owned by Private stockholders. And these stockholders are just who?

Well by this stage of things you can probably guess..

Eustace Mullins;

"An examination of the major stockholders of the New York City Banks shows clearly that a few families related by blood, marriage or business interests, still control the New York City Banks, which in turn hold the controlling stock in The Federal Reserve Bank of New York."

In his 1983 book 'Secrets of The Federal Reserve', Mullins shows charts connecting the Fed and its member banks to The Morgans, Rothschilds, Rockefellers, Warburgs and so on....

They've been controlling and printing money which the U.S. Government pays interest on ever since. They control the U.S. Money Supply! This means they can decide exactly when you are going to have a recession in America in order to achieve their own financial ends.

Here is the real long term bankers' goal achieved by the Federal Reserve Act;
Taxpayer liability for the losses of private banks!

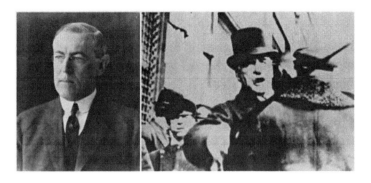

President Woodrow Wilson   JP Morgan

A while ago at an event near Austin, Texas, Congressman Ron Paul was asked a very direct question by Eric Rainbolt;

"Could you tell the people in this room any information you may have of an international and deceptive conspiracy to overthrow the American Republic and its Constitution and Bill of Rights in order to set up and usher in a totalitarian World Government likely espoused under the U.N. also?"

Congressman Paul:

"The answer is 'Yes'. I think there are 25,000 individuals who have used offices of power, and they are in our Universities and they are in our Congresses and they believe in One World Government. And if you believe in One World Government then you are talking about undermining the National Sovereignty and you are talking about setting up something that you could well call a Dictatorship. And those plans are there!"

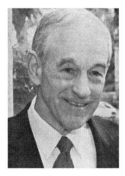

Senator Ron Paul

The modern factions of the Illuminati have a Global agenda for our time which draws upon;

- Ancient Babylonian mystery religion for its satanic root and inspiration.
- The fathers of Modern Freemasonry and Illuminism like Francis Bacon and Adam Weishaupt for its form.
- The philosophy of men like Georg Friedrich Hegel for its ruthless methods in implementing 'The Grand Scheme.'

Hegelian Dialectic.

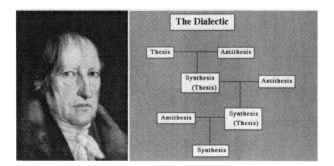

Georg Friedrich Hegel was a brilliant thinker who put forward a series of ideas building on the work of Immanuel Kant. At the mention of philosophy, many people throw up their hands and say; "I can't understand that stuff – it's way beyond me!" What follows is important and <u>not</u> hard to understand.

Even if you grasp it in this simplified form, it will give you some insight into the way many world events are presently being set up and brought to a predicted conclusion.

Until Hegel's ideas took hold, most people took for granted the idea of 'absolutes'.

Traditional or classical thinking runs along lines like these;
'A' cannot be 'Non-A'.

In other words if one thing is absolutely true, then the opposite is absolutely false.

This can take the form;
Thesis (True) – Antithesis (False)
Hegel's thinking attacked the basis of absolute truth.

In his method an assertion is made which finds resistance in its opposite. The conflict between them gives rise to a new viewpoint. Thus, we no longer have a system which accommodates unchanging truth. The THESIS in the clash with its opposite ANTITHESIS produces a SYNTHESIS.

Synthesis

↑

One can view this too like a triangle; Thesis→ ▲ ← Antithesis

Instead of the linear approach we have a situation whereby a relative truth clashes with an opposite and their collision results in a new relative truth.

This, in its turn stands for a while until a clash with its opposite gives rise to yet a new viewpoint.

Synthesis – This becomes the new Thesis etc…

↑

Synthesis → This becomes the new *Thesis* ▲ *Antithesis*
Thesis ▲ Antithesis

When you reason this way you no longer ask "What is Right?"
Rather, you ask "What is right for now?" or "What is right for this situation?"
Thus history progresses in a triangular series of steps….You are now in a position where you no longer even search for absolute truths. The basis for their existence has been cut away.
The 'fallout' from this settled into political thinking and has invaded every area of life. Hegel has been referred to as the 'Philosophical Dictator' of Germany.
His thinking was picked up by Karl Marx and formed the Communistic economic and political outlook. Hitler's National Socialism was founded on Hegelian thought.
The whole nineteen-sixties idea of 'Whatever gets you through the night!" "Whatever floats your boat" "Whatever

feels good – do it!" These dispositions all flow out of this approach to truth. Herein lie the seeds of 'Situation Ethics' as we encounter them today. Relative thinking rapidly became an accepted way of looking at life.

As this approach permeated the Universities, the results were obvious. The more 'educated' people became, the less time they had for the very idea of a God or absolute moral ideas.

How many times have you heard the cliché 'Well, if it works for you then fine.' As Dr Francis Schaeffer pointed out in his book 'The God Who Is There', it was subtle because it wasn't that truth was being directly attacked – rather it was the pre-suppositional basis for truth that was under siege. It was rather like the Trojan horse. Once a person started to reason in terms of relative thinking it invaded the way they thought in every area of life. What Hegel did in philosophical terms was earth-shaking. It is idiotic to dismiss philosophy without understanding it. Why?

Because.... Belief Informs Action!

Hegel glorified the State and taught that it was above obeying moral laws. Governments were not obliged to keep promises. Hitler followed Hegel's line of thought perfectly. Human beings were the 'hand of God' in history and no progress was made without conflict. The conflicts led to forward progress. Take a few minutes and reflect on that. This philosophy has been, and is being, used time and again on an International basis to create and resolve conflicts.

1. Pick the factions and create the conflict
2. Finance both sides in the conflict using carefully chosen 'fronts'
3. Steer and control the outcome
4. Count your profits and repeat the process

For the highly placed Puppet Masters and their willing minions, it is the preferred method of manipulation for profit.

If one can direct the flow of a conflict, the outcome can be determined and there are huge profits to be made.

Rehoisting the Jolly Roger

In 1823 Samuel Russell, son of the Wall Street banking establishment, founded 'Russell & Company', the largest Opium smuggling operation in the world. Based in Connecticut, they transported Chinese tea and silk along with their other 'specialty product' which they acquired in Turkey and took to China.

In 1830 they bought out their chief competitor, the Perkins syndicate and set up Boston as the capital of the illegal opium trade. By means of the staggering wealth generated by this trade and his connections to Wall Street, Russell's company grew as a centre of illegal and secretive political power.

President Franklin Roosevelt's grandfather served as Chief of Operations at Russell and Co. later becoming a partner.

A year later, William Huntingdon Russell, Samuel's half brother, left Yale University for a year of study in Germany. Germany was seen as a place brimming with new ideas in psychology, philosophy and educational reform.

Children were being educated within the framework of the 'Scientific Method'.

They were taught what to think and a total obedience to the state.

Hegel held the chair in Philosophy at the University of Berlin until his death in 1831.

Hegel's ideas were in full circulation by then and when he died, the ideas we now call Hegelian Dialectic were already being applied to education as well as every other area of human endeavour. Through this so-called 'new scientific method' it was possible to create a pre-determined 'synthesis' and thus the most desirable pre-determined outcomes.

Russell, like many others was fascinated by the ideas of dialectic. The state was all powerful; individuals were allowed freedoms based on their obedience to the state. Conflict, created and controlled by an intellectual elite produced a pre-determined outcome.

Russell rapidly grasped the possibilities as applied to his own sphere. Hegelian ideas could be put to use for him in banking. Through controlled conflict it would be possible to produce a synthesis of vast wealth. The bankers provided the finance to those involved in the conflict. Secrecy was needed to ensure that the adversaries never realised that the same banks were providing financial support to both sides.

Russell wasn't the first to understand that secrecy was a key ingredient in applying these principles to banking. If you have huge sums of money generated through international crime and drug trafficking, you have to manage these funds under a cloak of absolute secrecy.

So taken was he with Hegelian method that he enrolled at the University of Berlin and while there joined 'Skull and Bones', a secret society incorporating Hegelian ideas. Berlin's order of 'Skull and Bones' were from the privileged and aristocratic class, from bankers' families and the moneyed elite. Russell mixed in effortlessly and formed many close friendships. He gained permission to open an American Chapter of the Order and, on his return to America and Yale University he and Alphonso Taft became founding members of the German society of 'Skull and Bones, Chapter 322, The Brotherhood of Death' along with thirteen other members of the Wall Street elite's offspring.

(Alphonso Taft was the father of future President Howard Taft who then became Chief Justice – yes, 'Justice'! - of the Supreme Court!)

Chapter 322 turned into a super secret society for the children of the Anglo-American Wall Street banking establishment at Yale University.

This was no ordinary University fraternity house for just fooling around and pulling student pranks. Its purpose is now, and has always been, to apply the Hegelian method to the creation of power and wealth. This is accomplished through setting up conflicts and then systematically controlling the outcome. It operates on a micro level, in commerce and on a macro level, influencing the affairs of entire countries.

It is also geared to promote the success of its members in their future careers. Membership is for life. New members are given a clock along with a large sum of money to remind them that The Order is timeless. As Anthony Sutton points out the 'timeless' nature of this brotherhood has provided it with capacity to build up both vertical and horizontal chains of influence.

This ensures the success of its members' schemes, whether it is financing both sides in a revolution, vast drug smuggling operations or getting elected as President of The United States like the two Bush presidents we have seen. Prescott Bush, George H.W. Bush and his son George W. Bush are all alumni of Yale University and all members of Order 322 'Skull and Bones'.

'The Tomb' at Yale University

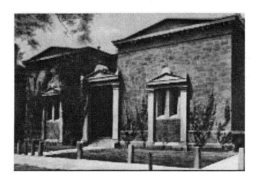

The home lodge of 'The Order' is known as 'The Tomb' and stands in the grounds of Yale University. Three generations of the Bush family have been initiated into the ranks of 'The Order'.

In 1856, 'The Tomb' as it is known, was erected. A vine – covered windowless brown stone building, this saved The

Order having to hire outside venues and provided secrecy for the rites that were held inside.

Campus publications couldn't get anything in print which questioned the activities of the Lodge. In October 1876 an article investigating the 'Skull and Bones' was published in 'The Iconoclast'. It was published in New Haven 'because the college press is closed to those who dare to openly mention Bones.'

The article reported that there was evidence of Satanism. Uninvited guests had discovered the black walls and pentagrams.

"On the west wall, an old engraving representing an open burial vault, in which on a stone slab are placed four human skulls, grouped about a fool's cap and bells, an open book, several mathematical instruments, a beggar's script and a royal crown." Article in' The Iconoclast.'

On the arched wall above the vault is the explanation;

'We War Thor, Wer Weiser, Wer Bettler Oder, Kaiser?'

Underneath the vault is engraved;

'Ob Arm, Ob Beich, im Tode gleich'

'Who was the fool, who the wise man, beggar or king?'

'Whether poor or rich, all's the same in death.'

In other words – there are no such things as morals, no right and no wrong!

The end justifies the means and everything ends 'in death'.

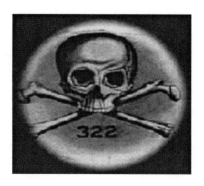

The Death's Head Insignia of Yale's Order 322.

This Lodge is the American Chapter of Hitler's Home Lodge in Germany which was the inspiration for its formation at Yale. It has had a manipulative and corrupting influence on American politics ever since its inception.

After the founding of this cancerous society at Yale University, Russell and friends hoisted up a Skull and Bones pirate flag. Remember the renegade Templar's sailing flag? A symbol of death and destruction, the skull and bones was the pirate's sign that they were cut-throats, thieves, terrorists, were totally outside the law and had no morals whatsoever. This is the stock from whence American Chief 'Justices' like Taft sprang. It's appalling but it gets worse.

For the next thirty years members of the Order in America made 'pilgrimages' to Germany and visited the University. This was almost holy ground to them.

Hegel's method had seeped out from here like a plague to infect government, education, business, psychology and the acquisition of wealth and power.

The State in Germany had taken over complete responsibility for the education of children. Young minds were moulded into the shape required by the Government.

Obedience was paramount.

The Americans took it all in and applied it at home.

Timothy Dwight – class of 1849, became Professor of

Divinity at Yale Divinity School! Yes, I did say Professor of Divinity. He went on to become 12th President of Yale University. Can you imagine how many young minds this man twisted as a respected authority on Divinity?

Daniel Coit Gilman – class of 1852 became the 1st President of The University of California, 1st President of the Johns Hopkins University and 1st President of the Carnegie Institution.

Andrew Dickson White – class of 1853 became 1st President of Cornell University.

For these brothers in the Occult, the whole purpose of an education was to mould the thoughts, ideas and prejudices of the generation of future leaders.

They had little time for the children of the masses. It was only the progeny of the rich and powerful who needed to be schooled in the application of Hegelian Dialectic in order to take forward the creation of the New World Order they envisaged; an Order ruled over and completely controlled by a mega-rich elite. Thought conditioning in education had taken root and the roots were going deeper and deeper.

The American Civil War – First Steps In Applying The Theory

Bankers Take Their First Steps in Hegelian 'Skullduggery'

The Civil War offered one of the first grand opportunities to apply the principles of controlled conflict. The synthesis would erode localised democracy, eliminate the State chartered 'Free Banking' and establish banks that could be owned and controlled by a few select families.

From the very first shot, these private national banks as well as the 'Free' banks, loaned money to both Union and Confederacy.

Bankers funded 'Death Squads' on both sides who specialised in torture and assassination. Private militias killed for 'fun' and often at random.

Even the unarmed were fair game as neighbours were picked off one by one.

Each side saw the atrocities and vowed even worse bloodshed on enemies who could commit such crimes. Scalpings, castrations, mutilations and the burning out of private homes were paid for by the banks in the shadows, to keep the 'pot boiling'.

Brutal, heartbreaking conflict pleased the bankers no end.

By the end of hostilities $6.6 Billion had been consumed in direct costs, by civil war and the government of Union and Confederacy.

Abraham Lincoln rightly referred to these Death Merchants as the enemies of mankind and of the U.S...

"more despotic than a monarchy, more insolent than autocracy, more selfish than Bureaucracy. It denounces...all who question its methods or throw light upon its crimes...... I have two great enemies, the Southern army before me and the bankers in the rear. Of the two, the one at my rear is the greatest foe.....corporations have been enthroned and an era of corruption in high places will follow, and the money power of the country will endeavour to prolong its reign by working upon the prejudices of the people until the wealth is aggregated in the hands of a few and the Republic is destroyed."

Thomas Jefferson said; "I sincerely believe that banking Institutions are more dangerous to our liberties than standing armies"

The secret lodges of the international brotherhoods have been used as a network to subvert the economy of entire nations. Whoever controls the money controls everything.

One of the famous sayings of the house of Rothschild runs: "Give me control of the banking system of a country and I care not who makes it's laws!"

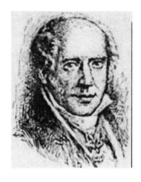

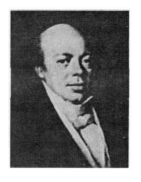

Mayer Amschel-Rothschild   Nathan Rothschild

PART TWO

The Modern Faces of
The Globalist Scheme

There are many other individuals and associations we could list who have had a part in laying foundations for what is set to happen in the next few years.

Who have the players been in more recent history? What about the present?

In place throughout the world right now is a network so powerful and well entrenched, it makes the Templar control of finances look puny. The power lines run out of sight, controlled through the network of lords, down through the top Illuminati/Masonic networks with control of International Banks.

The picture only starts to come into focus when one appreciates the way that the various societies behind these world events lock together.

Ever come across 'couch weed' in your garden? You start to dig out what you think is the main network only to find you uncover a myriad of other hidden root networks running all over your property. You are left exhausted and wondering whether you will ever be totally free of its chokehold. These societies are very similar. They have taken great trouble to conceal themselves from view while all the time systematically subverting governments.

Lower down the ladder are those want to get on board but perhaps don't have the exact credentials. If they are favoured by their overlords, they are given the positions they are hungry for. They can be assisted up the pyramid so to speak. They will never have the absolute power but they can be used as important chess pieces in the Illuminati game of bringing about 'The New World Order'.

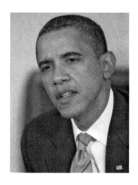

In the early 80s, a young man called Barak Obama was spotted at University by Zbigniew Brzezinski. Anyone who lived through the Carter years of the presidency U.S. should remember Brzezinski's terrifying foreign policy tendencies. He taught at Columbia University from 1960 to 1989 and was the Head of The Institute for Communist Affairs, as you might expect, a hot bed of anti-Soviet thinkers.

Obama did two years at Occidental College in California before transferring to Columbia where he majored in political science with a specialty in international relations – Brzezinski's territory. He got his B.A. in 1983.

In his book, 'Dreams From My Father' Obama describes a conversation with Frank Davis, his communist mentor prior to leaving for Occidental during which Davis tells him;

"*College is an advanced degree in compromise.*" Davis lays out for him the 'real price of admission' as he sees it; "*The real price is leaving your race at the door. Leaving your people behind. Understand something boy, you're not going to College to get educated. You're going there to get trained. They'll train you to want what you don't need. They'll train you to manipulate words so they don't mean anything anymore.*

They'll train you to forget what it is that you already know. They'll train you so good that you'll start believing what they tell you about equal opportunity and the American way and all that sh*t. They'll give you a corner office and invite you to fancy dinners and tell you you're a credit to your race. Until you want to actually start running things and then they'll jerk *your chain and let you know that you may be a well trained, well paid n****r but you're a n****r just the same...."*

It is an illuminating passage. As Webster Griffin Tarpley observes, he is in effect telling the reader what was about to take place...through meeting Brzezinski he was to become a wholly owned asset with a career sponsored by networks of the Trilateral Commission, The Bilderberg Group and The Council On Foreign Relations! *"He describes a process of training and indoctrination so thorough that it should be described as brainwashing. The personal identity of the individual is largely erased resulting in a kind of automaton or zombie. Obama has now passed beyond the stage of brainwashing into the phase of spouting slogans to get ahead. He knows that what awaits him is a phase of nominal authority masking the reality of his role as abject puppet and stooge of his masters"*.

Like Clinton and the others, he had been spotted, recruited and trained for the role he was selected to play in the elections following Bush Jnr. His entire campaign was coordinated and run by Brzezinski.

I followed this latest American 'election' circus as closely as I could stomach.

The media showed street scenes and the reactions of ordinary Americans. It was a dreadful sight. Many African-American faces tearstained with joy as they thought they were seeing a real political shift. Obama was welcomed as a black messiah. Ordinary people saw what they thought they had wanted – they saw what they were meant to see. I got emotional too, but for different reasons as I watched the new face of corporate fascism 'enthroned' as U.S. President. Another chapter in this ongoing deception was about to begin. On his 'election' his appointees give a direct insight into the might of his masters. As Webster Tarpley says; *"It's Government by Wall Street for Wall Street"*.

In the short time since his election, Barak Obama has broken just about every promise he made to the trusting U.S. population.

President Bill Clinton, another example, wasn't the sharpest intellect to arise from his lineage, which ties to the Russell family, but he was a 'Rhodes scholar'. *(see 'Skull and Bones' Lodge 322 –Yale University)* and is said to have more British blood than any of the other American Presidents. One of the first errands that he performed for his masters was to become a key member of an anti-Vietnam war student group at Oxford. He proved an obedient lap dog and carried out his little spying assignments as bid. Later, as Fritz Springmeir reports, while Governer of Arkansas he was involved in large covert drug smuggling operations. Arkansas is Rockefeller's 'back yard' – Clinton's most prominent backer. Clinton's brother served time for involvement in these activities which ran out of hangars at Mena and Nella. Fritz Springmeir and others, in the course of their investigations, have found that his wife Hilary Clinton outranks him in the occult/political hierarchy as she occupies the rank of 'Illuminati Grande Dame' ascending to this rank from 'Mother of Darkness' at age forty years. Cathy O'Brien tells of her abuse at the hands of Hilary Clinton and members of Clinton's inner circle in her heartbreaking book 'The Tranceformation of America'.

(Fritz Springmeir – 'Bloodlines of the Illuminati',
O'Brien and Phillips – 'The Tranceformation of America')

On Hilary Clinton's campaign flag few noticed the stars had been shifted to form pentagrams. A printing accident? No, it was intentional. See also illustration of EEC propaganda poster.

The modern factions of the Illuminati already had twenty years invested in 'Slick Willie' as he is known, when he took Presidential Office. The elite behind him gave him special training and he can lie and manipulate with the best on the world stage. *Remember? "I did not have sexual relations with that woman."*

As a Rhodes scholar, he was offered opportunities to serve the N.W.O. way back in his University days. Being faithful in the discharge of these duties can open the door to the lower rungs of the Illuminati network. He was also easily controllable and disposable to his handlers due to his criminal background and sexual perversions. He made an ideal and willing puppet for Illuminati control.

See Rhodes Scholarship Notes Under Section on United Nations

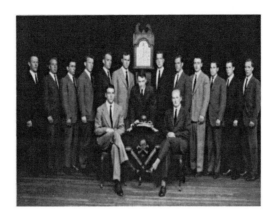

<u>George Bush Snr. shown here posing with his</u>
<u>fellow initiates in 'The Tomb'</u>

He stands to the left of the clock in the back row. On a table draped with the Order's Death's Head insignia a human skull is placed. The clock is a reminder that they are sworn to serve the interests of The Order for all time. On initiation each candidate is presented with a clock as a reminder of this.

Each time a member of this brotherhood 'swears in' to a public office they have already given their superior allegiance to The Order. This makes a mockery of any vows they may make to uphold the interests of those who have elected them.

The Rhodes Scholarship

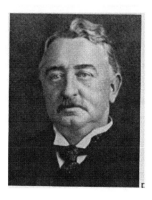

Cecil Rhodes 1853-1902

On his death in 1902 the millionaire Cecil Rhodes left a vast fortune in gold and diamonds. Rhodes founded yet another secret society, mentioned in the first five of his seven wills. One of the brainchildren of his legacy was The Rhodes Scholarship fund in England;

"In the fifth will it was supplemented by the idea of an educational scholarship, whose alumni would be bound together by common ideals – Rhodes's ideals.

The Rhodes scholarships were merely a façade to conceal the secret society, or more accurately, they were to be one of the instruments by which members of the secret society could carry out his purpose. This purpose as expressed in the first will (1877) was the 'extension of British Rule throughout the world, the perfecting of a system of emigration from the United Kingdom and of colonisation by energy, labour and enterprise....the ultimate recovery of the United States of

America as an integral part of a British Empire, the consolidation of the whole Empire...."
Carrol Quigley – 'The Anglo-American Establishment from Rhodes to Cliveden'
(Note; Quigley was a mentor to Bill Clinton – A Rhodes Scholar)

The objective is to educate men and women from around the world who are not necessarily the brightest, but who are made of the right stuff to fulfil offices which advance the programme. The Rhodes programme envisages a New World Order built around the oldest and most established throne in the world - the British throne. In his writing Carol Quigley overrates the participants' Anglophile devotion. Many researchers believe that he deliberately does this to divert attention away from the more important connections to satanic societies held by those involved.

The Business Of War

By 1900 Germany was leading the world as an industrial nation.

On June 28th 1914 Arch Duke Franz Ferdinand, the heir to the Austrian/Hungarian throne was assassinated while in a motorcade. Responsibility was claimed by the Serbian secret society 'The Black Hand, a group with known links to British and French intelligence. Here was the touch paper to ignite World War One.

In Germany, England, France and Austria armament manufacturers, heavily financed by Rothschild-controlled banks, swung eagerly into action to produce the hardware. Twenty million lost their lives in this needless conflict as the bankers counted their vast profits in blood money.

Throughout this 'war to end all wars' the Globalist elite had in mind the opportunities it would create as a bridgehead towards their eventual goal;

1. Vast fortunes in interest on loans to all concerned.
2. A springboard on the way to establishing Globalism by putting forward the 'League of Nations' camouflaged as a solution.

A history of conquest, domination and exploitation gave the British vast experience in concealing their empire behind puppet regimes. Surely for a nation to join with this new 'League of Nations' could only be of benefit in ensuring that there was no repeat of this dreadful scale of war, couldn't it?!

Rhodes's trustees, who were members of the British aristocracy came up with the idea of a 'League of Nations' which fulfils the 'Imperial Parliament' requirement in which all countries would join under the banner of Peace'.

The League convened in Paris in 1914. Many of the shrewder statesmen at that time foresaw the dangers to their sovereignty which lay behind the rhetoric and they rightly refused to participate.

Neither would the U.S. senate ratify the treaty and so, for a period, the League was forced into obscurity in Switzerland.

The Council On Foreign Relations

Frustrated by this temporary upset to their scheme, but ever resourceful in pursuing their goals, British Intelligence with aid from the Rockefeller family set up 'The Council On Foreign Relations' in 1921 in New York City. The Rockefellers are another key bloodline in the NWO. This Council head-hunted the best candidates they could find to support and advance the growth of The Anglo-American Empire. It remains one of the most powerful engines behind the Globalist agenda.

The stated aim of the The Council On Foreign Relations is to abolish all Nation States in favour of a One World Government to be administered by a tiny ruling elite.

By 1930 the elites with a Globalist agenda had split into two main camps;

The Communist faction and the Fascists.

These enclaves of opinion spread across international borders but England had a powerful group in the Fabian Socialists based in London. The most influential Fascists were in Italy and Germany.

In the United States and in England, the most zealous Fascists wanted to see the military utilised to transform society into a New World Order. The more subtle activists favoured the use of stealth and incrementalism to bring about World domination.

Major General Smedley Butler and the American Takeover Plot

In America in 1934, Major General Smedley Butler exposed a plot by some of the most powerful men in America to bring about a military coup. He testified to the McCormack-Dickstein committee in the U.S. Congress that he had been approached to lead a military force of 500,000 troops in a revolution to establish National Socialism in The United States of America.

War Is A Racket

A speech delivered in 1933, by Major General Smedley Butler, USMC.

"WAR is a racket. It always has been. It is possibly the oldest, easily the most profitable, surely the most vicious. It is the only one international in scope. It is the only one in which the profits are reckoned in dollars and the losses in lives.

A racket is best described, I believe, as something that is not what it seems to the majority of the people. Only a small "inside" group knows what it is about. It is conducted for the benefit of the very few, at the expense of the very many. Out of war a few people make huge fortunes.

In the World War [I] a mere handful garnered the profits of the conflict. At least 21,000 new millionaires and billionaires were made in the United States during the World War. That many admitted their huge blood gains in their income tax returns. How many other war millionaires falsified their tax returns no one knows.

How many of these war millionaires shouldered a rifle? How many of them dug a trench? How many of them knew what it meant to go hungry in a rat-infested dug-out? How many of them spent sleepless, frightened nights, ducking shells and shrapnel and machine gun bullets? How many of them parried a bayonet thrust of an enemy? How many of them were wounded or killed in battle?

Out of war nations acquire additional territory, if they are victorious. They just take it. This newly acquired territory promptly is exploited by the few – the selfsame few who wrung dollars out of blood in the war. The general public shoulders the bill.

And what is this bill? This bill renders a horrible accounting. Newly placed gravestones. Mangled bodies. Shattered minds. Broken hearts and homes. Economic instability. Depression and all its attendant miseries. Back-breaking taxation for generations and generations.

For a great many years, as a soldier, I had a suspicion that war was a racket; not until I retired to civil life did I fully realize it. Now that I see the international war clouds gathering, as they are today, I must face it and speak out.

Again they are choosing sides. France and Russia met and agreed to stand side by side. Italy and Austria hurried to make a similar agreement. Poland and Germany cast sheep's eyes at each other, forgetting for the nonce [one unique occasion], their dispute over the Polish Corridor.

The assassination of King Alexander of Jugoslavia [Yugoslavia] complicated matters. Jugoslavia and Hungary, long bitter enemies, were almost at each other's throats. Italy was ready to jump in. But France was waiting. So was Czechoslovakia.

All of them are looking ahead to war. Not the people – not those who fight and pay and die – only those who foment wars and remain safely at home to profit.

There are 40,000,000 men under arms in the world today, and our statesmen and diplomats have the temerity to say that war is not in the making. Hell's bells! Are these 40,000,000 men being trained to be dancers? Not in Italy, to be sure. Premier Mussolini knows what they are being trained for. He, at least, is frank enough to speak out. Only the other day, Il Duce in

"International Conciliation," the publication of the Carnegie Endowment for International Peace, said:

"And above all, Fascism, the more it considers and observes the future and the development of humanity quite apart from political considerations of the moment, believes neither in the possibility nor the utility of perpetual peace... War alone brings up to its highest tension all human energy and puts the stamp of nobility upon the people who have the courage to meet it."

Undoubtedly Mussolini means exactly what he says. His well-trained army, his great fleet of planes, and even his navy are ready for war – anxious for it, apparently. His recent stand at the side of Hungary in the latter's dispute with Jugoslavia showed that. And the hurried mobilization of his troops on the Austrian border after the assassination of Dollfuss showed it too. There are others in Europe too whose sabre rattling presages war, sooner or later.

Herr Hitler, with his rearming Germany and his constant demands for more and more arms, is an equal if not greater menace to peace. France only recently increased the term of military service for its youth from a year to eighteen months.

Yes, all over, nations are camping in their arms. The mad dogs of Europe are on the loose. In the Orient the maneuvering is more adroit. Back in 1904, when Russia and Japan fought, we kicked out our old friends the Russians and backed Japan. Then our very generous international bankers were financing Japan. Now the trend is to poison us against the Japanese. What does the "open door" policy to China mean to us? Our trade with China is about $90,000,000 a year. Or the Philippine Islands? We have spent about $600,000,000 in the Philippines in thirty-five years and we (our bankers and industrialists and speculators) have private investments there of less than $200,000,000.

Then, to save that China trade of about $90,000,000, or to protect these private investments of less than $200,000,000 in the Philippines, we would be all stirred up to hate Japan and go to war – a war that might well cost us tens of billions of dollars, hundreds of thousands of lives of Americans, and many more hundreds of thousands of physically maimed and mentally unbalanced men. Of course, for this loss, there would be a compensating profit – fortunes would be made. Millions and billions of dollars would be piled up. By a few. Munitions makers. Bankers. Ship builders. Manufacturers. Meat packers. Speculators. They would fare well.

Yes, they are getting ready for another war. Why shouldn't they? It pays high dividends. But what does it profit the men who are killed? What does it profit their mothers and sisters, their wives and their sweethearts? What does it profit their children? What does it profit anyone except the very few to whom war means huge profits? Yes, and what does it profit the nation?

Take our own case. Until 1898 we didn't own a bit of territory outside the mainland of North America. At that time our national debt was a little more than $1,000,000,000. Then we became "internationally minded." We forgot, or shunted aside, the advice of the Father of our country. We forgot George Washington's warning about "entangling alliances." We went to war. We acquired outside territory. At the end of the World War period, as a direct result of our fiddling in international affairs, our national debt had jumped to over $25,000,000,000. Our total favorable trade balance during the twenty-five-year period was about $24,000,000,000. Therefore, on a purely bookkeeping basis, we ran a little behind year for year, and that foreign trade might well have been ours without the wars.

It would have been far cheaper (not to say safer) for the average American who pays the bills to stay out of foreign entanglements. For a very few this racket, like bootlegging and other underworld rackets, brings fancy profits, but the cost of operations is always transferred to the people – who do not profit."

At this time, there was also a strong Fascist base in England. However, the Fabian Socialist bloc managed to retain overall control in the United States, Russia and England. In the build up to the Second World War, the Banking fraternities again readily financed all participants.

Let's Trade With The Enemies!

During the 1930s the grandfather of President Bush snr. Along with Harriman and Rockefeller went into business with Adolf Hitler!

"The general consensus at the bankers' meetings was that the only way to free Germany from French financial clutches was by revolution – either Communist or National Socialism. Rockefeller argued that the money should go to Hitler. After some negotiation, 10 million dollars was transferred to the Nazis. During subsequent meetings it was explained that Hitler's storm troopers and S.S. were insufficiently equipped and badly needed machine guns, revolvers and carbines. Hitler explained that he had two plans for takeover in Germany. a) Revolution b) Legal Takeover Plan. Hitler is quoted as saying "...revolution costs five hundred million marks. Legal takeover costs two hundred million marks – what will your bankers decide?" Legal takeover thus offered the best deal......After further negotiations Rockefeller and the American banking and oil interests offered an additional $15 million which would help finance the legal takeover. Revolution would be too expensive and destructive. In the months after Hitler took power, in 1933, Warburg delivered yet another payment from Rockefeller and Carter and their associates in banking, industry and oil, i.e. $7 million....."

Antony Sutton – from Warburg's 'Financial Sources of National Socialism'.

Bush was still in business with the Nazis when Hitler declared war on America and several of his companies including the Hamburg-Amerika shipping line were confiscated by the U.S. Government. After Hitler came to power, the Hamburg-Amerika line started financing Nazi Propaganda and subsidizing pro-Nazi newspapers in the United States.

The purpose of the propaganda was clear. The men of Lodge 322 'Skull & Bones' were not only seeking to support Nazi Germany, but were seeking to undermine the constitutional government of the United States. The 'Bonesmen' were – and are, sworn enemies of democracy and the American Republic.

May 25th 2004. Source; Gary Indiana – 'The Village Voice'

"....*the necessary proof of such a conspiracy, if we choose to call it that, often turns up 25 or 50 years after the fact, when the release of classified documents churns up no public outcry or indictments. Such was the recent case with the de-classified revelation that the late Connecticut Senator Prescott Bush, grandfather of the current President, along with his Law partners W. Averill Harriman, a former Governor of New York, managed a number of concerns on behalf of Nazi industrialist Fritz Thyssen. These included the Union Banking Corporation, seized under the Trading With The Enemy Act on October 20th, 1942 (Office of Alien Custodian, Vesting Order 248), Seamless Steel Equipment Corporation (Vesting Order 259) and The Holland –American Trading Organisation (Vesting Order 261).*

The Union Banking Corporation financed Hitler after his electoral losses in 1932; the other Bush–managed concerns have been characterised as "a shipping line which imported German spies; an energy company that supplied the Luftwaffe with high ethyl fuel and a steel company that employed Jewish slave labour from the Auschwitz concentration camp....." *confirmed John Loftus, a former Prosecutor in the Justice*

Department's Nazi War Crimes Unit. Since only the Nazi partners in the Bush-Harriman interests were permanently deprived of their frozen stock, Prescott Bush and his father-in-law, George Herbert Walker, waltzed off with $1.5 million when the Union Banking Corporation was liquidated in 1951.

(This was, in effect, the foundation of the Bush family fortune.)

Briefly picked up by the Associated Press and buried deep in the pages of American Newspapers, this half-century late disclosure led to no media follow-up and left no impression on the potential electorate for the 2004 U.S. Presidential contest.

The Fabian Socialists

The Insignia of the Fabian Socialists is a wolf disguised in a sheep's fleece! A Wolf in Sheep's' Clothing!

Most people in Britain have no idea of how deeply their leading politicians are involved in these treasonous plans to undermine national sovereignty.

<u>Recent British Prime Minister Tony Blair was actually the Chairman of the present Fabian Group!</u>
 These people plot and pursue their goals 'incrementally'.
 They work by stealth, hence the Logo – successfully pulling the wool over most peoples' eyes!

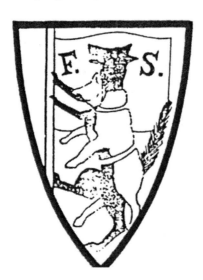

The Fabians have included the author HG Wells who wrote eloquently about The New World Order, creating its Utopian image. The reality is to be brutally different.

In 1945 amidst the shocking devastation left in the aftermath of World War Two and the obvious desire for peace, representatives from all over the world started working furiously on the 'Charter of the United Nations'.

The 'Trojan horse' was decked with new colours and different grooming. Then, in its new guise it was trotted out from the obscurity of its Swiss stable back into worldview. Its livery now was that of the United Nations.

The U.S. Senate passed the 'United Nations Charter' in August 1945.

The European Economic Community has got you used to the economic idea but the United Nations is the template to get you used to the scale: World Military, World Police, World Government.

The British Royal family drive many agendas through the U.N. Prince Charles plays a major part of which most people are ignorant.

He carries out his role behind the scenes. Those who think he is a lightweight, polo playing heir-in-waiting should think again. This man is not in a hurry to be crowned the king of England – He's already a king in a realm that wields the real power behind the scenes in today's world.

All Charles's activities reinforce Clinton's phrase "Reinventing Government" along with the rest of U.N. Agenda 21 –

"Sustainable Development" and "Public-Private Partnerships".

When Prince Charles called for a conference on "Stakeholders – The Challenge in a Global Market", over one hundred Chief Executive Officers of Multi-National Corporations from thirteen countries attended.

This impetus was behind the formation of the 'Prince of Wales Business Leaders Forum' (PWBLF).

This Forum consists of over two hundred Multi-National and Trans-National Corporations that have set up "Public Private Partnerships around the world.

The thrust of the argument is that national Governments cannot do it all.

Why not partner with those who can provide the funds for worthy schemes?

Like many other of these agendas, it seems to be reasonable to the average person –why not?

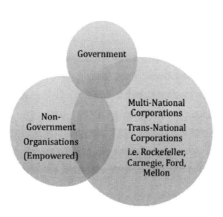

Re-Invented Government

When you bring these agencies together where does the
<u>real</u> power lie? It lies in the deepest pockets! Is that likely to
be government? No! Business Interests rule to the eventual
extent that representative government disappears in all but
name.

That's re-invented Government all right!

Benito Mussolini defined fascism as the situation where
government takes over and runs business. The Fascism in play
now differs only in that business has taken over and runs
government! Corporate Fascism is its flavour for our time.

The wealthy bloodlines who want to re-structure
Government are pushing through the agendas of the <u>U.N.</u>, <u>The
Trilateral Commission</u> and <u>The Council on Foreign Relations</u>
to accomplish their own ends. Some of the initial undertakings
might seem good to you but think carefully about the
outcomes!

The agenda being pursued is not 'Independence' but rather
'Interdependence'.

By means of massive loans which have <u>severe</u> conditions
attached to them, World Bankers have ensnared Governments
in their agenda.

Once they have opened the way for foreign investments to take over huge chunks of their enterprise, the conditions begin to bite. Each nation is assigned a task in the grand scheme. For example, as Barry Smith points out in his excellent observations, New Zealand was known for its lamb exports. In the New World Order Scheme it is charged with producing lumber as it has the quickest growth and drying rate for certain trees.

This Globalist scheme sets up a scenario wherein each country produces a resource needed by its neighbours. It doesn't matter that your nation might have a proud history of say, agriculture – if your region is on the checklist for something else, then something else is what <u>you will</u> do! It is vital to understand that your national politicians are puppets and have no power whatsoever to stand in the way.

The philosophy behind this is that you are unlikely to go to war with neighbour nations in the scheme who produce what you need – by this means you create the required INTERDEPENDENCE. It is a Key part of The Globalisation Plan.

Remember that the tearing down of sovereignty and National borders is the aim towards creating the global, borderless New World Order.

What about this other buzz phrase "Sustainable Development?"

Again the reality behind the 'U.N. - speak' is chilling.

It was Jacques Costeau who said something to the effect that three hundred and fifty thousand people would need to die each day in order to get the population figures down to where those behind this New World Order think they should be!

Prince Phillip is reported to have said that if he were re-incarnated (please let us hope not!) he would come back as a virus to reduce the population.

Why isn't more done to ease the misery of starving millions?

The phrase is that they are 'useless eaters'. In the economy of the New World Order you are what you produce. Much is made of the ecological arguments and many, if not most, of our young people are swayed by the 'Mother Earth' propaganda. The real issue for those who finance the world is 'zero population growth'. How much 'human cargo' can be sustained against acceptable profit margins? Remember Thomas Malthus?

The people who come through the Rhodes Scholarship are schooled for key office in their respective countries and to push forward the New World Order agenda. For example, once Bill Clinton took the Presidential Office in America, he appointed numerous other Rhodes scholars to his cabinet. The successor organisation to Rhodes trustees is known today as the <u>Royal Institute for</u> <u>International Affairs</u>. Its foreign relatives include the <u>Council on Foreign</u> <u>Relations</u> in the U.S.A. and others around the globe. These organisations are steered by powerful men and members occupy key positions in manufacturing, media, education and the military.

The push towards World Government is funded by corporations such as;

The Carnegie Endowment for International Peace,

The Rockefeller Foundation,

The Ford Foundation and The Mellon Foundation.

(This was borne out by the Reese Commission, a special committee to investigate Tax exempt foundations.)

To rise to a certain level on the stage of International Politics, one has to be prepared to 'get with' the Globalist Programme or that's where it ends. The power of the controlling dynasties is beyond what many, (perhaps most) people can even begin to appreciate.

Though it is now reaching 'critical mass', I hope I have made it clear that the bloodlines and dynasties behind these unfolding events plan generationally. The changes necessary to bring about their envisaged New World Order are arranged to take place incrementally and often over many years.

The United Nations

On March 19^{th,} 1970 The United States Senate voted to give the United Nations; "Full diplomatic recognition as being a Sovereign World Government."

The most ambitious part of Rhodes's vision had been carefully nurtured and patiently assembled piece by piece. At that moment his trustees saw his 'League of Nations', which would fulfil the role of 'Imperial Parliament', become a reality!

When the journalist Joan Veon started to cover U.N. conferences, she was shocked at the agendas. What is even more shocking is seeing the U.N. agendas made reality as International Laws which are being adopted by those under its vast umbrella.

Whenever the U.N. General Assembly meet they pass resolutions which help to expand the field of International Law. Article 13 of the U.N. Charter gives the General Assembly the duty of initiating and promoting International political cooperation and encouraging the development of International Law.

Types of International Law include;

- Municipal Law
- Rules of Jurisdiction (extradition and immunity)
- International Environmental Law
- Human Rights Law
- International Court of Justice - which renders opinions
- Laws of War and Laws of Force
- International Laws governing the sea, waterways, polar regions and even outer space!
- International Economic Law – such as International Monetary Fund, World Bank

- International Labour Organisation
- Civil Aviation
- International Communication
- Postal Law

Many of us are frankly sick of hearing the term Democracy applied to this vast template for World Government. American friends are justifiably infuriated – the Laws of their REPUBLIC – yes, the term is REPUBLIC, are being thrown aside to accommodate U.N. ideas on how things should be done. The United States Constitution and Bill of Rights are being replaced with the United Nations Charter and the United Nations Declaration of Human Rights.

Under President Bill Clinton, Executive Order 13107 implemented U.N. Human Rights Law into the American system. America is being used to fulfil the role her shadowy mentors intended from the very beginning.

We have been constantly told that the United Nations was born out of two World Wars and a desire for peace. What the U.N. means by peace is; 'no opposition to the U.N. agenda!'

We have been sold the lie that the U.N. was set up as a forum within which countries could discuss their differences. The use of Hegelian Dialectic ensures that the individual arguments are dissolved into a United Nations 'Synthesis'. Controlling the discussions and conflicts means that the outcome can be pre-determined - the outcome being a solution along the lines of U.N. policy as it unwinds.

In fact the United Nations is the brainchild of people who wish to bring about a One World Government. Most of their objectives have been met to date....

- The U.N. already sets out Global Policy for all countries to follow!
- Agreements coming out of the U.N. General Assembly become International Legal Code, which transcends National Law.

- Every member state contributes annual dues based on complex calculations as to its wealth, income, economic power and population among other things.
- Each country has an Ambassador appointed to handle its affairs and vote at the U.N.
- The United nations has its own Army composed of troops from all its Member States.
- The United Nations structure is vast and comprised of the same sort of Commissions, Agencies and Committees you would find in any national Government. Why?

Because it is a Government! It is set up for World Government!

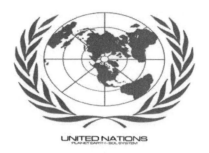

The United Nations Insignia

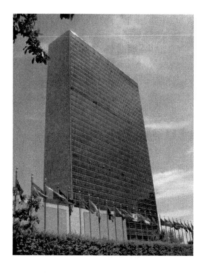

The United Nations Headquarters Building

Let's look at the reality of Government Structure alongside the U.N.;

A Government has a 'Ruler' or 'Head of State';

The U.N. has a Secretary General – These people are elected in secret!

They are not elected by the whole body or by the ballot!

Governments have 'A Governing Body';

The U.N. has The General Assembly and The Security Council.

The U.N. has the ability to create International Law.

Since its inception it has been the primary originator of International Law.

The U.N. has the power to make treaties;

Examples of those made so far in U.N. history;

Human Rights

The Declaration of Human Rights

The U.N. Rights of the Child

The Declaration to Eliminate All Forms Of Discrimination against Women

Environmental Rights

The Rio Declaration

Agenda 21

The Law Of The Sea

The Convention On Climate Change

Peace Instruments

Salt I and Salt II

The Outer Space Treaty

Nuclear Non-Proliferation Treaty of 1968

Equitable and Environmentally Sound Development

ie. The Programme of Action of the U.N. International Conference on Population and Development 1994

Sources of Income
The Dues of Member States

Currency
The International Monetary Fund has Special Drawing Rights.
This is a form of Liquid Money created in the 1960s and used among Members.

Treasury/Banking System
World Bank and International Monetary Fund.
The Bank for International Settlements oversees the control of the World's Monetary System. This is the Central Bank's Bank!

Court and Legal System
International Court of Justice – World Court!

Policing
Interpol and U.N. Peacekeeping Troops

Military Force
U.N. Peacekeeping Forces
Fighting wars to keep the world at peace!

Bureaucratic Agencies
Every level of bureaucracy in any government is matched within the U.N. set up.
World Health Organization, United Nations Conference on Trade Development
World Food Council, World Intellectual Property Organisation,
World Meteorological Organization, International Atomic Energy Agency, International Postal Union, International Maritime Organization,

United Nations Childrens' Fund,
United Nations Education, Scientific and Cultural
Organization
and so on and so forth…..

Flag
The United Nations Flag

Oath of Allegiance
Every U.N. Employee takes an oath of allegiance to the
U.N.!

Charter
The U.N. Charter

Constitution
Current actions under way on the 'Earth Charter'

If it looks like a Government, is set up like a Government and
behaves like a Government – guess what?!

IT'S A GOVERNMENT!

In the Book of Psalms the term 'Selah' occurs repeatedly.
It means to pause and reflect on what you've just read.
Let it sink in….
World Government is already here.

The Bilderbergers

'It is difficult to re-educate people who have been brought up on nationalism to the idea of relinquishing part of their sovereignty to a supra-national body'

Prince Bernhard – Former SS Officer and Founder of The Bilderberg Group

'......A clique of the richest, economically and politically most powerful and influential men in the Western World, who meet secretly to plan events that later appear just to happen...'

The Times of London 1977

'World events do not occur by accident. They are made to happen, whether it is to do with national issues or commerce; and most of them are staged and managed by those who hold the purse strings'...

Denis Healey –Former British Defence Minister
    (and himself a member of the Bilderberg group!)

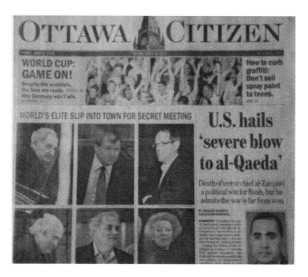

Prince Bernhard of The Netherlands was an Officer in The Nazi Reiter S.S. Corp. The Dutch royal family carefully suppressed this part of Bernhard's history as he went on to become a senior official in Royal Dutch Shell, an Anglo-Dutch organization. To this day the inner circle of the Bilderberg Group contains members of this rich European oil company. Bernhard was also once Secretary to the Board of Directors of the infamous Nazi chemical giant I.G. FARBEN, the firm who serviced the Nazis with lethal Cyclon gas for their concentration camps.

It was Bernhard who convened the first Bilderberg meeting at the Bilderberg Hotel in Oosterbeek, Holland between May 29th and 31st 1954.

The Bilderberg Group were and are a gathering of the world's most powerful figures in the industrial, political, economic and military spheres.

The first Bilderberg meeting closed with the agreement to form a secret association.

Author Georgos Hatton in his book 'Rape of the Constitution; Death of Freedom' makes the claim that Bernhard drew upon his Nazi background in bringing the group together and he encouraged this 'super-secret policy-making group' to call themselves The Bilderbergers. Their name comes partly from the original meeting place and partly as a reference to the late Farben Bilder, an IG Farben executive who had organised Heinrich Himmler's 'Circle of Friends'. This circle consisted of elite, wealth-building leaders who gave massive financial kickbacks to Himmler in return for his protection throughout the war years right up to Hitler's defeat.

The over arching intention was to form 'an aristocracy of purpose' between the United States and Europe and come to agreement on questions of policy, economics and strategy in jointly ruling the world. The NATO Alliance was a main theatre for subversion as it provided them with an umbrella for their plans for 'perpetual war'.

Jim Marrs has written extensively on what he rightly calls 'The Rise of The Fourth Reich'. The Nazi blueprint for a world dominated by a Master Race elite was not abandoned after WW2. Hitler was defeated – not the vision of a Global Empire!

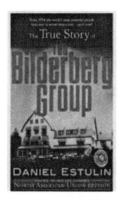

Daniel Estulin's 'Bilderberg Group'

Long before the war ended the 'ratlines', escape routes and strategies were put into place. Prominent Nazis saw the writing on the wall and used the staggering wealth that had been amassed to buy boltholes abroad. All over the world Nazi loot was used to set up 'front' companies and businesses, erase records, create new identities, and purchase property and influence. Anyone discovering for the first time the sheer extent of operations such as 'Operation Eagle Flight' or the very real 'Odessa' is staggered by the scale of the subterfuge.

People raised with the 'shop window' image of England or America are dumbstruck when they discover how the elites of these nations fought to recruit and re-accommodate these men who had often been party to mass murder.

If they had some cash and or skills to offer then the West desperately wanted them.

From scientists and mathematicians to medics who had destroyed thousands of people in hideous experiments, they were all welcomed into new lives, often with new names and frequently appointed to government or military posts.

In 1951 the Treaty between BELGIUM, FRANCE, ITALY, THE NETHERLANDS, LUXEMBOURG and WEST GERMANY was a provision for shared coal and steel production.

An early example of the doctrine of Interdependence, it was thought by many to be a preventive measure against future conflicts between these nations.

(As writer and investigator Jim Marrs points out, it might also be seen as a means of consolidating the massive Nazi business holdings of the Bormann organization after World War 2).

The European Economic Community or Common Market was established in 1957 by the TREATY OF ROME. It was signed by those same nations as in 1951.

Bilderberg member George McGhee who was a former U.S. Ambassador to West Germany agreed that *"the Treaty of Rome which brought the Common Market into being was nurtured at the Bilderberg meetings."*

As was to be the case with all that followed, it was styled as a step toward equalizing trade balances and tariffs. Significantly, with the signing of the Maastricht Treaty, the word 'economic' was dropped.

The French President Charles de Gaulle realized The Bilderbergers intentions very early on. The French faction of the Bilderberger camp were opposed to De Gaulle's nuclear policy. P.M Georges Pompidou along with other Ministers in the French Government including Antoine Pinay and Guy Mollett were pushing against de Gaulle because one of the Group's main goals was to undermine the sovereignty of free European nations and subject them to a Bilderberg – controlled, British-American One World Government. The nuclear threat was the ace in the hole and in order to control Europe it was crucial to the Bilderbergers to have eliminated France's nuclear deterrent even in the face of the perceived Soviet nuclear threat. Jean Lacouture, de Gaulle's biographer put it this way;

"de Gaulle had to establish an incontrovertible position of strength in Europe against Britain's free trade orientation toward a New World Imperial Order. This is why France had to be one of the three pillars of the free world as opposed to one of the columns of the European Temple."

Daniel Estulin observes that analysis of the Bilderberg agendas since 1954 shows the attempt to manage and control differences in ideology between the American and European aristocracies as to just how these two groups could go about looting the planet! When the Bilderbergers sweep into town for a summit, you won't be allowed anywhere near the building. The outer hotel perimeter is protected by hired security guards.

The hotel itself bristles with armed secret service from the homelands of the attending elitists. While they keep you at bay they will be discussing just how they see fit to steer the world you and your children will have to live in. If that doesn't make you angry you must be in a coma.

The Modern Templars Take Control....

As far back as 1863, following attempts to bring the Banks under government control, President Lincoln and Congress took the advice of his Secretary of Treasury and the Northern banking establishment and created a uniform banking system and a uniform national currency. This was to be issued only by 'national banks'. The National Banking Act of 1863 was superseded by the National Banking act of 1864 just one year later. The new Act also established federally-issued bank charters, which took banking out of the hands of state governments. Prior to the Act, charters were granted by state legislatures who were under an immense amount of political pressure and could be influenced by bribes.

The goal of the Act was that free banking was established on a uniform, national level and charter issuance was taken out of the hands of discriminating and corrupt state legislatures. The granting of charters led to the creation of many national banks and a national banking system which grew at a fast pace. The number of national banks rose from 66 immediately after the Act to 7473 in 1913. Initially, this rise in national banking came at the expense of state banking—the number of state banks dwindled from a 1466 in 1863 to 247 in 1868. Though state banks were no longer allowed to issue notes, local bankers took advantage of less strict capital requirements ($10,000 for state banks vs. $50,000-200,000 for national banks) and opened new branches en masse. These new state banks then served as competition for national banks, growing to 15,526 in number by 1913.

A later act, passed on March 3, 1865, imposed a 10 percent tax on the notes of state banks. Like previous taxes, this effectively forced all non-federal currency from circulation.

It also resulted in the creation of demand deposit accounts, and encouraged banks to join the national system, greatly increasing the number of national banks.

Despite the intended safeguard, gradually, the control of money fell under the control of a handful of individuals, as private companies printed the banknotes under contract to the Federal Government.

The Guaranty Trust Company was one of the national banks which emerged during the Wars between the States. Established in 1864, it was almost entirely controlled by families whose sons were, or would become members of the Skull and Bones Order: Vanderbilt, Whitney and Harriman.

With the vast sums coming in to the Guaranty Trust Company, the Harrimans bought the bankrupt Union Pacific Railroad. It went on to set up the W.A. Harriman investment firm. Bert Walker, George W. Bush's maternal great grandfather was a principal partner. He had run for but lost, the Republican Presidential nomination. However, in the process, he had become accepted into the Republican power elite. Bert Walker and his son George were not only partners with the Harrimans, but through their Republican credentials, could influence the administrations of successive republican Presidents. The Harrimans were also partners with the Rockefellers. The Harriman railroad shipped the oil pumped out of the ground by John D. Rockefeller who founded Standard Oil.

Samuel P. Bush the father of Prescott, was also in business with the Harriman-Walker-Rockefeller circle. Bush owned Buckeye Steel Castings making parts for the Harriman Railroad Company.

This is what Abraham Lincoln was driving at when he spoke of "money powers who prey upon the nation in times of peace and conspire against it in times of adversity.....until the wealth is aggregated in the hands of a few and the Republic is destroyed.."

During the 1960s British born Antony Sutton was a fellow of Stanford's Hoover Institute when he discovered that, in spite of the cold war, the U.S. was supplying the U.S.S.R. with its technology including weapons used against the American soldiers in Vietnam! Sutton was shocked but as he dug deeper and deeper he found that Wall Street had sponsored both the Bolshevik revolution and the rise of Hitler in Nazi Germany! *(Remember what you read earlier about the application of Hegelian dialectic.)*

International Dialectic

Woodrow Wilson and a Passport For Trotsky

"You will have a revolution, a terrible revolution. What course it takes will depend much on what Mr. Rockefeller tells Mr. Hague to do. Mr. Rockefeller is a symbol of the American ruling class and Mr. Hague is a symbol of its political tools."

Leon Trotsky, in New York Times, *December 13, 1938. (Hague was a New Jersey politician)*

In 1916, the year preceding the Russian Revolution, internationalist Leon Trotsky was thrown out of France, officially because of his participation in the Zimmerwald conference but also, probably because of the inflammatory articles he had written for *Nashe Slovo,* a Russian-language paper printed in Paris. During September 1916 Trotsky was escorted across the Spanish border by French police. A few days later Madrid police arrested him but lodged him in a "first-class cell" at a charge of one-and-one-half pesetas per day. After that he was taken to Cadiz, then to Barcelona. Finally he was put on board the Spanish Transatlantic Company steamer *Monserrat,* on which he and his family crossed the Atlantic Ocean landing in New York on January 13, 1917.

"He soon discovered that there were wealthy Wall Street bankers who were willing to finance a revolution in Russia...." wrote Journalist William T. Still.

"At times capitalism and communism would appear to be in conflict, but this writer is confident that their interests are in

common and will eventually merge for one-world control."
A.K. Chesterton (right wing British journalist and politician
writing in his magazine 'Candour')
  John Schiff, grandson to the banker Jacob Schiff, reckoned
that 'the old man had sunk around twenty million dollars into
the triumph of Bolshevism in Russia'. *(New York Journal*
–American)

According to the congressional record of Sept. 2nd 1919,
Senator Elihu Root, attorney for the Federal Reserve co-
founder Paul Warburg's 'Kuhn, Loeb & Co.' put up around
twenty million dollars.

Arsene de Goulevitch, a witness to the early days of the
Bolsheviks wrote later:

"In private interviews I have been told that over 21 million
rubles were spent by Lord (Alfred) Milner in financing the
Russian revolution." Milner was a prime mover behind Cecil
Rhodes's Round Tables, a precursor to The Council On
Foreign Relations.

The American International Corporation which was formed in
1915 also aided through their directors representing the
interests of the Rockefellers, Rothschilds, Du Ponts, Kuhns,
Loebs, Harrimans and Federal Reserve Co-Founder Frank
Vanderlip. George Herbert Walker, who was the maternal
grandfather of President George W. Bush, was also a
benefactor to the cause of the revolution.

It wasn't just Trotsky and family who made their way
westward across the Atlantic. One Trotskyite group acquired
sufficient immediate influence in Mexico to write the
Constitution of Querétaro for the revolutionary 1917
Carranza government. This actually made Mexico the first
government in the world with a Soviet-type constitution !!

Trotsky knew only German and Russian, so how did he get by in America? According to his autobiography, *My Life; "My only profession in New York was that of a revolutionary socialist."*

Trotsky wrote occasional articles for *Novy Mir,* the New York Russian socialist journal. Yet we know that he and family lived in an apartment boasting both a refrigerator and a telephone. Keep in mind when this was! On top of that, the family occasionally travelled in a limousine complete with chauffeur. Their standard of living was way beyond Trotsky's reported earnings. The only funds that Trotsky admits receiving in 1916 and 1917 are $310, and, said Trotsky, "I distributed the $310 among five emigrants who were returning to Russia." Yet Trotsky had paid for a first-class cell in Spain, the Trotsky family had travelled across Europe to the United States, they had acquired an excellent apartment in New York - paying rent three months in advance - and they had use of a chauffeured limousine. All this on the earnings of an impoverished revolutionary for a few articles for the low-circulation Russian-language newspaper *Nashe Slovo* in Paris and *Novy Mir* in New York!

Joseph Nedava estimates Trotsky's 1917 income at $12.00 per week, "supplemented by some lecture fees." (*Nedava –'Trotsky and the Jews'*) Trotsky was in New York in 1917 for three months, from January to March, so that makes $144.00 in income from *Novy Mir* and, say, another $100.00 in lecture fees, for a total of $244.00. Of this $244.00 Trotsky was able to give away $310.00 to his friends, pay for the New York apartment, provide for his family - and find the $10,000 that was taken from him in April 1917 by Canadian authorities in Halifax. Trotsky claims that those who said he had other sources of income are "slanderers" spreading "stupid calumnies" and "lies," but unless he had come up lucky at the races, it simply doesn't figure. Trotsky obviously had a secret source of income.

Arthur Willert in 'The Road To Safety' puts forward the story that he worked as an electrician at Fox Film Studios! There are various other theories but there is no evidence that he did anything for income but to write and speak during this period. When he left New York in 1917 for Petrograd, to organize the Bolshevik phase of the revolution, Trotsky had in his possession $10,000.

In 1919 the U.S. Senate Overman Committee investigated the links between the tide of Bolshevik propaganda and German money in the United States. When Overman questioned Colonel Hurban, Washington attaché to the Czech legation, regarding Trotsky's $10,000 the replies were as follows:

"COL. HURBAN: Trotsky, perhaps, took money from Germany, but Trotsky will deny it. Lenin would not deny it. Miliukov proved that he got $10,000 from some Germans while he was in America. Miliukov had the proof, but he denied it. Trotsky did, although Miliukov had the proof.

SENATOR OVERMAN: It was charged that Trotsky got $10,000 here.

COL. HURBAN: I do not remember how much it was, but I know it was a question between him and Miliukov.

SENATOR OVERMAN: Miliukov proved it, did he?

COL. HURBAN: Yes, sir.

SENATOR OVERMAN: Do you know where he got it from?

COL. HURBAN: I remember it was $10,000; but it is no matter. I will speak about their propaganda. The German Government knew Russia better than anybody, and they knew that with the help of those people they could destroy the Russian army.

(At 5:45 o'clock p.m. the subcommittee adjourned until the next day, Wednesday, February 19, at 10:30 o'clock a.m.)

(United States, Senate, Brewing and Liquor Interests and German and Bolshevik Propaganda (Subcommittee on the Judiciary), 65th Cong., 1919.)

How remarkable that the committee was adjourned so abruptly before the source of Trotsky's funds could be placed into the Senate record.

When questioning resumed the next day, Trotsky and his $10,000 were no longer of interest to the Committee! We learn from a British Directorate of Intelligence report that Gregory Weinstein, who in 1919 was to become a prominent member of the Soviet Bureau in New York, collected funds for Trotsky in New York. These funds originated in Germany and were channelled through the V*olks-zeitung,* a German daily newspaper in New York and subsidized by the German government.

(Special Report No. 5, The Russian Soviet Bureau in the United States, July 14, 1919, Scotland House, London S.W.I. Copy in U.S. State Dept. Decimal File, 316-23-1145.)

While Trotsky's funds are officially reported as German, Trotsky was actively engaged in American politics immediately prior to leaving New York for Russia and the revolution.

Woodrow Wilson – A Passport for Trotsky

President Woodrow Wilson actually provided Trotsky with the passport he used to return to Russia. Once there he was able to "carry forward" the revolution. Alongside his American passport, Trotsky also had in his possession a Russian entry permit and a British transit visa.

Jennings C. Wise, in *Woodrow Wilson: Disciple of Revolution*, makes the pertinent comment;

"Historians must never forget that Woodrow Wilson, despite the efforts of the British police, made it possible for Leon Trotsky to enter Russia with an American passport."

President Wilson facilitated Trotsky's passage to Russia at the same time careful State Department bureaucrats, concerned about such revolutionaries entering Russia, were unilaterally attempting to tighten up passport procedures. The Stockholm legation cabled the State Department on June 13, 1917, just *after* Trotsky crossed the Finnish-Russian border, "Legation confidentially informed Russian, English and French passport offices at Russian frontier, Tornea, considerably worried by passage of suspicious persons bearing American passports."

(U.S. State Dept. Decimal File, 316-85-1002.)

The State Department replied the same day;

"Department is exercising special care in issuance of passports for Russia"

The Department also authorized expenditures by the legation to establish a passport-control office in Stockholm and to hire in "absolutely dependable American citizens" for employment on control work. But it was too late. Trotsky with Lenin's Bolsheviks was already in Russia to "carry forward" the revolution.

Somewhat tardily, in mid-August 1917 the Russian embassy in Washington requested the State Department (and State agreed) to "prevent the entry into Russia of criminals and anarchists... numbers of whom have already gone to Russia."

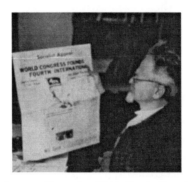

Trotsky reading the U.S. Socialist Appeal

Thanks to preferential treatment, when the S.S. Kristianiafjord *left* New York on March 26, 1917, Trotsky was on board with a U.S. passport. Fellow passengers were other Trotskyite revolutionaries, Wall Street financiers, American Communists, none of whom were engaged in 'above board' errands of business.

This mixed bag of passengers has been described by Lincoln Steffens, the American Communist:

"The passenger list was long and mysterious. Trotsky was in the steerage with a group of revolutionaries; there was a Japanese revolutionist in my cabin. There were a lot of Dutch

hurrying home from Java, the only innocent people aboard. The rest were war messengers, two from Wall Street to Germany."

(Lincoln Steffens, Autobiography (New York: Harcourt, Brace, 1931), p. 764. Steffens was the "go-between" for Crane and Woodrow Wilson.)

Lincoln Steffens was en route to Russia at the specific invitation of Charles Richard Crane, a backer and a former chairman of the Democratic Party's finance committee. Charles Crane, vice president of the Crane Company, had organized the Westinghouse Company in Russia, was a member of the Root mission to Russia, and had made no fewer than twenty-three visits to Russia between 1890 and 1930.

Richard Crane, his son, was confidential assistant to then Secretary of State Robert Lansing. According to the former ambassador to Germany William Dodd, Crane "*did much to bring on the Kerensky revolution which gave way to Communism." And so Steffens' comments in his diary about conversations aboard the S.S. *Kristianiafjord* are highly pertinent: ** " . . . all agree that the revolution is in its first phase only, that it must grow. Crane and Russian radicals on the ship think we shall be in Petrograd for the re-revolution.!"**

*(*William Edward Dodd, Ambassador Dodd's Diary, 1933-1938 pp. 42-43.)*

*(** Lincoln Steffens, The Letters of Lincoln Steffens p. 396)*

Crane returned to the United States when the Bolshevik Revolution (that is, "the re-revolution") had been completed and, although a private citizen, was given first hand reports of the progress of the Bolshevik Revolution as cables were received at the State Department! So Charles Crane, a friend and backer of Woodrow Wilson and a prominent financier and politician, had a known role in the "first" revolution and travelled to Russia in mid-1917 in company with the American Communist Lincoln Steffens, who was in touch with both Woodrow Wilson and Trotsky. The latter in turn was carrying a passport issued at the orders of Wilson and $10,000 from supposed German sources. On his return to the U.S. after the "re-revolution," Crane was granted access to official documents concerning consolidation of the Bolshevik regime.

Anthony Sutton in his meticulously researched book 'Wall Street and the Bolshevik Revolution' dedicates large portions to exposing the ongoing link between Soviet development and secret American finance. There has been a constant flow of support which runs through successive Presidencies. Soviet truck plants, Jet engine development and advancement in Chemical Warfare capability are just some areas in which the puppet masters in the States have made money from playing both sides. While the tension between Super Powers was being sold to us, behind the scenes money and technical expertise poured out of the West to Russia in secret.

A Dynasty of Mass Murderers -
The Bush Family

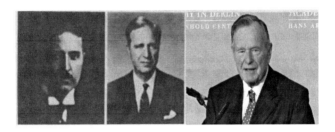

George Herbert Walker operated with criminal overlords to devour companies and peoples' life works for his own gain. His collaborators and sometime business partners included John D. Rockefeller (founder of Exxon way back then under the name of Standard Oil of New Jersey), E.H. Harriman (Railroad Owner) and William Rockefeller (who financed Harriman's railroad through Rockefeller's 'Citibank' predecessor).

Samuel Prescott Bush – Son of an Episcopalian preacher converted to the dark side by George Herbert Walker. Walker and Bush each contributed one child to the union of Dorothy Walker and Prescott Bush to produce grandson George Herbert Walker Bush and great – grandson George Walker Bush.

Prescott Sheldon Bush – became Hitler's Banker through Fritz Thyssen. He collaborated with the Nazis from before the 2nd World War broke out and through the year after Pearl Harbour. Auschwitz Death Camp was sited where it was because of its proximity to Thyssen's coal, steel and railroads. The Bush family and their allies grew enormously rich from exploiting mass murder. Their factories used these resources of slave labour in their production programmes. It is so mind numbing that many simply refuse to believe the facts even when they are clearly backed with historical evidence.

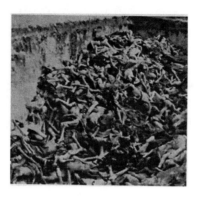

<u>A Mass Grave of Slave Labourers at Auschwitz</u>

The S.S. – Deal Genocide and Make Money

When Hitler had got his grip on power in Germany, the dreaded S.S. was turned loose on the German people. The S.S. was not just a terrorist organisation, but deeply involved in espionage and big business. Long term goals included the establishment of business monopolies in all countries conquered by the Nazis.

Himmler's men of the S.S. had a huge network of friends throughout the international business community who also hoped to benefit from the spoils of their conquest. They gave Himmler and the S.S. staggering amounts of money which, in effect, made them stockholders in this moneymaking terrorist organisation.

Like its later American twin, the German 'Order' of Skull and Bones, the Thule Society, was out to make money for its elite inner circle.

Initiating Adolf

As far back as 1919, Dietrich Eckhart, an occultist and member of the Thule Society had been introduced to Adolf Hitler.

He believed from then on that Adolf Hitler was the dark messiah he had looked for: the one who would lead Germany to meet her destiny. Driven by this belief, he took him under his personal direction and initiated Hitler into the deepest satanic rituals, sparing him nothing. At certain points during these ceremonies, the demonic energy is as tangible as electricity surging through the initiate's body. The procedures involve extremes of sexual depravity which may have been the reason behind Hitler's impotence.

Before he died, Eckhart said;

"Follow Hitler; he will dance, but it is I who have called the tune. I have initiated him into the secret Doctrine, opened his centres of vision and given him the means to communicate with the powers."

Hitler viewed his mentor as the 'spiritual founder' of the Nazi Party.

"He shone in our eyes like the polar star" (Hitler -Table Talk)
   "He was one of the best, who devoted his life to the awakening...."
   (Hitler - Mein Kampf)

Prescott Bush became vice president of W.A. Harriman and Co. in 1926.

That same year, Wall Street banker Clarence Dillon, a friend of Prescott Bush's father Sam Bush, organised the German Steel Trust for their client Fritz Thyssen, Hitler's principal sponsor. It was Germany's largest industrial corporation.

Another prominent member of the Thule Society was Rudolf Hess who had introduced Thyssen to Hitler in 1922. His reaction was the same as Eckhart's.

He was certain that he had met the German saviour. Thyssen rightly believed that the New World Order was making advances and that it would be ruled by the 'kings of banking and commerce'. Thyssen and Harriman's financial relationship had given rise to the international investment firm 'Union Banking Corporation'.

"by personal agreement between Averill Harriman and Fritz Thyssen in 1922... the Union Banking Corporation has since its inception handled funds chiefly supplied to it through the Dutch bank by the Thyssen interests for American investment....transferring funds back and forth between New York and the Thyssen interests...."

The Union Banking Corporation and Thyssen's bank acted as Nazi fronts, laundering funds for Thyssen and the Nazis. These were used to buy guns, publicity and dozens of U.S. senators, congressmen and newspaper editors.

(See W. G. Tarpley and A.Chaitkin - 'George Bush: The Unauthorised Biography')

According to the United States Government, Prescott Bush's Union Banking Corporation worked as a front for the "Thyssen family – nationals of a designated enemy country.."

As summed up by John Loftus, U.S. Department of Justice Nazi War Crimes Prosecutor;

"Thyssen (and the Nazi Party) obtained his early financing from Brown Brothers Harriman and its affiliate, the Union Banking Corporation. Union Bank, in turn, was the Bush's holding company for a number of other entities, including the Holland-America Trading Company. The Bush's Union Bank bought the same corporate stock that the Thyssens were selling as part of their Nazi money laundering...."

These Nazi-front companies 'Brown Brothers, Harriman' and 'Union Banking Corporation' were almost entirely controlled by members of the American chapter of 'Skull and Bones'. Prescott Bush and associates along with Standard Oil provided not only loans, but also executive expertise and petroleum related products to I.G. Farben. Farben used that expertise to develop poison gas and petroleum to drive the hellish war machine of Nazism and to run death camps like Auschwitz where 83,000 people worked as slaves. In the camps alone Himmler's S.S. worked to death and murdered over 10 million men and women. Their favourite murder weapon – deadly gas developed by I.G. Farben with American aid and expertise.

Prescott Bush and Harriman were also in business with several other leading Nazis, including Friedrich Flick, who became Hitler's Minister of the Interior.

The Flick-Harriman partnership was managed by Prescott Bush.

The closest and most loyal supporters of the Reich were known as the "Circle of Friends" or "Friends of the Reichsfuhrer S.S." Prescott Bush's Hamburg-Amerika line was also counted as a "Friend of the Reichsfuhrer".

Standard Oil, the Bush-Harriman associations and Rockefeller not only provided finance and technological assistance to the Nazis, but further they assisted his terror campaign to the detriment of the U.S.

"In two years we will be manufacturing enough oil and gas out of soft coal for a long war. The Standard Oil Company of New York is furnishing millions of dollars to help" Commercial Attache', U.S. Embassy in Berlin, Germany, January 1933.

Death's Head

The diabolic symbolism of the Skull and Bones is intended to invoke fear and warn of death. For precisely that reason, the gruesome crest was used to decorate the black uniforms of the Nazi S.S. They were the Order, the Brotherhood of Death.

Like the members of Lodge 322 'Skull and Bones' at Yale University, the members of the S.S. were drawn from the elite and privileged classes of Germany. These were the bankers and aristocracy of the land. Even before the Nazis seized power, certain 'great' names had been added to the list of members; Grand Dukes, Counts and Princes.

As Heinz Hohns reveals in 'The Order of the Death's Head';

"In spring 1933 came a further infusion of blue blood. Many of the senior S.S. posts were occupied by the nobility... and the ruling class elite. The primary requirements in the S.S. were money and officer material, and they could come only from one source – the old-established ruling class elite - the nobility, the world of commerce and financiers....Germany's captains of industry."

Those who were to belong to the higher ranks in the S.S. underwent initiation rites and ceremonies parallel to the American Order. Ceremonies took place at midnight in a Castle, beneath the dining hall where lay a stone crypt and 'the realm of the dead'. "A flight of steps in the middle of the crypt led down into a well-like cavity; in the centre of the cavity were twelve stone pedestals." Bones and relics including the skull and skeletons of noble men and kings were also kept within the 'holy of holies' including the bones of "King Heinrich". Initiates would commune with spirits of the dead, who might appear and even speak. The S.S. initiate by means of this journey would be 're-born' as a member of the Secret Order.

These rituals ran along the same lines as Yale's American Order, where the initiates are required to undergo a variety of Occult and bonding rituals. These occur at midnight in 'The Tomb'. The initiate is taken on a journey through the underworld to re-birth.

The American 'Tomb' contains a little Nazi shrine.

On re-birth, the newborn is given his special garments. The implication is that henceforth, he will tailor himself to the Order's mission on earth.

For many years in the Order, to prove mettle and perhaps to bond them in corporate guilt over an illicit act, each class of 15 new initiates were required to dig up the skull of a famous person and bring it to the tomb to be enshrined in its skull collection.

The leading Native American newspaper has run articles on the Order and their grave robbing. '60 Minutes' ran a programme which addressed the Order's alleged possession of the skull of Geronimo, the Native American Chief. The media exposure led to activists pressing for return of the skull and whatever else was taken.

Robert McNamara - Prolonging War for Profit

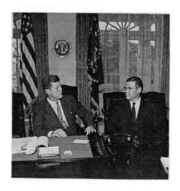

Robert McNamara was Secretary of Defense under Presidents Kennedy and Johnson before 'steering' the World Bank for thirteen years as its President. He steered it all right! Like a drunk driver!

"As a result of our superiority over the Russians, Walt Whitman Rostow, who served in the Kennedy administration as Chief of the State Department's Policy Planning Council, and Jerome B. Weisner, then Director of MIT's Electronic Research Laboratory, agreed that it was time to help Russia catch up to our weapons superiority. It was McNamara who in June 1964 eliminated or shelved a whole array of America's most effective or promising weapons...such as the Skybolt and Pluto missiles...The X-20 Dynasoar, The B-70 Bombers, 195 Bomarc-A missiles, Nike-Zeus ABM defense system and the Navy's Typhoon frigates and weapons systems...the 129 Atlas missiles which had alone cost £5.4 billion......"

William J. Gill 'Trade Wars Against America'

While Secretary of Defense this man issued "Rules of Engagement" that actively disadvantaged U.S. soldiers in combat in Vietnam!

These combat troops were;

"....not permitted to fire until their situation became desperate. This kind of suicidal warfare was an everyday occurrence in Vietnam. Yet McNamara's Rules of Engagement were themselves covered up and it was not until 1985 – ten years after the fall of Vietnam – that the Defense Department declassified them at the behest of Senator Goldwater who then inserted them into the Congressional Record. Goldwater remarked that 'these layers of restrictions, which were constantly changing and were almost impossible to memorize or understand, although it was required of our pilots, granted huge sanctuary areas to the enemy. Although we lost hundreds of our pilots over North Vietnam, they were never permitted to bomb really strategic targets. Airmen contended that one bomb could have knocked out a huge hydro-electric dam, cutting off most of the communist country's power, flooding its food supply and probably forcing an end to the war. But that bomb was never dropped on that critical target."

William J. Gill 'Trade Wars Against America

Further Examples;

Robert McNamara and sustaining the Vietnam War

It was McNamara who covered up the Soviet's vast involvement in supplying Communist forces. American casualties multiplied and mounted. Still McNamara refused to remove the 'classified' tag he had put on years of reports of Russian ships off-loading weapons and materials at Haiphong. McNamara, with the full co-operation of the media, continued to conceal these facts from the American people who were sending their young men off to be slaughtered. The American Military-Industrial Complex was in for the long haul and maximum profits! The death toll of young American men didn't matter to them one jot!

Manipulating The World's Finances

McNamara's next post was President of the World Bank.

Bruce Rich wrote 'Mortgaging the Earth: The World Bank, Environmental Impoverishment and the Crisis of Development'. In it he spends a lot of time on McNamara's evil tactics while in this powerful position. McNamara's stated dream was that of eliminating poverty through World Bank development projects. The reality was that this 'dream' intentionally drove countries into social, economic and environmental chaos.

The Bank prepared five year master–plans for lending. These contained priorities and targets for all bank lending in a country. These reports were kept so confidential that even the ministers of a nation's cabinet were not permitted access. These became the planning documents for the Bank's entire lending portfolio. When this level of stark insanity is reached there is no accountability – certainly not to a Board of Directors!

Rich points out;

"The Bank prepared a development document for 'every relevant aspect' of a 'nation's social framework'. The Bank would go on to lead scores of governments in formulating these plans, which it goes without saying would attempt to regulate 'every relevant aspect of society'. Based on the Bank's gathering, filtering and organizing of information, other international agencies would help to finance the elements of the development blueprints formulated under the Bank's aegis.

The Bank would guide the generation of such knowledge in order to plan; implicit in the planning is control, and in control domination – over the evolution of human beings and nature on a planetary scale. It is no exaggeration to call such a project Faustian."

The conclusion according to Rich is that;

"Bank poverty-oriented agricultural lending actually promoted the destruction of smaller local farms and the displacement of hundreds of millions of peasants around the world. McNamara's poverty strategy in practice only accelerated a process of agricultural modernization and integration into the global market that, in the view of many researchers, increased inequality and produced poverty and underdevelopment by displacing rural people formerly rooted in traditional subsistence-farming communities."

Central banks were founded in Sweden in 1668, England 1694, France 1803, Italy in 1861 and Germany in 1870. Look at the situation now;

Every country has a central bank, i.e. a private corporation controlled by the same group of banks and individuals who own the Banks of England, France, Italy, Germany, Canada, Japan, Russia etc etc.

All of these Banks own some of every country's currency. We have examined previously how these banking dynasties seek to subvert and control the currency of nations. It should be easy by now to see how straightforward international control by the banks and their shadowy puppeteers becomes. All that needs to be done in order to bring a country into line with the financiers' agenda is for all central banks to sell that country's currency at the same time.

For example, Malaysia, Thailand and South Korea did not want to sign the 'World Trade Organization's Financial

Services Agreement'. Just to help their decision along a little, their currencies were de-valued!

"Power corrupts – absolute power corrupts absolutely." Lord Acton.

As the Washington Post observed in an article on Dec 2 1996;

"Hans Teitmeyer may wield greater power than any President or Prime Minister in Europe. He has never been elected to public office and yet he can make or break the fortunes of governments as well as investors......"

As stated in the above article;

- Teitmeyer or any other central bank manager actually has more power than Presidents or Prime Ministers although bank Governors <u>are not elected officials.</u>
- Every country has borrowed money from these private banking corporations
- It follows that every country is beholden to them

"Politicians..... must take political de-accession."

In other words politicians rank under the central bank chairman in terms of actual power!

The central banks, corporations and financial markets are in the process of consolidating this awesome power. This was first observed when the individual central banks all coalesced into one united central bank of Europe. (ECB) The European Investment Bank, its predecessor (EIB) paved the way for a United Europe by helping to standardize the currencies between countries joining the EEC. The 'Euro' was traded as early as 1998 in the bond markets.

The Bank of England received radical new powers as of May 6th 1997.

These included the Power to set interest rates without permission from the Government. They were also allocated a separate pool of foreign exchange reserves by the Treasury which they could, at their discretion, use to intervene in the currency markets.

These powers are viewed as;.

"the most radical internal reform to the Bank of England since it was established in 1694"

Gordon Brown – then British Chancellor of the Exchequer quoted in the Washington Times May 1997.

The article further explains that Brown was modelling the Bank of England much more closely after the Federal Reserve which can adjust rates even if that causes short term political discomfort for the White House.

The Bank of Japan

In 1997 Japan's Central bank was given more powers to determine monetary policy.

Under these reforms the policy making body was restructured to mirror the same membership as the U.S. Federal Reserve and the Bank of England. This new policy making board would draw six of its members from business and academia alongside the Bank's Governor and two vice governors. The stated purpose here was to provide more autonomy in line with international standards and the plans for the de-regulation of the financial markets in 2001.

The Bundesbank, Bank of Japan, Bank of England, Federal Reserve Bank and The EIB all have freedom to set interest rates apart from Government opinion.

The Bank for International Settlements (BIS)

Until recently the BIS was seldom mentioned in the press. Based in Basle, Switzerland it operates in great secrecy. Its power is immense and it is the 'Central Banks' Bank'. On a Global level it coordinates with the local Central Bank in each country regarding material changes in domestic law which are needed to bring the world economy into harmony.

Over a period of years it has gained greater and greater control over the Global Monetary System.

According to Dr. Quigley;

"The powers of capitalism had another far-reaching aim, nothing less than to create a world system of financial control in private hands able to dominate the political system of each country and the economy of the world as a whole.....The apex of the system was to be The Bank for International Settlements in Basle, Switzerland, a private Bank owned and controlled by the World's Central banks, which were themselves private corporations. Each Central Bank...sought to dominate its government by its ability to control.... The BIS was generally regarded as the apex structure of financial capitalism whose remote origins go back to the creation of the Bank of England in 1694 and the Bank of France in 1803.....It was set up rather to remedy the decline in London as the world's financial Centre by providing a mechanism by which a world with three chief financial centres in London, New York and Paris could still operate as one."

Ten times a year, the heads of the World's major central banks meet at their 'supranatural second home, the BIS ...they are;

"International freemasons possessing a natural second allegiance to the often lonely interest of international monetary order..." 'Steve Solomon – The Confidence Game'

177

The Stock Market crash of 1987 empowered the BIS to find support for its 'Basle Capital Accord' which extended;

"Basle guidelines into comprehensive harmonized global rules and oversight for all financial firms" Steve Solomon- The Confidence Game

Many of the necessary changes in national law have already been affected in most countries in order to facilitate the BIS agenda. In the U.S. the law no longer restricts the free flow of money in or out of the country. The Monetary Control Act removed all of the restraints on the U.S. banking system such as the interest rate ceiling or Regulation Q – the amount of interest a Bank could pay on deposits. It also erased Regulation D, which set a minimum amount of reserves to be held by commercial banks. The door is open for the Globalized economy we are seeing today.

A year before the United Nations Charter was signed, over seven hundred delegates from forty four countries met to construct a World Monetary System which would be used to govern the world after the War. The gathering was sponsored by the United Nations. The 'Bretton Woods' Conference had two objectives;

1. To reduce obstacles of International Trade
2. To bring about the harmonization of national policies of member states

Two key figures at that conference were John Maynard Keynes, the British Socialist who stated that what was agreed at 'Bretton Woods' was the opposite of the Gold standard, and Harry Dexter White, Assistant Secretary of the Treasury. White was later named by Whittaker Chambers and Helen Bentley as a deep cover Soviet agent. He drew up the plans for the International Bank for Reconstruction and Development which is now known as the World Bank. This was stated originally as a means of helping war-torn countries re-build after the war. In 1947 the loans became 'developmental loans'. The International Bank for Reconstruction & Development, The International Development Agency, The International Finance Corporation and the Multilateral Investment Guarantee Agency are some of the faces the World Bank wears. In these guises it becomes much more than just a bank involving itself in water reform policy, agriculture, forestry, urban and industrial management as well as social issues. As Joan Veon points out, many third world countries are so indebted to the Bank that they are unable to build schools, roads, hospitals and other infrastructure as a result of the crippling debt. At the same time Bruce Rich identifies what can be termed 'white elephant' projects which are instrumental in creating this level of debt. (*Bruce Rich – 'Mortgaging the Earth'*)

The International Monetary Fund

Another of 'Harry the Spy's' little brainchildren was the International Monetary Fund! This has expanded alongside the World Bank. In the 1960s the IMF created a form of liquid money called Special Drawing Rights –SDRs. This is basically money printed out of thin air whenever money is needed.! It puts money in the system without accountability and is thus extremely inflationary.

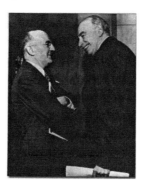

Harry Dexter White with John Maynard Keynes

Henry Ford and Hitler

Dialectic in the Driver's Seat

If you ask any one what they know about Henry Ford they'll be able to tell you about the model 't' motor car and his approach to mass auto production. Henry's factories worked day and night turning out American vehicles for the war against Germany. What the history books aren't so open about is the fact that he had factories in Germany which were also working day and night turning out vehicles for the Nazis to use in their war against the allies! Hitler was a big fan of good ol' Henry Ford. He decorated Ford with a medal and had a photograph of him in his personal office! He was awarded the Grand Cross of The Supreme Order Of The German Eagle.

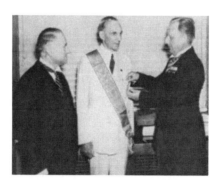

Ford and his medal reward

I trust that certain things are clear from what has been set down so far;

- It is a mistake to think in the terms many of us have been brought up and brainwashed with, such as 'Left' Wing and 'Right' Wing. They are both wings on the same scrofulous bird!

- The New World Order is a plan to abolish all national sovereignty, all national borders and to abolish all authority save that of the Global elite. It has participants at the highest levels of government in every country who share this common vision. Behind it are the most powerful people on the planet.

- The Banking System is controlled by an elite and in turn controls the world. There is absolutely no limit to the level of its corruption. Anyone who is very successful in finance or in gaining a high level of control in the area of technology is targeted for recruitment. If they do not eventually come on board they are destroyed.

- Like a beast with numerous tentacles, it has its eyes, ears and claws into every human network. It subverts even sincere Christian ministries through finance and blackmail. It will recruit and control those in the media and show business to further its plans. (I grew up listening to the veteran reporter Walter Kronkite, for example. I now know that he became one of many media fronts, the present crop of which includes the actor Arnold Schwartzenegger and singers such as Kris Kristofferson and Jerry Reed).

- The elite adherents have a satanic belief system. One of their stated aims is to destroy Christianity. The system intends to persecute the Christian faith out of existence. Only the trappings will be allowed to survive and woven into a syncretised 'World Faith'.

It should be clear to anyone who has read up to this point that practically everything is in place for the last push into real global Government. Any one who glibly says 'Okay, so what – it doesn't concern me - bring it on!" hasn't taken account of the nature of those who will be in control. Behind the manoeuvring of finance and political appointments lies the same ruthless, satanic spirit that has inspired and possessed tyrants right back as far as ancient Babylon. The original 'Goals for Control' envisaged by those occupying the top of the pyramid are all but met. This has been achieved through decade after decade of careful manoeuvring, worldwide espionage and the subversion of the highest political offices in the world. As stated earlier, the mechanisms are all in place for the United Nations to take up its role as the first Phase of the New World Order. Mark that this will be only the 'first chapter'. The exact shape of things beyond that will be argued out between the European elite and the present American factions. However the details are worked out, the checklist for success is almost complete. The economic crisis referred to cannot be that far off. We have already felt the first warning tremors. When fully activated, it will result in utter catastrophe for most people as banks demand payment of mortgages, loans and overdrafts. The social chaos which will follow has been well planned for and extensive measures are already in place for control of an outraged populace.. However, though these plans are now on the table they can be stalled and delayed. Of course, you can dismiss all this as paranoia - I am well beyond wanting to argue the point. All I would urge is that you look into these matters for yourself. If you insist on being 'comfortably numb' to what is actually going on around you that's up to you. Biblical prophecy makes it clear that the plans for a One World Government will be allowed to succeed on a short term basis.

"Well what am I supposed to do? It's too big to fight....." is a common reaction. Well, first of all, pray - not last of all pray! Intercessory prayer can and does change things. Those who know the grace of God through Jesus Christ are not praying to some inert idol. If you are a Christian, begin to ask God what your role is. Whatever sphere you operate in; business, the arts, medicine, law, journalism, agriculture, media, banking – whatever your occupation, how can you make a stand for the values of God's kingdom where you are? The trouble with so many Christians today is that they retreat into church culture instead of seeking God about being salt and light just where they are in the world's marketplace. God asked Moses "What is in your hand?" (Exodus 4 v 1-4). In other words, what do you have at your immediate disposal? Moses had only a wooden staff but God used it to demonstrate that the simplest of things, once surrendered to Him, can work miracles. What are your gifts and talents? If God can do miracles with just a simple stick, what changes can He bring about as you present yourself in His service? At every stage of history God seeks for men and women who will stand for Him. The sorry truth is so often that 'Many are called but few get up.' Retreating into church culture makes you invisible in the world. Jesus didn't teach us to do that. His prayer was not that His disciples be taken out of the world but that they be in the world but not 'of it'. Elsewhere He taught us to pray to God that 'Your Kingdom come, Your will be done on earth as it is in heaven." (Luke 11). How many times do you hear people berate the sorry state of the Arts or corruption in politics when these are areas churchy-minded Christians have almost totally retreated from. God is there and He is not silent! He can and does act into human situations to change things.

Prophetic Warnings

The Book of Amos Chapter 3 verse 7 says "Surely the Lord will do nothing without revealing it to his servants the prophets."

- God warned Noah of the coming flood in Genesis 6.
- God warned Abraham and Lot of the coming destruction of Sodom in Genesis 18.
- God warned Joseph that there was to be a seven year famine in Genesis 41.
- God told Moses of the seven plagues that were to befall Egypt in Exodus 7.
- God warned Jonah of the destruction of Nineveh (Jonah 1:2 3:4)
- God warned Amos of the downfall of Syria, Philistia, Tyre, Edom, Ammon, Moab, Judah and Israel. (Amos 1 & 2).

Various prophets were told about the captivity of the chosen people – every one was fulfilled in startling detail. God forewarns His people of the larger world events because he loves them and does not wish that they be taken by surprise.

Christ's coming was foretold throughout the Old Testament from Genesis to Malachi and we read in Luke 19 v 37- 44 that Jesus judged the people for not knowing the time of their visitation! They had all the prophecies and still did not understand the significance of His coming. Because they had not understood, there was to be disaster. Of course that prediction was also fulfilled to the very letter when the Romans tore into Jerusalem. Exactly as Jesus had said, they threw up a siege embankment and got quickly on with their horrible task.

The difficulty in introducing Globalism to people for the first time is to get them to understand the extent to which it has been planned for generations. Its scope is huge and it is very far advanced. The dynasties behind it are patient people and a year or two here or there doesn't usually matter to them. Although there are some among them who would gladly force their way to control, the majority of them see the advantages of incrementalism. They prefer tactics of stealth to gain control. They can see it working effectively while the majority of people remain completely unaware of the changes taking place all around them.

As they control every major media outlet from newspapers to TV Networks, they show you what they want you to see and hear. Take a look for yourself at just who is in control of the major outlets – it will shock you to the core. When you trace things back you find the same dynasties, personalities and foundations.

However, we are living in the days of Joe Sixpack when it has become possible for the architects of the New World Order to hasten things against the background of a severely 'dumbed-down' populace.

In Genesis 11 we read the account of the tower of Babel.

The Jewish Historian Josephus gives the same account in his 'Antiquities of the Jews' ...

"Now the sons of Noah were three – Shem, Japhet and Ham, born one hundred years before the Deluge. These first of all descended from the mountains into the plains and fixed their habitation there; and persuaded others who were greatly afraid of the lower grounds on account of the flood, and so were very loath to come down from the higher places to venture to follow their examples. Now the plain in which they first dwelt was called Shinar. God also commanded them to send colonies abroad, for the thorough peopling of the earth – that they might not raise seditions among themselves, but might cultivate a great part of the earth and enjoy its fruits after a plentiful manner: but they were so ill instructed that they did not obey God; for which reason they fell into calamities and were made sensible, by experience, of what sin they had been guilty; for when they flourished with a numerous youth, God admonished them again to send out colonies; but they imagining the prosperity they enjoyed was not derived from the favour of God, but supposing that their own power was the cause of the plentiful condition they were in, did not obey Him. Nay, they added to this their disobedience to the Divine Will, the suspicion that they were therefore ordered to send out separate colonies, that being divided asunder they might be more easily oppressed.

Now it was Nimrod who excited them to such an affront and contempt of God. He was the grandson of Ham, the son of Noah, - a bold man and of great strength of hand. He persuaded them not to ascribe it to God, as if it were through His means they were happy, but to believe that it was their own courage which procured that happiness. He also gradually changed the government into tyranny – seeing no other way of turning men from fear of God but to bring them into a constant dependence upon his power. He also said he would be revenged on God, if He should have a mind to drown the world again: for that he would build a tower too high for the waters to be able to reach! And that he would revenge himself on God for destroying their forefathers!

Now the multitude were very ready to follow the determination of Nimrod and to esteem it a piece of cowardice to submit to God; and they built a tower neither sparing any pains nor being in any degree negligent about the work; and by reason of the multitude of hands employed in it, it grew very high, sooner than anyone could expect; but the thickness of it was so great and it was so strongly built that thereby its great height seemed upon the view to be less than it really was.

It was built of burnt brick, cemented together with mortar made of bitumen, that it might not be able to admit water. When God saw that they acted so madly He did not resolve to destroy them utterly since they were not grown wiser by the destruction of the former sinners, but he caused a tumult among them by producing in them diverse languages and causing that, through the multitude of these languages they should not be able to understand one another.

The place wherein they built the tower is now called Babylon because of the confusion of that language which they readily understood before.

For the Hebrew mean by the word Babel – Confusion!"

Josephus 'Antiquities Of The Jews' Chapter IV

Here was the prototype New World Order as referred to by Margaret Thatcher; *who commented; "At least they spoke the same language when they began..."* The story of Babel is an account of a scheme visionary and vast in its scope. Those involved were committed to their task until God decided to rain on their ambitious parade.

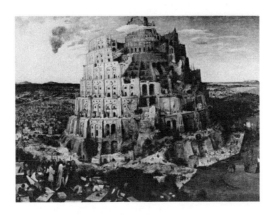

Pieter Bruegel's famous painting of The Tower of Babel

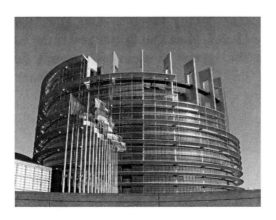

European Parliament Building – Strasbourg.
Yes – it is a deliberate architectural image
of the unfinished Tower of Babel!

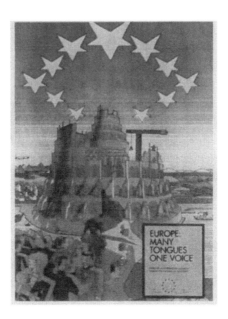

An E.E.C. Propaganda Poster actually uses
the Tower of Babel with the caption
'Europe – Many Tongues, One Voice'.

The poster shows the people of Europe rebuilding the Tower
that God destroyed in the Book of Genesis.

The statement - 'Many Tongues – One Voice' inverts God's
judgement on Babel. Note that in this poster the normal stars
are inverted Pentagrams. A close look reveals the intended
image over the Tower. Also see shot of Hilary Clinton's
campaign flag which featured the same device.

Europa

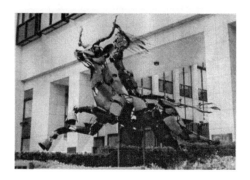

The image of the 'Woman riding the Beast'. This large
sculpture sits outside the European Union Council
of Ministers Offices in Brussels, Belgium

Many are unaware that Europe takes the name from Europa.
In the legend, Zeus lusted after Europa and transformed
himself into a giant white bull in which guise he was able to
mingle among her father's herds. While Europa and her female
attendants were gathering flowers, Europa saw the bull and
began to caress his flanks. Eventually she climbed upon his
back. Zeus took this opportunity to run into the sea, raping
Europa.

Europa again, this time riding the beast on the Greek 2 Euro Coin.

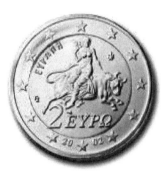

An image chosen by the European Union:
The Woman Riding The Beast'

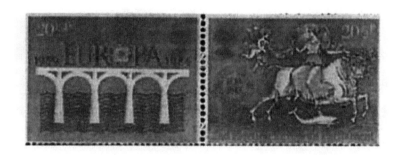

Europa is depicted riding the beast on this
1984 centenary stamp.

The Biblical texts of Daniel and Revelation

The prophetic book of Daniel gives a historic overview, from the prophet's time, of world empires which arise in the course of human history. Some critics dismiss this and would explain the empires as those within a limited time frame of the prophet's lifespan. The crux of the matter is whether you actually believe in Biblical prophecy!

On one hand many people today are publicly dismissive of any belief in a spiritual dimension. On the other hand they flock to movies characterised by demons, wizards, witchcraft, time-travel and sorcery. It is one of the great contradictions of our time. What lies behind this fascination with all things paranormal? The fact is that the spiritual world is very real and most people, deep down, despite their public attitudes, know it.

A while ago the Rock group U2 did a series of concerts featuring massive back screens. Onto these were rapidly projected a number of verbal messages. One read; 'Everything You Know is Wrong'. For the last few years of my life I have realised how close to the truth that is. The actual nature of our reality is very different from the picture of life we are sold from infancy.

Everything You Know Is Wrong!
Re-Thinking Reality

In the film 'The Matrix' the character Neo realises that there is something wrong with what he has hitherto accepted as 'reality' and begins to seek the truth. The character Morpheus offers him enlightenment; "I imagine you are feeling a bit like Alice, tumbling down the rabbit hole" he says, quoting from Lewis Carroll. "You have the look of a man who accepts what he sees because he is expecting to wake up. Ironically, this not far from the truth." Morpheus offers him a choice; "You take the blue pill and you wake up in your bed and believe whatever you want to believe. You take the red pill, you stay in Wonderland and I show you how deep the rabbit hole goes."

For us, like the character Neo, examining the present geo-political reality requires setting aside much of what we've believed as true. This also applies to our outlook on the nature of the wider universe we live in, including the reality of the spiritual dimension and the true nature of biblical prophecy.

We can start with the sort of assumptions we were taught to accept in the science classes at school. For instance in our classes in plane geometry we are taught that the angles of a triangle all add up to 180 degrees. This classroom theory becomes useless when we encounter triangular measurements on a larger scale – for example in oceanic navigation where we encounter the curvature of the earth.

Plane geometry is just that – useable in a two dimensional setting on a desktop. The reality is very different. In the same way, many need to start expanding their thinking to appreciate the far more complex nature of the universe, as well as the verity and relevance of the prophetic books in the Bible.

The Finite Universe and The Microcosm

The Boundaries Of Our Existence

The Macrocosm

Two of the most important discoveries of the twentieth century have been that:

The universe we inhabit is finite – it has a definite beginning and a definite boundary. Laws of Thermodynamics demonstrate that energy travels from hot to cold. All the processes taking place in our universe make a contribution to the ambient temperature. If the universe went on infinitely, then the present ambient temperature would be uniform. It is not; hence it had a beginning and it's demise will be characterised by what is known as 'heat death' when the ambient temperature becomes uniform and no further transfers of heat are taking place. We exist between the massive event that started it all and a certain sentence of termination.

The Microcosm

At the other end of our reality is another boundary – the finiteness of the Microcosm. For example, let's say we take a length of something like a piece of string and begin to cut it in half. We then take one of the remaining pieces and again cut it in half. Our assumption is that, in theory at least we might go on doing this infinitely. It turns out that this is not so. As we cut down to the tiny length of 10-33 centimetres we find that it cannot be further divided. This is termed the Planck Length by Physicists. At this point we have cut down to the size of one of the 'building blocks' of our reality. More astonishing still is the fact that if we attempt to further divide it, it loses 'locality'. This is true as we explore virtually every other measure. It is true for our three spatial dimensions, for mass, for energy and even for time itself. For example, there is no briefer time than 10-43 seconds!

Quantum Thinking

We find that the measures we investigate are 'Quantised'. Things break down to 'quanta' or indivisible units, hence this area of study is termed 'Quantum Physics'.

As we break things into smaller and smaller sections we reach a point where these tiny pieces, the electrons, protons etc. stop displaying the traits associated with objects. They literally possess no dimensions, though they sometimes complicate matters further by behaving like small particles.

A sub atomic particle such as an electron can show itself as a particle or a wave. An electron fired at a T.V. screen while the set is turned off, will show a small point of light when it hits the phosphorescent materials in the screen. This single point of impact shows the electron manifesting as a particle. However, the electron can also manifest itself as a wave and in this guise it behaves differently. Fired at a barrier in which two slits are cut, it will go through both slits simultaneously.

Whaaat!?? Yes, both at exactly the same time. As Danish Physicist, Niels Bohr put it; "Anyone who is <u>not</u> shocked by Quantum Physics has not understood it!"

In 1906 J. J. Thompson received the Nobel Prize for proving that electrons are particles. In 1937 his son was awarded the Nobel prize for proving that electrons were waves! Both were correct. All subatomic particles have these strange abilities, being able to show themselves as either waves or particles. But, things get stranger still. There is astonishing evidence that the only time quanta show themselves as particles is when we are observing them. As Bohr pointed out, if subatomic particles only come to exist in the presence of an observer, then it is meaningless to talk about a particle's characteristics as actually existing before they are observed. Give yourself a minute to ponder that. This rabbit hole goes pretty deep!

Further still, some subatomic processes give rise to the creation of paired particles with what seem identical properties. Quantum physics predicts that efforts to measure the complementary characteristics on the pair would be futile – even when they are travelling in opposite directions. This carries the implication that they are somehow interconnected so as to be able to instantaneously communicate with each other.

Albert Einstein, despite his founding role in Quantum theory, was extremely troubled by some of the conclusions of the young science. His Special Theory of Relativity asserted that nothing could travel faster than the speed of light. This assertion would appear to be violated if there was instantaneous communication between these paired particles. Einstein and his camp were convinced that 'no reasonable definition' of reality would allow communication at speeds exceeding that of light. On this basis, surely the assertion must be wrong. In 1935 they voiced their reservations in a paper, "Can Quantum-Mechanical Description Of Physical Reality Be Considered Complete?" (Einstein, Podolsky and Rosen).

Niels Bohr sidestepped the extremes of the controversy by saying that if subatomic particles don't come into being until they are observed, one could not legitimately think of them as independent 'things'. These were, rather, parts of an indivisible system and should not be thought of otherwise.

In the 1950s Physicist David Bohm from the University of London, who had worked with Einstein, put forward evidence to suggest that our world and everything within it was a projection of a much greater reality beyond space and time. His work was in plasma physics. Plasmas are gases made up of high density electrons and positive ions. He had noticed that in plasmas the particles ceased their individual behaviour and started to act as if they were part of a greater interconnected whole. Their actions were highly organised as if they were actually aware of what the trillions of other individual particles were doing. Bohm concluded from his observations that, at a subatomic level, location just ceases to exist. All points in space become equal to all other points in space. It becomes meaningless to speak of anything being separate from anything else. Physicists now call this property 'nonlocality'.

As JBS Haldane observed; "The Universe is not only queerer than we imagine, it is queerer than we <u>can</u> imagine."

The work was taken forward by John Stewart Bell of CERN, the European Centre for Atomic Research In Geneva. Bell set out the conditions needed to verify the assertions about particle communication. In 1964 he formulated the 'Bell Inequality'.

Bell's conditions demanded that the experiment be performed in time frames the equipment of that era wasn't capable of performing to. Finally, in 1982 a team at the Institute of Theoretical and Applied Optics in Paris were in a position to carry out the landmark experiment. They produced a series of twin photons by heating up calcium atoms with lasers. Each photon was allowed to travel in opposite directions through 6.5 metres of pipe. Special filters directed them toward one of two possible polarization analysers. It took each filter ten nano-seconds to switch between one analyser and the other. This was about thirty nano-seconds less than it took light to travel the thirteen metres of pipe separating each set of photons. Each photon was still able to correlate its angle of polarization with its twin just as Quantum theory had predicted. The success of this experiment ruled out the possibility of the photons communicating by any known process. Either Einstein's ruling that nothing travels faster than light was being violated or these photons were connected 'Non-locally'.

In the last three hundred years the speed of light has been measured 164 times by 16 methods. In 1987 Barry Setterfield and Trevor Norman presented an analysis of the previous research indicating that the speed of light was actually slowing down. Canadian mathematician Alan Montgomery came to the same conclusion. It was travelling between 10% and 30% faster in the time of Christ, it was twice as fast around the time of King Solomon, four times faster at the time of Abraham and ten million times faster prior to 3,000 B.C. Similar trends have been noted in 475 measurements of 11 other atomic quantities tested in 25 methods.

Our universe is like a giant clock that is gradually winding down.

Ten Dimensions

The very fabric of the universe we live in is at odds with the picture we have been given. Part of that fabric is time itself. People were comfortable with the familiar dimensions of Height, Depth and Breadth as directly measurable. It is only comparatively recently that Albert Einstein managed to show time as the fourth dimension. We refer to Einstein's work in this sphere as 'The Theory of Relativity' but it has been confirmed 14 ways to 19 decimal places!

The twelfth century Hebrew scholar Nachmonides concluded from his studies in the book of Genesis that we actually dwell in a universe of ten dimensions of which only four are 'knowable' to us in the ordinary sense. Particle physicists have only now come to the same conclusions: that we live in ten dimensions, of which four are knowable in the ordinary sense. The three spatial dimensions can be directly measured and so can time. The six other dimensions are curled up in less than 10-33 cm and can only be inferred by indirect means.

Time is NOT a Constant

The very way we think about time is often flawed. It was drummed into us in early education that time was a constant. In reality time varies just the same as the other measurable dimensions.

Atomic clocks are accurate to better than 1 second in a million years. Their incredible accuracy enables the performance of global positioning satellites.

There is one of these clocks at the National Institute of Standards and Technology in Boulder, Colorado in the United States. There is another at the Royal Observatory at Greenwich, England. Yet, the N.I.S.T. clock is faster than the one in England by 5 microseconds per year. So, which is correct? They are both correct! Time is different in Boulder, Colorado at an altitude of 5,400 feet above sea level than it is at Greenwich which is at 80 feet above sea level. Time is different at these altitudes due to the differing gravity.

In 1971 one of many verification tests was carried out. Two aeroplanes were sent flying around the world in opposite directions. One flew Eastward and other Westward and each carried one of these clocks. The Eastern flight lost 0.059 milliseconds while the Western flight gained 0.273 microseconds just as theory predicted.

An oft-quoted illustration of Time dilation is that of twin brother astronauts born at the same instant. One is sent on a mission to Alpha-Centuri while the other stays on earth. On the trip the outgoing brother takes a clock. If he could travel at 99.9% the speed of light the journey out would take $4\,^1/_2$ years and the return trip the same. The total would be 9 years spent on the mission. The clock on his journey would read very differently from his brother's earthbound timepiece and on his return he would find himself the younger of the twins by 2 years and 5 months!

Remember at school, the familiar 'timelines' to pinpoint historic events? In that context these can be helpful study aids. Outside of that context this idea of time as linear is not helpful at all: it can actually hinder a more accurate view. We can develop an idea of infinity as just a very long 'timeline'. Again this ties us into thinking of time as a constant. A minute three thousand years ago actually wasn't the same as one of our minutes today. Again, give that a moment to sink in...

The definition of time changed in 1967 when one second was defined as 1/31,556,925,99747 of one earth orbit around the sun. This was Orbital Time. After 1967 Atomic Time defined a second as 9,192, 631,770 oscillations of the caesium -133 atom –Atomic Time.

In 1981 T.C. Flanders of the United States Naval Observatory noted Atomic Clocks slowing their time in relation to Orbital Clocks.

When the biblical prophet Isaiah refers to God as 'inhabiting eternity', he is not referring to a situation where the Creator just happens to have an awful lot of time on His hands! God is outside of the dimension of time altogether.

One way to try and illustrate this is to imagine a parade you have watched from the sidelines. To you it is a series of floats and bands that come into your view and pass one at a time in procession. The commentator up in his helicopter can see the start as well as the finish in one glance. He observes the various participants getting ready and mounting their horses and float vehicles at the starting point. At the same time he can see the procession winding through town and the people in the end enclosure disembarking and packing up their costumes. What you see in series, he observes as one event.

One way to express Biblical prophecy is to view it just that way – it is history told in advance.

Daniel – God's Man At The Courts Of Kings

The prophet Daniel had been taken captive to Babylon as a young man. He was a man of uncompromising principle and great integrity. God gifted him with exceptional prophetic insights . God gave Daniel a snapshot of the world empires that would arise one after the other in history when He gave him the following interpretation of king Nebuchadnezzar's dream. The king of Babylon had been greatly troubled by a dream and had set almost impossible conditions for his astrologers, magicians, enchanters and sorcerers to interpret it. He wasn't even prepared to recount the dream to them. He instructed that they recount the dream to him and <u>then</u> interpret it. Failure would mean them being cut into pieces and their houses being turned into piles of rubble. You might say ol' Neb was a pretty tough boss for your average soothsayer! The 'wise men' told the king it was an impossible task 'except for the gods and they do not live among men'. Enter Daniel who gets his two friends praying with him about the matter. In a vision of the night God reveals the mystery to Daniel. He tells the king that no mortal is capable of such insights but that there is a God who has shown him both the dream and its interpretation.

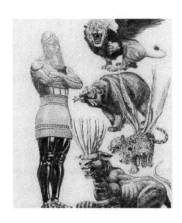

DANIEL 2 verse 29 - 47

"As you were lying there, O king, your mind turned to things to come and the revealer of mysteries showed you what is going to happen. As for me this mystery has been revealed to me, not because I have greater wisdom than other living men, but so that you, O king may know the interpretation and that you may understand what went through your mind.

You looked, O King and there before you stood a large statue – an enormous, dazzling statue, awesome in appearance. The head of the statue was made of pure gold, its chest and arms of silver, its belly and thighs of bronze, its legs of iron, its feet partly of iron and partly of baked clay. While you were watching, a rock was cut out, but not by human hands. It struck the statue on its feet of iron and clay and smashed them. Then the iron, the clay, the bronze, the silver and the gold were broken to pieces at the same time and became like chaff on a threshing-floor in the summer. The wind swept them away without leaving a trace. But the rock that struck the statue became a huge mountain and filled the whole earth.

This was the dream and now we will interpret it to the king. You, O king are the king of kings. The God of heaven has given you dominion and power and might and glory; in your hands he has placed mankind and the beasts of the field and the birds of the air. Wherever they live he has made you ruler over them all. You are that head of gold.

After you, another kingdom will arise, inferior to yours. Next a third kingdom, one of bronze, will rule over the whole earth. Finally there will be a fourth kingdom, strong as iron – for iron breaks and smashes everything – and as iron breaks things to pieces, so it will crush and break all the others. Just as you saw that the feet and toes were partly of baked clay and partly of iron, so this will be a divided kingdom, yet it will have some of the strength of iron in it, even as you saw iron mixed with clay. As the toes were partly iron and partly clay, so this kingdom will be partly strong and partly brittle. And just as you saw the iron mixed with baked clay, so the people will be a mixture and not remain united, any more than iron mixes with clay.

In the time of those kings, the God of heaven will set up a kingdom that will never be destroyed nor will it be left to another people. It will crush all those kingdoms and bring them to an end, but will itself endure forever. This is the meaning of the vision of the rock cut out of a mountain, but not by human hands – a rock that broke the iron, the bronze, the clay, the silver and the gold to pieces.

The great God has shown the king what will take place in the future. The dream is true and the interpretation is trustworthy.

Then king Nebuchadnezzar fell prostrate before Daniel and paid him honour and ordered that an offering and incense be presented to him. The king said to Daniel "Surely your God is the God of gods and the Lord of kings and the revealer of mysteries, for you were able to reveal this mystery."

In Matthew 24 Jesus Himself refers to Daniel as a prophet of the end times and quotes him. That's good enough for me.

- The golden head of the statue was Nebuchadnezzar himself – head of the Babylonian Empire.
- The Medo-Persian era is illustrated by the chest of silver
- The Hellenic era of Alexander the Great and his successors is represented by the belly of brass.
- The Roman Empire is typified by the crushing legs of iron. Many forget that the Roman Empire was divided into two!
- The symbol of the feet of the statue being made of iron mixed with clay typifies the era we now live in. The 'revised' Roman Empire. Remember we were roped into the signing of the 'Treaty of Rome' when joining the EEC.

References –

Babylonian Empire .... Daniel 2 v 37-38
Medo-Persian Empire............................. Daniel 5 v 28
Grecian Empire....................................... Daniel 2 v 39
Two Legs Of The Roman Empire................. Daniel 2 v 33
Ten Toes – Revived Roman Empire .... Daniel 2 v 41- 43

God, who is outside time, has created us as verbally communicating beings.

He is able to communicate verbally and propositionally to us in time and reveal history in advance.

Just as Daniel prophesied, Babylon fell to the Persians who, in turn were conquered by the Greeks. The Greeks were ultimately defeated by the Romans whose empire emerged in two successive phases – remember the two legs of iron. God, from outside time, communicated the order of things to His servant Daniel.

Herodotus tells how the Persians diverted the Euphrates River into a canal up stream so that the water level dropped down to a height level with the middle of a man's thigh. The Babylonian defences were based on the depth of water and so the invading troops simply marched through the riverbed in the exposed space beneath the gates under cover of night. There was virtually no bloodshed or battle and therefore no real damage to the city of Babylon itself.

In the 'Antiquities of the Jews' the historian Josephus tells of how the conquering Persian Cyrus made his triumphal entrance to Babylon and was confronted by a 'letter from God' addressed personally to him but written around a hundred and fifty years earlier. The letter was contained in the writings of another biblical prophet, Isaiah. Can you imagine his reaction?

"This is what the Lord says – your redeemer who formed you in the womb:

I am the Lord who has made all things, who alone stretched out the heavens, who spread out the earth by myself, who foils the signs of false prophets and makes fools of diviners, who overthrows the learning of the wise and turns it into nonsense, who carries out the words of his servants and fulfils the predictions of his messengers, who says of Jerusalem 'It shall be inhabited', of the towns of Judah 'They shall be built', and of their ruins, 'I will restore them', who says to the watery deep, 'Be dry and I will dry up your streams', who says of Cyrus 'He is my shepherd and will accomplish all that I please; he will say of Jerusalem, 'Let it be rebuilt', and of the temple, 'Let its foundations be laid.'

This what the Lord says to his anointed, to Cyrus, whose right hand I take hold of to subdue nations before him and to strip kings of their armour, to open doors before him so that gates will not be shut: I will go before you and will level the mountains; I will break down gates of bronze and cut through bars of iron.

I will give you the treasures of darkness, riches stored in secret places, so that you may know that I am the Lord, the

God of Israel who summons you by name.....” Isaiah from 44 v24 to 45 v3.

“I am the Lord and there is no other, apart from me there is no God: I will strengthen you, <u>though you have not acknowledged me</u>, so that from the rising of the sun to the place of its setting men may know there is none beside me.” Isaiah 45 vs 5-6

“I will raise him (Cyrus) up in my righteousness: I will make all his ways straight. He will rebuild my city and set my exiles free, but not for a price or reward says the Lord Almighty.” 45 v13

As I mentioned before, biblical prophecy is history told in advance. God, who is outside time, has created us as verbally communicating beings. He is able to communicate verbally and propositionally to us in time and reveal history in advance. So, one hundred and fifty years before Cyrus walked through the gates of Babylon, God had dictated a personal letter to him through the pen of Isaiah. It is addressed to him by name! So astonished was Cyrus with this whole section of Isaiah’s prophecy that he arranged for the freeing of the Hebrew captives and their return to Jerusalem.

Daniel lived through the subsequent rulers of Babylon after Nebuchadnezzar and up until around the third year of the reign of Cyrus.

Just before Babylon fell to the Persians, although he must have known there was a military threat on the horizon, Belshazzar, the Babylonian regent decided he would have a big party! He was confident in the defences and in the sheer scale of the obstacle Babylon presented to an attacking force. The city was around fifteen miles square with walls 87 feet thick. Herodotus tells us that a four-horse chariot could turn around on top of the wall. Babylon was thought to be unassailable.

He sat in the vast banqueting hall and in his arrogance ordered the vessels captured from the Jewish Temple by his grandfather, Nebuchadnezzar, to be brought out for the booze. Bad move! We don't know quite how drunk he was when supernatural fingers appeared and began to write on the plaster of the wall in full view of the revellers. We do know that he messed his pants in sheer terror so I guess he sobered up fairly rapidly.

"In the same hour came forth the fingers of a man's hand and wrote over against the candlestick on the plaster of the wall of the king's palace: and the king saw the part of the hand that wrote. Then the king's countenance was changed and his thoughts troubled him so that the joints of his loins were loosed and his knees smote one against another..." Daniel 5 v5-6.

Daniel is summoned out of retirement and offered rewards to translate the words on the wall. He tells the king to keep his gifts but translates the awful message; 'Mene, Mene, Tekel, Peres.' "God has numbered the days of your reign and brought it to an end. You have been weighed on the scales and found wanting. Your kingdom has been divided and given to the Medes and Persians." That very night Balshazzar met his death.

Jeremiah, another biblical prophet had written specifically that the captivity of the Jewish people in Babylon would last seventy years. Daniel had been there since the beginning and, upon reading the prophecy, realised that the time span was approaching its end. He began an intense time of prayer and fasting to enquire of God what was to happen next. His prayer was interrupted by the angel Gabriel who gave to him probably the most amazing prophecy in the entire Bible.

"Seventy sevens are decreed for your people and your holy city to finish transgression, to put an end to sin, to atone for wickedness, to bring in everlasting righteousness, to seal up vision and prophecy and to anoint the most holy.

Know and understand this: From the issuing of the decree to restore and rebuild Jerusalem until the Anointed One, The Ruler comes, there will be seven 'sevens' and sixty two 'sevens'. It will be rebuilt with streets and a trench, but in times of trouble. After the sixty two 'sevens', the Anointed One will be cut off and will have nothing. The people of the ruler who will come will destroy the city and the sanctuary. The end will come like a flood. War will continue until the end and desolations have been decreed. He will confirm a covenant with many for one 'seven'. In the middle of the 'seven' he will put an end to sacrifice and offering.

And on a wing of the temple he will set up an abomination that causes desolation until the end that is decreed is poured out on him" Daniel 9 v 24 – 27.

The 'sevens' referred to are weeks of years - 'Shabu'im. Seventy weeks of years are reckoned (*hatak*) upon Daniel's people and the city of Jerusalem. The important thing to note is that the focus of this prophecy is not on the Gentile world or the church to come but specifically on the Jewish people.

There are six major things on the list that are not yet fulfilled;

1. The finishing of transgressions
2. Making an end of sins
3. Making reconciliation for iniquity
4. The bringing in of everlasting righteousness
5. The sealing up (*closing up the authority of*) the vision
6. The anointing of the Holy of Holies (*Godesh Godashim*)

Ancient calendars were all based around a year of 360 days, *the Assyrian, Chaldean, Egyptian, Hebrew, Persian, Greek, Phoenician, Chinese, Mayan, Hindu, Carthaginian, Etruscan and Teutonic.*

These years were typically of twelve thirty day months.

The ancient Chaldean calendar was structured on this and it

is from this ancient Babylonian tradition that we have 360 degrees in a circle, 60 minutes in an hour with sixty seconds in each minute.

Under Numa Pompilius, Rome's second king, the calendars were re-drawn by adding five days a year. Taking account of this, Hezekiah, the Jewish king of that time reorganised the Jewish calendar by adding a month in each Jewish leap year. This was on a cycle of seven every nineteen years.

The 3rd, 6th, 8th, 11th, 14th, 17th and 19th years were leap years although this was not revealed to the people until the Fourth Century.

(Arthur Spier – The Comprehensive Hebrew Calendar)

The Biblical Calendar uses a 360 day year throughout.

At the time this prophecy was given, the city of Jerusalem was, of course lying in ruins. God had destined it to be rebuilt and here was a mathematical map telling him that from the time of the decree going forth to rebuild the city to the advent of the Messiah would be 173,880 days *(7 + 62) >< 7 >< 360 = 173,880 days)*

Scholars differ over just why the 69 weeks was separated into 7 + 62. Some suggest that seven weeks of years was the timespan for rebuilding the temple at Jerusalem.

Between the decree for the rebuilding of Jerusalem and the presentation of the Messiah would be a period of 173,880 days.

There were several decrees allowing for the re-building of the Jerusalem temple but the prophecy was specifically about the city.

The decree which triggered this amazing prediction was given by Artaxerxes Longimanus on March 14th, 445 BC.

This granted authority to rebuild the city walls. The trials accompanying the rebuilding of the temple are recorded in the Book of Ezra but in the book of Nehemiah we have the account of the rebuilding of the actual walls.

The milestone for the completion of the sixty nine weeks prophecied was the presentation of the Messiah King. But when was Jesus presented as King?!

(Note: The English Bible translates the word Nagid as 'Prince'. However it should be 'King'. The word 'Nagid' is first used of King Saul)

There are several references in the New Testament to the people wanting to appoint Jesus as their King. On these occasions we read the accounts of his refusal on the grounds that "My hour is not yet come."

John Chapter 6:

'After the people saw the miraculous signs that Jesus did they began to say "Surely this is the Prophet who is to come into the world." Jesus, knowing that they intended to come and make him king by force, withdrew again to a mountain by himself..'

Just before attending the Passover feast Jesus does something remarkable in suddenly permitting what He has hitherto sidestepped.

John 12 vs 12- 15. "The next day a great crowd that had gathered for the feast (Passover) heard that Jesus was on his way to Jerusalem. They took palm branches and went out to meet him, shouting 'Hosanna! Blessed is he that comes in the name of the Lord!' 'Blessed is the king of Israel!' Jesus found a young donkey and sat upon it, as it is written, "Do not be afraid O daughter of Zion; see your king is coming seated on a donkey's colt." At first his disciples did not understand all this. Only after Jesus was glorified did they realise that these things had been written about him and that they had done these things to him."

On this day and only this day, He allows Himself to be hailed as king! He rides into the city, fulfilling an ancient prophecy by Zechariah from five hundred years before.

'Rejoice greatly, O daughter of Zion; shout O daughter of Jerusalem: Behold thy King cometh unto thee: he is just, and having salvation: lowly and riding upon an ass, and upon a colt, the foal of an ass." Zechariah 9 v9.

While the people were presenting Passover lambs for their sacrifices, Jesus, the Christ was presenting Himself as the perfect sacrifice for the salvation of all mankind. This took place on the 10th of Nisan (April 6th) 32 A.D.

Converting the Hebrew text to our calendar reveals that there were exactly 173,880 days between the decree of Artaxerxes Longimanus and Jesus presenting Himself as the Messiah King. The prophecy Gabriel gave to Daniel was fulfilled to the exact day!

The Maps They Are A-Changing

This is a time of great questioning about the make up of the universe. It is time also to re-think one's attitude to the inspiration of scripture and the God who inspired it.

As the late Dr Francis Schaeffer once put it "There is nothing back of God!" He brought our universe into being and is well able to speak into it. The question is 'Are we listening?'

I have tried to give just a few examples of those things we need to be clear on. The play of history is in its closing act. Jesus made it clear that we are held accountable to understand the signs of our times.

Luke's gospel tells us;

"As He approached Jerusalem and saw the city He wept over it and said; 'If you, even you had only known on this day what would bring you peace – but now it is hidden from your eyes. The days will come when your enemies will build an embankment against you and encircle you and hem you in on every side. They will dash you to the ground, you and the children within your walls. They will not leave one stone upon another because you did not recognise the time of God's coming to you."

Jesus held them accountable to recognise the significance of this special day. They had failed to realise the significant events of their times and He knew the terrible events that awaited them in their ignorance. Thirty eight years later His words came true as the 5th, 10th 12th and 15th Legions of Rome led by Titus Vespasian laid siege to the city of Jerusalem. They laid a siege embankment just as Jesus had said and proceeded to slaughter over a million men, women and children. During the battle for the city, a torch lit a fire inside the temple. The intense heat of the blaze melted the gold fixtures and furnishings. Titus ordered every stone to be taken down to recover the melted gold.

"They will not leave one stone upon another".

In the terrible autumn of AD70 the words of Jesus were fulfilled exactly.

To most of the people of Jerusalem the day of Jesus's 'triumphal entry' as it has become known, was just another day. Biblical prophecy is not to be taken lightly by us either. David Pawson observes that the Bible as a whole predicts 735 specific events. 27 % of these verses focus on the future while 593 (that is 81%) of these predictions have already been fulfilled! We have the warnings and notification of the signs to look for in our day and age. How many of us are aware of the signs of our times? The Bible's God-given insights are intended to let us know what is on the horizon. Some of what was revealed to Daniel could not possibly have been understood until this stage in history.

In Daniel 12 v 8 we read;

"I heard but I did not understand. So I asked, "What will the outcome of all this be?" He replied "Go your way, Daniel because the words are closed up and sealed until the time of the end..."

Feet Of Iron Mixed With Clay

If ever there was an apt picture of what is happening right now it is this image of powerful people trying to force through an agenda which mixes iron with clay. The fact is that 'one size fits all' doesn't work! Never has! Never will!

Whereas Christians worship a God who creates, loves and nurtures individuals, the present powers want to create a single, uniform Fourth Reich. Each of us at this point in history must ask which kingdom they align themselves with. The Globalist agenda is not just political. Even if you just take the crop of people who have recently jostled for places within its hierarchy, you get an idea of the kind of world they are constructing. Satanic bloodlines, high masonic mystery religion and occult blood rituals along with a lust for total control link those involved at the highest level. These people are preparing to enthrone their king – the one the Bible speaks of as 'The Man of Sin' or the 'Antichrist'.

Historian Arnold Toynbee held the view that modern nationalism was a 'false god'. Nonetheless he could observe that; "The stage is being set for the deification of any future Caesar who will promise World Peace."

The North American Union and The Demise of Britain

As I write this, new developments are already coming into view.

The presidents of America, Mexico and Canada have created the North American Union which will take its place alongside the European Union, The African Union and The Asian Union as parts of the New World Order jigsaw.

The Illuminati hierarchy and royal bloodlines, Committee of 300, World Banks, The Bilderbergers, The Council on Foreign Relations, The United Nations, The Trilateral Commission and the rest of the architects with backing from The Rockefellers, Rothschilds, Ford, Carnegie and the other key financial players are re-drawing the world around you right now.

Under the guise of 'Trade Agreements' nations are being erased and put into blocs. England has been newly mapped into three sections for the new regions of Europe (Cornwall, Devon, Dorset, Hants, Sussex, Kent, Essex, Suffolk and Norfolk now lumped with Seine Maritime, Somme, Calvados, Manche, Ille-et-Villaine, Cotes D'Armor and Finistere to form the MANCHE REGION).

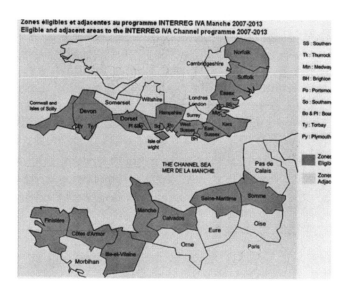

The first stage of re-mapping what was Britain – The Manche Region.

Many in Britain are still unaware of the fact that their country has literally disappeared into new sectors carved up by those behind The New World Order.

The Lisbon Treaty actually abolished Britain on the 1st January 2010!

This was the last of six treaties signed and ratified treasonously by the Prime Minister and Queen of England.

Whether people voted for The Conservatives, The Labour Party, The Liberal Democrats, The British National Party or saddest of all, The United Kingdom Independence Party, they were actually voting for a EU dictatorship. All five Party Leaders are controlled and run by the EU. Three are members of The Bilderberger Group. In order to occupy any significant office in the present party 'vetting' system, a candidate for any significant senior political appointment <u>must</u> hold a pro EU stance. The Conservatives have been EU controlled since the 1960s, Labour and Liberal Democrats since 1985. UKIP and BNP are also under EU control.

Those who thought they were actually striking a blow for freedom by voting UKIP were taken in perhaps even more cruelly than the others as this party is actually a 'honey trap' operation.

David Noakes, who is <u>genuinely</u> opposed to the EU, ran for the leadership of UKIP. Needless to say, he was not selected. He found that any really effective strategy tabled in opposition to the EU agenda was stifled.

UKIP leader Malcolm Pearson is not only a high-ranking Freemason but also has links to Common Purpose. From the elitists' point of view it's rather like watching with amusement the excitement among the crowd as they place their bets on one of five horses, knowing that, despite different public colours, they are all owned and run by your stable! A good illusionist will always get your attention to go where he wants it directed while he pulls off the real trick.

The Bilderberg group runs all these puppets in bright and seemingly different livery colours. At grassroots level organisations such as 'Common Purpose' serve as the foot soldiers, and have successfully planted their people into thousands of positions controlling local Councils and Media outlets throughout Britain. You will only be told what those pulling the strings wish you to hear.

As George Orwell put it;

"In a time of universal deceit, telling the truth is a revolutionary act."

The Late U.S.A.

America is finished. Canada and Mexico have also disappeared. In their place has risen one massive country – The North American Union. Bordered by the Bering Sea to the North and Guatemala to the South, the Pacific Ocean to the West and The

Atlantic to the East, the currency of this new country is the 'Amero' and its flag shows the western Hemisphere.

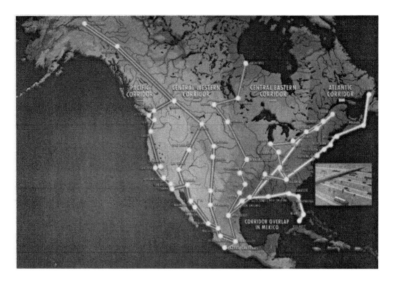

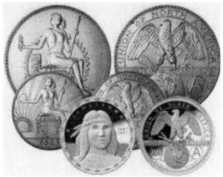

The Proposed Currency of 'The North American Union'
THE 'AMERO'

The Trilateral Commission – New Steps In Stealth

Once again this stage has been reached through a series of 'enabling steps' by those working carefully out of sight. This particular chapter in 'steering' America began in 1973 with the creation of The Trilateral Commission by David Rockefeller and Zbigniew Brzezinski. Its membership – 300 powerful elitists from North America, Europe and Japan.

Its goal was to foster a 'New Economic Order' to supplant the historic economic order. Under Brzezinski's tutelage Jimmy Carter, on his election appointed one third of the entire Trilateral Commission to his cabinet. As journalist Lou Dobbs expressed it – the Trilateralists had established a headlock on the Executive branch of the US Government! As Reagan took office, he appointed Trilateralist George Bush as Vice President and continued to select key appointments from the ranks of The Trilateral Commission. Fellow Trilateralist Bill Clinton followed and during his eight years appointed no less than 14 Trilateral members to his administration. Next in the carefully presented parade came Bush Jnr.

Under the thumb of his father and other ruthlessly powerful men, his administration featured the odious Trilateralist Dick Cheney whose wife Lynne was also a member in her own right.

The 'Trade Agreements' such as GATT (General Agreement on Trade and Tariffs) and the arrangements that followed were all carefully engineered phases leading up to the present dissolution of America. Richard Gardner was an original member of the Trilateral Commission and a principle architect in the 'New Economic Order'. He wrote an article in 'Foreign Affairs' – the magazine of The Council on Foreign Relations.

Its tone sums up the total disdain he and his fellows have for anyone holding nationalistic views.

"…an end run <u>around</u> national sovereignty, eroding it piece by piece, will accomplish much more than the old-fashioned frontal assault."

Anthony Sutton said something about letting your resistance find a thousand forms. You must find your own way to resist the advance of the evil these people wish to force upon you and your children. Many are finding ways of delaying and sometimes de –railing the agenda.

Under Clinton and Bush the American people have been betrayed in the worst ways. Now it's time for Obama to play out his assignments. But it's not just in America – this is happening globally. They are working towards all national borders coming down and all sovereignty being replaced by allegiance to a Global Government.

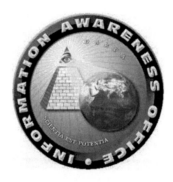

"....he also forced everyone, small and great, rich and poor, free and slave to receive a mark on his right hand or forehead so that no one could buy or sell unless he had the mark which is the name of the beast or the number of his name.

This calls for wisdom. If anyone has insight, let him calculate the number of the beast for it is man's number. His number is 666...."

Revelation 13 v 16 – 18.

When The Book of Revelation speaks of not being able to buy or sell unless you bear the 'mark' of the system or the 'mark of the beast' it is giving an accurate representation of the way it is going to be shortly. The way it almost is now!

Ever lost your Credit Card? Ever been on the wrong side of the System?

You become like one of the characters in George Orwell's writings: -

You are an 'un-citizen', an 'un-customer' – an 'un-person'.

As far as the checkout is concerned –you have ceased to exist!

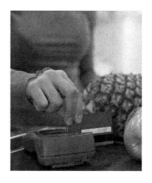

"Well, you know me, I shop here all the time. Couldn't you let me have the groceries and I'll get this sorted out and come back?"

"Sorry, I couldn't do that. Got to stick to the System! Your number is either right or wrong – yours is wrong! NEXT!"

It's pointless trying to reason with a machine or the person who works for the machine.

The Microchip Agenda

Think of a cash point fouling up or a mechanised Gas Station.

You may be stranded hundreds of miles from home but unless your 'mark' is recognised by the System – that's the end of the story!

Credit cards are all very well but they can be easily ruined, de-magnetised, duplicated and so on. Personal Identity chips are the next phase in the plans of the New World Order and they are here. Already used to keep track of pets, Identi-chips are inserted beneath the skin and can be easily read by a hand held scanner. Driving Licences carrying more and more personal details are being employed right now, despite resistance. If you are stopped without the correct type of Driver's Licence in New Zealand right now, your vehicle is confiscated then and there and you have to find alternative means to get home. This is just the thin end of the wedge but it gives you some idea of where it is all leading.

The more sophisticated RFID Identi-chips for human beings are not just scanner friendly! They give off a signal which is trackable anywhere.

These are being manufactured in massive numbers.

They are about the size of a grain of rice and automatically re-charge with the person's natural biological rhythms. A great deal of money has been spent in locating the best place for these to be located in the body.

The two sites agreed are; 1) Back of the hand
2) Under the skin on the forehead

(See Revelation 13 v 16-18 - above)

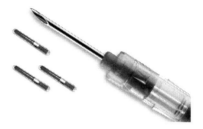

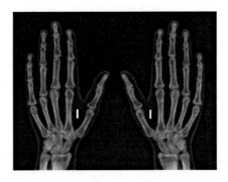

While many in the West scoff at these observations as 'Paranoia' or 'Conspiracy Theory', millions and millions of people in China already have implanted chips!

The implants are used to police draconian restrictions on travel between the Chinese provinces in that vast country.

One school in Rhode Island has cast aside all notions of civil liberties and has implanted RFID chips in students in a programme to keep track of their movements at all times! Sections of the Western Military routinely use them. As more advanced versions are available they will be brought into service. Many people have volunteered to take part in 'pilot' schemes to try out these devices because they have been convinced of their value in personal security.

Piece by piece the System for World Government is being assembled.

In Britain, the planned programme for personal ID cards is to be axed we are told. Briefing notes suppressed for two years show that the Labour Government, despite its assurances that the ID system would be 'Voluntary' always intended them to be compulsory. A table illustrating the unfolding of the scheme in terms of its savings on fraud shows compulsory IDs by 2014. The first were scheduled for 2009 to anyone applying for a Passport. Extensive personal details, face scan, details on second homes, health information, driving licence number, insurance numbers would have been required. Without the required type of passport you would forfeit the right to travel. The new British passports already have an Identity chip placed in the cover. Again, a small setback for those behind these plans but we wait to see what their <u>next</u> step will be. As I've said, they are patient and cunning and prefer incrementalism to direct conflict wherever it is possible.

Whatever methods are employed, at the end of the process is a code system straight out of Biblical prophecy:

No one knows for certain exactly what form this will take but variations on several present systems could be employed.

The late Barry Smith suggested the following as an easily envisaged possibility based on the research he had done;

Date of Birth – 2 Digits for Year, 2 Digits for Month and 2 Digits for Day

Grid Location Code – Satellite Location - 2 Digits for Major Region, 2 Digits for Area and 2 Digits for Exact Location Point (i.e. England, London. Street and House Number.

Person Identity Number – Again - 2 Digits, 2 Digits. 2 Digits.

Put them together and you have 666 – The Biblical 'Number of the Beast'.

Once again, I stress I am <u>not</u> saying that this is what will be implemented. It's just one way of executing the scheme that is being planned. The exact methods are less important than the known intent to impose this sort of control.

Aaron Russo and Nick Rockefeller

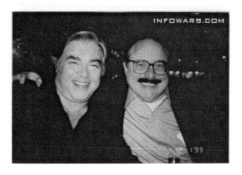

The well known filmmaker Aaron Russo had the power brokers' intentions laid out to him directly by Nick Rockefeller himself. Because of his powerful work in exposing the intentions of the New World Order, Russo was courted with a view to recruitment on to the 'Council on Foreign Relations' by Nick Rockefeller. Rockefeller became friendly with Russo and was genuinely puzzled by this man who opposed the Master Plan. He couldn't understand why Russo didn't view ordinary people as 'cattle' which needed to be controlled. He advised Russo to 'just look after your own'. During their numerous conversations, Rockefeller was quite clear that the intention was to get everyone implanted with a microchip ID – that way their finances as well as their movements could all be more easily monitored. He told Aaron that he didn't have to worry for himself because if he came 'on board' his chip would have a 'KMA' status. When Russo asked what that meant he was told 'Kiss My A**!' In other words – he would be one of the elite untouchables and any authority scanning his identity chip would know enough to leave him well alone!

(See DVD recording of 'Interview With Aaron Russo' on 'infowars.com')

In Britain, mainstream newspapers have carried articles about biometric information being taken from schoolchildren for future use. Illegal or not – the NWO don't care what you think about it; they're going to do it anyway.

As part of a 'Pilot Plan', children in the UK are being tracked by means of RFID chips attached to their school uniforms. A growing number are fingerprinted for administrative and security purposes. Since 2001 almost 6,000 pupils have been fingerprinted and new schools embrace this practice every week.

At a time when we should be telling our children to guard this data carefully, they are being brainwashed into thinking that divulging these details for a central record is a safeguard for freedom against terrorists and so forth....

Even your nightly news is carefully controlled by these people to suppress that which they do not wish you to be aware of.

I was given to understand that CNN for instance was set up as a genuine alterative to the broadcasting monopoly of the airwaves. This didn't last long as an independent voice and CNN has, for some time, been under their control.

In America, attacks perpetrated against the American people by their own leaders such as the dreadful truck bombings and the destruction of the twin towers on 9/11, have been set up to frighten the American populace into giving up its liberties. 9/11 was sold to the American people as a good excuse to go thundering into Iraq under the banner of a 'war on terror.' If you still doubt that the collapse of the towers was planned, do some investigation of your own – read the reports of those who were there, study the film footage carefully. There are several excellent full length DVD reports currently available in which eye witnesses, top architectural, explosive and structural experts demonstrate what <u>actually</u> happened that terrible day. One newswoman can be seen 'reporting' the collapse of one of the structures still clearly standing behind her. She faithfully says what she has been briefed to say, unaware at that moment of the contradiction. There are other examples we could quote but the point is – check for <u>yourself</u> and don't expect the BBC or Fox or any of the others to tell you the truth.

Just as Hitler had his agents set fire to the Reichstag as a ruse to gain more power – so the American leaders have used the 'War on Terror' to push through the Patriot Acts I and II. These dreadful documents have robbed the American citizens of all the rights they had under their Constitution. 'The War on Terror' is a giant hoax and many Americans are only just now waking up to it – too late!

The American Shadow Government has cultivated Black Operations or 'False Flag Operations' throughout its history including allowing horrors such as Pearl Harbour despite clear knowledge beforehand. News shots and reports of American service men being killed stir up the desired emotions in the duped populace and children being blown up is even better fuel on the fire.

An angered, fearful citizenry become very willing to go to war or give up more and more of their liberty when promised protection in exchange! The lives of ordinary people, who do not begin to understand this hellish agenda, mean nothing to these ruthless Globalists who are determined to tear down every vestige of sovereignty and nationhood in pursuit of their goals.

The Shape Of Things To Come

So here is their glistening vision;

- One Absolute World Ruler – 'The Strong Man' or 'Antichrist'
- A small hierarchy of World Ministers bred from generationally satanic bloodlines
- 80% World Population Reduction – by Malthusian or chemical/viral means
- Industrial Cessation and a return to Feudalism
- A One World Currency
- A One World Police Force
- World Citizens all Chipped and given a Personal Identity Number (P.I.N.) You are either 'in the system' or not. If not, even getting a bag of groceries becomes impossible. You won't be able to pay cash because the system will be 'cashless'. In truly Orwellian terms you will become an 'un-person'.
- No Individual Citizen Rights – Resources centrally controlled
- Forced Urbanisation for easier control of the population – Huge areas closed for 'Re-Wilding'
- Constant surveillance
- Severe restrictions on Travel – Citizens must be tracked
- One approved World Religion – A synthesis which does not allow for specifically Christian faith

Do your own research into some of these areas and decide; Is this what you want for your children? It's up to you!

We have discovered that our universe is limited and is moving from a beginning towards a definite end. Not only does biblical prophecy speak volubly on this, but we have the authoritative words of Jesus Christ himself. It is clear from scripture that the Globalists will be successful in fulfilling their objectives for a short time. Just as Belshazzar's kingdom was judged and its days numbered, so the Bible makes clear that God has already judged this emerging would-be World Government and set His divine boundaries on it.

'Mene, Mene, Tekel, Peres.' "God has numbered the days of your reign and brought it to an end. You have been weighed on the scales and found wanting."

I am indebted to the many sources who have supplied information on the planning and development of the New World Order. I would need a separate book to mention you all, but 'Thank You'. Here are just some of many references and some reading for those wishing to do their own research but not knowing where to start:

The Holy Bible – *Thomson Chain Reference, New International, King James, New King James, Amplified and New English Versions*

The Antiquities Of The Jews – Josephus

The Wars Of The Jews - Josephus

Daniel's Seventy Weeks – DVD C. Missler

Europa Rising – C. Missler

The Coming Prince – Robert Anderson

The Rape Of Europe –David Hathaway

The Rise of The Fourth Reich – Jim Marrs

Rule By Secrecy – Jim Marrs

The Bilderberg Group – Daniel Estulin

The New Rulers Of The World - John Pilger

The Secret Teachings Of All Ages – Manly P Hall

Lectures On Ancient Philosophy – Manly P Hall

The Antiquities Of The Jews – Josephus

The Wars Of The Jews – JosephusCriteas –Plato

Svali – Complete notes and Radio Interview Transcript

Timaeus – Plato

The Grand Chessboard _Zbigniew Brzezinski

The Late Great U.S.A. – Jerome R. Corsi

Confessions Of An Economic Hitman - John Perkins

Synthetic Terror/Made In The USA –Webster Grifin Tarpley

Barak Obama –The Post Modern Coup – Webster Griffin Tarpley

Obama – The Unauthorised Biography – Webster Griffin Tarpley

Obama – The Mask Comes Off – Film Alex Jones

George Bush – The Unauthorised Biography – Webster Griffin Tarpley

Shock Doctrine – Naomi Klein

Cults and Isms – J. Oswald Sanders

Daniel – Joyce Baldwin

George Bush – A Charge To Keep

The New Economic Disorder – Larry Bates

The United Nations Straightjacket – Joan Veon

Prince Charles, The Sustainable Prince – Joan Veon

The Prince and The Paranormal - *thanks to Pauline Ruffles for the copy*

Dumbing Down – Ivo Moseley

Lost Colony Of The Templars – Steven Sora

The Templars and The Holy Grail – Karen Ralls

The Knights of The Quest - Karen Ralls

The Rosicrucians – Chris Mcintosh

Templar Treasure and The Secrets of Renne Le Chateau – L & P Fanworth

Babylon – Mystery Religion – Ralph Woodcock

The Confidence Game – Steve Solomon

Distraction – Mark Curtis

Who's Who In Mythology – Michael Senior

Perpetual war for Perpetual Peace – Gore Vidal

Dreaming War – Gore Vidal

The Order of the Death's Head – Heinz Holns

Morals & Dogma - Albert Pike

Wall Street and the Rise of Hitler - Anthony Sutton

Wall Street and The Bolshevik Revolution - Anthony Sutton

The Queen's Conjuror – Benjamin Wooley

Imperial Ambitions - Noam Chomsky

Hegemony or Survival? - Noam Chomsky

Deterring Democracy - Noam Chomsky

1984 – George Orwell

Animal Farm – George Orwell

Brave New World – Aldous Huxley

Tragedy and Hope – Carrol Quigley

One Nation Under Siege - Kleist

Wise As Serpents – Fritz Springmeier

The Bloodlines of the Illuminati – Fritz Springmeier

Better Than Nostradamus – Barry Smith

The Devil's Jigsaw – Barry Smith

Warning - Barry Smith

Final Warning - Barry Smith

Revelation TV – Supplied all Studio Interviews with Barry Smith

Unlocking the Bible – David Pawson

Mein Kampf – Adolf Hitler

The Lion Handbook to the Bible

E.U. Final World Empire – Alan Franklin

End Game – DVD Alex Jones

Terror Storm – DVD Alex Jones

Dark Secrets at Bohemian Grove – DVD Alex Jones

America's Secret Beginnings I & II – DVD Antiquities Research Films

America/From Freedom to Fascism – Aaron Russo

America/Destroyed By Design – DVD Alex Jones

The MK Ultra Files (de-classified) *sent by Mark Phillips from America. Thank You, Mark.*

Templars and Assassins – James Wasserman

What We've Lost – Gaydon Carter

Mortgaging The Earth – Bruce Rich

The Brotherhood – Stephen Knight

The Great Deception/The Secret History of the E.U. – C.Booker & R.North

The Tranceformation of America – Cathy O'Brien and Mark Phillips

For Reasons of National Security – Cathy O'Brien and Mark Phillips

Lincoln Steffens – Biography

Lincoln Steffens – The Letters of Lincoln Steffens

Complete Works – Francis Schaeffer

9/11 and The American Empire – D.R Griffin & Dale Scott

Christian Faith And The Truth Behind 9/11- David Ray Griffin

The Money Masters – DVD Bill Still

63 Documents the Government does not want you to read - Jesse Ventura

Lightning Source UK Ltd.
Milton Keynes UK
UKOW052222020212

186552UK00001B/77/P